RUNNER'S WORLD®

Complete
Book of
Running

Everything You Need to Run for Weight Loss, Fitness, and Competition

EDITED BY AMBY BURFOOT

Editor at Large, **RUNNER'S WORLD** and Winner of the 1968 Boston Marathon

RODALE

Library of Congress Cataloging-in-Publication Data

Runner's world complete book of running : everything you need to run for weight loss, fitness, and competition / edited by Amby Burfoot.
    p.   cm.
Rev. and updated edition.
Includes index.
ISBN-13 978–1–60529–579–4 paperback
ISBN-13 978–1–60529–545–9 hardcover
    1. Running.   2. Running—Training.   I. Burfoot, Amby.   II. Runner's world (Emmaus, Pa. : 1987)
GV1061.R83365   2010
796.42—dc22
                                                                                          2009033150

Distributed to the trade by Macmillan

2   4   6   8   10   9   7   5   3   1   paperback

2   4   6   8   10   9   7   5   3   1   hardcover

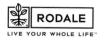

RODALE
LIVE YOUR WHOLE LIFE™

We inspire and enable people to improve their lives and the world around them
For more of our products visit **rodalestore.com** or call 800-848-4735

Contents

Part IV: Women's Running

Part V: Building Strength, Endurance, and Speed

Part VI: The Mental Side Of Running

Part VII: Cross-Training

Part VIII: Weight Loss For Runners

Part IX: The Half-Marathon

Part X: The Marathon

Introduction

Hello. And welcome to what I hope you'll find to be the most informative and friendly running book ever published. From the very beginning of this project, I have had just two simple goals: to gather, in one place, the best and most helpful running advice available, and to present it in the clearest, most user-friendly manner.

The first part was easy. The chapters in this book have been selected from the thousands of articles published in *Runner's World* Magazine, the world's biggest and most successful running magazine for more than four decades. These chapters aren't just the best, they're also the ones readers have responded to most enthusiastically. I should know, I've been a *Runner's World* editor for more than 30 years. During this time, I've read every word that has gone into *Runner's World*, and most of the letters from readers.

To keep the book friendly and personal, I've concluded each chapter with a short summary section called "Amby Burfoot's Running Round-up." In this modest essay, I comment on the chapter you've just finished reading. I might say something

like, "This is the most important nutrition advice I've ever read. Be sure to come back and review it often." Or I might expand the chapter, adding my own thoughts and experience to the primary author's. Either way, I'm trying to lead you through the book and its major conclusions the same way a historical tour guide might lead you through a civil war battlefield. I hope I've succeeded, and that you enjoy these "cool down" sections.

Some things in running don't change much decade-by-decade—sports drinks continue to use roughly the same formulations, running shoes still contain the same basic parts and materials, and long runs are still essential to marathon success. But the sport does and has changed, and this new edition of *The Runner's World Complete Book of*

Running reflects those changes. In particular, this revised edition includes three entirely new sections that would have been difficult to anticipate 10 to 15 years ago.

The first, "Weight Loss for Runners," strikes some people as an out-of-place topic. Aren't runners already the leanest, fittest slice of our society? To some extent this is true, and I strongly believe that the calorie-burning potential of a good running workout can help anyone lose fat or maintain their healthy body weight. But we live in a society where rampant obesity is almost the norm. Many runners gain unhealthy pounds in their midlife years. And many beginning runners are drawn to the sport for its promise of health, fitness, and pounds-lost. This section is for all these runners.

The second new part retains an old title, "Cross-Training," but is full of new material due to the rapid rise of core training. When I was a young runner, we did a lot of situps, but no other core exercises. We had never seen or heard of the exercises that have been perfected in recent years. I have a strong skeptic's streak, but core training makes complete sense to me. After all, when we run, we move our our legs and our shoulders and arms vigorously. To maintain a smooth, strong co-ordination between the lower-body movements and the upper-body movements, it makes total sense that we should develop our body's "core." The chapters in this newly-imagined section will help you do that.

The third new part is the "Half Marathon" section, devoted to the wildly popular distance that so many runners are using as a stepping stone to their first marathon (or as a major focus of their training and racing.) It wasn't long ago, I remember, that we used to sit around in the *Runner's World* offices bemoaning the half-marathon's lack of popularity. We thought the sport needed an in-between distance, but the half simply wasn't attracting much attention. We used to debate whether or not we could make the distance more enticing by calling it "the 21-K" or "the double 10-K" or some other equally laughable name. Happily, the half marathon caught on all by itself, and this section will show you how to be successful at it.

The other sections of this book have been organized according to the topics that always have been most important to successful running, and always will. We don't need new names for these sections like "Beginning," "Nutrition," "Injury Prevention" and "Women;" we simply need new material as it becomes available. And this revised book contains dozens of new chapters full of the newest and most relevant information on running.

I want to close this introduction on a personal note. Above, I talked about the "Round-Up" essays that I've written for the end of each chapter. I said I wanted to be your guide. But throughout this book, I also want to be your cheerleader. I want you to understand that the whole is greater than the sum of the parts. I want you to know that running is the best, most time-efficient health and fitness activity in the world; that the payoffs from a running lifestyle are greater than you can possibly imagine; and that you can do everything that's described in this book. Even a marathon.

I won't lie and say it's easy. I won't over-promise and say you might win an Olympic medal. I won't deny that you'll have occasional aches and pains, or days when you just don't feel like doing your workout. Those are inevitable. We're all tired or lazy at one time or another.

But I will guarantee you that any healthy person can run. After all, any number of physically and mentally challenged individuals have proven their courage through running. And running *is* simple, and it *will* produce positive changes in your life. Every day, more and more medical and scientific studies are proving the benefits of high-level fitness.

You might not run fast. You might not run far. You might have to mix walking with your running. But you can do it; and in the process you'll lose weight, lower your blood pressure, and reduce your heart disease and diabetes risks. And those are only the physiological changes. At the same time, you'll feel more energetic, less depressed, and more enthusiastic about your prospects in life.

Many runners take up the sport to lose a few pounds. But they continue running for the way it clears their mind, reduces stress, and helps them feel better every day.

Running is the ultimate individual sport.

You shouldn't worry about anyone else's pace. You should focus entirely on finding the pace that's most comfortable and productive for you. You can't lose this race because you're not competing with anyone else. You're only running against yourself, and as long as you *are* running, you're also winning.

Ultimately, I hope that's the message you'll get from this book. The advice is all here. Your cheerleader is at your side. You can hardly go wrong. So lace up those running shoes and get on with it.

Run long and healthy.

Amby Burfoot
Editor at Large
Runner's World *magazine*

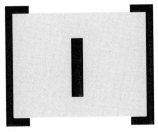

Beginning Running

Chapter 1

Get Started on the Right Foot

A Surefire Plan to Get You Running

All running programs for beginners are the same: They move you from walking, which anyone can do, to running, which anyone can do if they have the determination. The difference between walking and running isn't speed or biomechanics. It's determination.

If you have the determination to stick with the following program, you'll soon be a runner. Trust me. It won't be long before you learn that I'm right.

The beginning of your life as a runner just might be the most exciting time in your entire running career. Of course, you won't necessarily realize that at the time. It may take months or years before you can look back and see what you've achieved. But rest assured—you will.

Getting started...first steps...the beginning of a great adventure. In many ways, beginning to run is a declaration of personal independence. It's a statement that says, "In a world that confronts me with mechanical convenience and idle luxury at virtually every turn, I have decided, nonetheless, to improve my physical fitness."

Later, of course, you realize that running offers so much more than a flatter stomach, more muscle tone, and a longer and more energetic life.

For most of us, body and soul both tune in to this stimulating activity we call running. Running strengthens the body while it soothes the soul. So what are you waiting for? The sooner you get started, the better.

WALK BEFORE YOU RUN

More than a few training programs—especially the New Year's resolution variety—are doomed almost before they start. Why? Because the schedules are overly ambitious and complex. Or, in contrast, they are completely lacking in a goal. The first step for an exercise program (after you get a medical exam) is to ask yourself, What's realistic for me? Think "simple." Think "goal." Think "long term."

Unless you are coming from a strong (and recent) background in another physically demanding sport (such as cycling, martial arts, tennis, basketball, soccer, or cross-country skiing), don't jump right into a running program. Instead, begin with a run/walk program. An excellent goal for a run/walk program is four workouts per week, with each one lasting 20 to 30 minutes.

THE BEST PLACES TO RUN

One of the first questions that beginners ask is, Where should I begin my running? It's probably not best to start on the street right outside your door, though certainly many runners do, if for no other reason than convenience.

Running on a smooth, soft surface is the key, so even if you're relegated to the roads, try to run on the silt along the road's edge. Avoid roads with a steep camber to them; these can throw off your foot-plant, leading to sore muscles and injuries. Whenever possible, choose blacktop roads over concrete (concrete is harder), and always run against oncoming traffic. This makes you more visible to the driver (especially if you're wearing light or reflective clothing) and allows you to spot threatening situations before they develop.

Sidewalks may offer better safety from traffic, but concrete's hardness can provoke shinsplints and other aches and pains common to the beginning runner. Also, sidewalks often force you to run up and down the edges at intersections—not a great way to develop your running rhythm.

Top training tips

"If you're just beginning a fitness program, the best way to start is with walking," says Budd Coates, health promotions manager at Rodale Inc. in Emmaus, Pennsylvania, and four-time Olympic Marathon Trials qualifier.

Coates recommends that a person with absolutely no running background get started with eight straight days of walking. (See "Ease into This Running Program" on page 6.)

After that initial break-in period, introduce two minutes of running, alternating with four minutes of walking. Do this five times for a total of 30 minutes per workout. The runs should be slow jogs, not your fastest sprints.

"The biggest mistake that beginning runners make is they think in mile increments," says Coates. "They need to think in minutes of running, not miles."

"The other big mistake is that beginners run too fast," adds Coates. "They get out of breath, their leg muscles scream, and so running isn't fun. They get discouraged and quit. Instead, begin at a pace that is about the same as a fast walk."

The talk test is a simple way to judge your pace. Run at a comfortable pace that lets you talk with a training partner.

After 10 weeks Coates's program brings the beginning runner to a complete 30-minute run, without walking. Once you can comfortably run 30 minutes without stopping, then you can think in terms of miles per week. A reasonable goal is 9 to 14 miles, with three days of running and four days of rest, some of which might include some alternative exercise such as swimming, cycling, or strength training.

A good start: Track running

If you can, start on a well-maintained track at your local school or a path in a public park. Grass can be good, too, but make certain the field is cut close and even. A treadmill at the local health club can also supply a smooth beginning.

Although admittedly not always the most exciting locale, the track has its advantages, especially for the beginner. First, it's flat and soft. Also, you can judge exactly how far you have been running and at what pace. This constant feedback helps you progress with minimal risk and also makes it easy to chart your progress.

When you're running on the track, it makes good sense to run in the outer lanes and occasionally—perhaps every two or three laps—switch direction. Running on the tighter inside lanes and in the same direction can put unnecessary wear and tear on joints and tendons, especially if you're not accustomed to running the turns. Also, if there are advanced runners conducting timed sessions on the track, it's considered proper etiquette to leave the inside lanes open for them.

RUNNING HILLS

Eventually you will encounter hills. You won't consider them a friend at first, but they can actually help you improve your fitness. Physically, running hills builds muscular and cardiovascular strength. Mentally, hills add a challenging touch to an advanced workout and therefore can be a good weapon against boredom. But both uphills and downhills add entirely new and taxing elements to your running program.

Olympic Marathon gold medalist Frank Shorter once referred to hills as speedwork in disguise. Treat hills as such; you'll probably be ready to run a hilly course about the same time you might be ready to attempt an introductory pace and speed session on the track. Therefore, avoid hills in the very early stages of your training program and introduce them in very small doses (and sizes) after you have logged more than a month of flat running at a comfortable pace.

If you do eventually add hills to a program as you advance beyond the beginner stage, start with some slight rollers; save the mountains for the future. Be particularly careful to avoid pounding on the descents. As with flat running, hills that feature grass and soft paths are preferable to hard surfaces.

Regardless of where you decide to walk and run, do some light stretching before you begin the workout. Stretching reduces muscle tightness and allows for a more comfortable stride action.

Your first race

What's the best way to start? Look for a local, relatively low-key race. For example, sometimes a competitive race—such as a 10-K—is accompanied by a two-mile fun run. Start with the fun run. In a year's time you might well progress to the longer, more-challenging race, but the two-mile distance is perfect for testing the waters.

Also, pick a flat course and shoot for a day that's likely to feature pleasant weather conditions—particularly low heat and humidity. Convince a training partner to do the race with you for support and to share the experience. Women may want to try one of the growing numbers of women's-only races such as the "Race for the Cure" series that promotes breast cancer awareness.

THE NEXT LEVEL: RACING

The late running philosopher George Sheehan, M. D., once noted that the only difference between a jogger and a runner is an entry blank. There's much truth to that statement. Most local races contain a number of runners who are lined up primarily to finish the course, even if just slightly faster than they might run the same route during a typical training jaunt.

The point is, if you're curious about racing—and you sense improved fitness in your training runs—try it. It's natural to feel anxiety over where you might place or how fast you will (or won't) run, but recognize such thoughts as the self-imposed barriers that they are.

Ease into this running program

This running schedule was created by Budd Coates.

Each spring Coates leads a corporate running program for beginners that takes nonrunners and, in 10 weeks, gets them to the point where they can run 3.5 miles without stopping. You too can do the same. Before you start this schedule, get your legs ready with eight days of walking: Walk for 20 minutes a day for the first four days, then increase to 30 minutes a day for four more days. Now you're ready to begin with Week 1.

Each week of the program, do your run/walk workouts on Monday, Wednesday, Friday, and Saturday. Take a rest day or an easy walk on Tuesday, Thursday, and Sunday.

Week 1	Run 2 minutes, walk 4 minutes. Complete 5 cycles.
Week 2	Run 3 minutes, walk 3 minutes. Complete 5 cycles.
Week 3	Run 5 minutes, walk 2.5 minutes. Complete 4 cycles.
Week 4	Run 7 minutes, walk 3 minutes. Complete 3 cycles.
Week 5	Run 8 minutes, walk 2 minutes. Complete 3 cycles.
Week 6	Run 9 minutes, walk 2 minutes. Complete 2 cycles, then run 8 minutes.
Week 7	Run 9 minutes, walk 1 minute. Complete 3 cycles.
Week 8	Run 13 minutes, walk 2 minutes. Complete 2 cycles.
Week 9	Run 14 minutes, walk 1 minute. Complete 2 cycles. Note: After completing Week 9, if you feel tired, repeat this week of training before moving on to Week 10.
Week 10	Run 30 minutes.

In your first race, be careful, above all else, not to start too fast. The excitement and adrenaline that you feel will tend to make you run faster than your accustomed pace, but you won't notice it. At least, not at first. Then, after a half-mile or so, you might realize that you're gasping for breath and your legs are beginning to feel like anchors. To avoid this, concentrate on total relaxation at the start and during the early going. Breathe comfort-ably, settle into a moderate pace, and enjoy your-self.

There's an old running maxim that holds for everyone from beginners to Olympic champs: If you start too slowly, you can always pick it up later; but if you start too fast, your goose is cooked. It takes most runners several races to find their perfect pace—a pace that spreads out their reserves equally over the full distance.

Do's and Don'ts for Beginners

Running is a simple activity, but the following guidelines will help you succeed at it.

1. Don't begin a running program without a full medical exam.

2. Don't attempt to train through an athletic injury. Little aches and pains can sideline you for weeks or months if you don't take time off and seek medical advice.

3. Do dress correctly. If it's dark, wear white or, better yet, reflective clothing. If it's cold, wear layers of clothing, gloves or mittens, and a wool ski cap to retain heat. Sunblock, sun-glasses, a baseball cap, and white clothing make sense on hot days.

4. Don't run in worn-out shoes (check them for broken-down heels or very smooth areas where you push off on your strides). Don't run in shoes that are designed for other sports, such as basketball or tennis sneaks.

5. Do tell someone where you'll be running and when you expect to return. Carry some identi-fication and your cell phone.

6. Do some light stretching exercises prior to your run/walk workouts to reduce muscle tightness and increase range of motion. You should do even more stretching after the workout.

7. Do watch out for cars, and don't expect drivers to watch out for you. Always run facing traffic so that you can see cars approaching. When crossing an intersection, make sure you estab-lish eye contact with the driver before proceed-ing.

8. Do include a training partner in your program, if possible. A training partner with similar abili-ties and goals can add motivation and increase the safety of your running.

9. Don't wear headphones when running outside, whether you're training or racing. They tune you out from your surroundings, making you more vulnerable to all sorts of hazards: cars, bikes, skateboards, dogs, and criminals.

10. Don't run in remote areas, especially if you are a woman running alone. If you don't have a partner, run with a dog or carry a self-defense spray (first ensuring it's legal to use where you run). Don't approach a car to give directions, and don't assume all runners are harmless.

For more information on safety, send a request to: Road Runners Club of America, 1501 Lee Highway, Suite 140, Arlington, VA 22209. Visit their Web site at: rrca.org

WATCH OUT FOR THE BUG

With the possible exception of the very beginning of your running program, the next most dangerous time for a novice runner is just after completing that first race—especially if the initial racing experience has been both a successful and enjoyable debut.

The danger, of course, comes from being bitten by the racing bug. The temptation for some runners is suddenly to race every weekend, but this multiplies the possibility of injury or burnout.

Along the same lines, beware of "marathon fever." Some novice racers run a couple of local 5-K events and, flush with excitement, jump right into training for a mega-marathon, such as New York City or Los Angeles. Resist the temptation. The marathon has been around since the ancient Greeks. It will still be there when your running has progressed to the point that your first marathon experience can be an enjoyable one. It doesn't do you any good to enter a marathon that reduces you to a survival crawl punctuated by self-doubt and tagged with the postscript "I'm never running one of these things again!"

Instead, prepare yourself for the transition to marathon running with a gradual introduction of weekly or biweekly long runs. A long run, by definition, is what's long for you in relation to your present level of training. For runners training for their first marathon, the long run might start in the 10- or 12-mile range and gradually progress over several months to distances approaching 20 miles.

Also, some race experience at the 10-mile, 20-K, and half-marathon distances can serve as dress rehearsals for the big one. The long runs and the race distances between 10-K and 26.2 miles will

Amby Burfoot's Running Round-Up

The key to success with a running program for beginners is to start slow and stay slow. Speed kills. Don't even think about it. Patience rewards, so stick with it, stick with it, stick with it.

A few years ago I taught a running program for beginners in which I told my students over and over again that they should run as slowly as possible. "Don't breathe hard," I said. "Stay comfortable. Don't worry about how you look, and don't worry about how fast anyone else in the class is running. Just go slow."

A couple of people in the class seemed to be struggling, so I asked if they were sure that they were running slowly enough. "No problem," they gasped. "This is real comfortable." I knew they were pushing too hard, but that's a hard thing to tell someone, so I asked if I could take their pulses. After only 10 seconds of counting their pulses, I was able to inform them that they were running at about the same effort level as an Olympic champion. One of them was running at a pulse rate of 170 beats per minute. (Most beginning runners should be between 120 and 140, depending on many variables, including age.)

Armed with an objective measure, I was able to convince my students to relax and slow down. They did, they stuck with the program, and eight weeks later they graduated from the class.

You'll graduate, too, to whatever goals you seek, so long as you concentrate on slow and steady. Remember the tortoise and the hare? You want to be a tortoise.

prepare you mentally and physically for the marathon challenge.

You don't have to finish a marathon, however, to be a runner. There are lots of great runners who never run 26.2 miles. A runner is someone who runs; it's that simple—and that grand. Be that someone. Be yourself. Be your own runner, whether the challenge is four times around the junior high school track or qualifying and running in the Boston Marathon.

Chapter 2

Oprah Did It, So Can You

How Running Changed Her Life

In November 1994, when Oprah Winfrey sneaked into the Marine Corps Marathon in Washington, D.C., and successfully completed the 26.2-mile distance in a heavy rain, she became the biggest running story in America since President Jimmy Carter collapsed during a road race in 1979. She was on TV, she was in the daily newspapers, she was on the front page of the *National Enquirer* and the other tabloids, and she recounted the story on her own *Oprah Winfrey Show*.

Why did she create such a stir? Because Oprah Winfrey was the last person the American media expected to run a marathon. When she did it, and did it without stopping to walk a single step of the way, she proved that essentially anyone can be a successful runner. Her inspirational success motivated tens of thousands of other Americans, especially American women, to take up running and get in shape themselves.

In March 1993 Bob Greene received a phone call from Oprah Winfrey. At the time, Greene was head of the exercise program at Telluride Ski Resort in Colorado. Six months earlier, he had led Winfrey, who has a home in Telluride, on several strenuous mountain hikes.

Now she was calling to ask him to move to Chicago to become her personal trainer. Greene hesitated. "I like to sit down with potential new clients to make sure they're serious," he recalls. "With Oprah, that wasn't possible. Still, it was Oprah asking." So he agreed.

Like everyone, Greene (an exercise physiologist) knew about Oprah and her yo-yoing weight-loss problems. Seven years earlier, in front of a national TV audience, she had told the story of her successful weight-loss diet. But within months the pounds had crept back on. She now weighed 222 pounds and didn't seem able to lose more than a pound or two, despite her adherence to a low-calorie, low-fat diet.

Greene had to wonder about Oprah's commitment to an exercise program. Five minutes into their first session, however, he knew he'd made a good choice. "I could tell she was completely determined," he says. "And she never wavered."

Both Oprah and Greene had the same original goal: healthy weight loss. But how? "I made a decision from the very beginning to center Oprah's exercise program around running," Greene says. "There were other options, including swimming or cycling. But if you want quick weight-loss results, as Oprah did, running is the best."

GETTING DOWN TO BUSINESS

At their first training session, Oprah and Greene walked about two and a half miles. Slowly. "I wanted to assess her condition," Greene says. He found her healthy enough to begin mixing jogging and walking within a few days. Her initial pace worked out to about 17 minutes per mile. But two weeks into her program, Oprah was running and walking three to four consecutive miles at that pace.

Scheduling these workouts was not easy. Five days a week Oprah would rise at 5:00 a.m. to run before taping her show. Each afternoon, she would step onto a stair-climbing machine for 45 minutes, followed by a half-hour or so of weight training. "That might be too aggressive a program for some people," Greene admits, "especially the two-a-day training sessions. But I wanted to get her metabolism revved up."

By early summer Oprah was on a roll. "She was achieving a steady, sustainable, 8- to 10-pound weight loss every month, and she didn't have to change her diet," Greene says. By July Oprah was running five to six miles a day at a 10- to 11-minute-per-mile pace. By midsummer, she had lost more than 40 pounds. It was time to race.

"I believe in using races as motivators," Greene says. "Sometimes it's hard to keep going on an exercise program if you don't have a goal in sight." He had hoped to find a 10-K for Oprah to enter but couldn't locate one that matched her busy weekend schedule. Eventually he decided to be more ambitious, so in August 1993 he entered Oprah in the America's Finest City Half-Marathon in San Diego. Oprah completed the distance in a respectable 2:16.

With her finisher's medal triumphantly in hand, Oprah began pressing Greene to come up with a new challenge. "At one point she told me that she had always loved watching the marathon in Chicago," he says. "She'd cheer for the runners going past and think, 'I'd like to do that someday.'"

Greene downplayed the idea. First, he told her, she should concentrate on reaching her goal weight of 150 pounds. She was so close. And on November 10, 1993, she made it. That same morning, for the first time ever, she completed her 5-mile run at an 8-minute-per-mile pace. "I was so proud of her," Greene remembers. "Sometimes people will say to me, 'Oprah's got it easy because she has a personal chef and a personal trainer.' But that's baloney. No one can run for you. She was on the track every morning. She worked herself as hard as any athlete I've seen. She deserved the results she achieved."

A NEW GOAL

From that day on, the focus of Oprah's training program shifted dramatically. She had achieved

Top training tips

"About three weeks into our program, Oprah noticed that she'd actually gained weight, not lost it, which is a common phenomenon for people who start a serious exercise program," explains Greene. "But that weight rolls right off after another week or so. Unfortunately, many people quit exercising as soon as the weight comes on. It's a convenient excuse."

Oprah didn't quit. "She was so excited, because she soon began seeing dramatic results. The body abides by the laws of physics. The more weight you lose, the faster you run. And the faster you run, the more weight you lose."

her weight-loss goal. She had even run a half-marathon. What was left? "Obviously, we wanted to maintain the weight loss, first and foremost," Greene says. "But we also knew that Oprah was ready to begin running more seriously. We decided to move from a weight-loss program to a training program. We decided that in 1994 she'd run a marathon."

So, beginning in January 1994, Oprah stepped up her training. Curiously, she began by running less, but this was part of the plan. "We stopped the two-a-day workouts," Greene says. "I even cut back somewhat on her mileage. Instead, I put her on a much more intensive strength-training regimen, because I knew training for a marathon would be hard on her body. I wanted to make sure that her joints were strong and healthy."

By midsummer 1994, Oprah was running as much as 50 miles a week, which included long-distance runs on weekends. At times, she complained. "This is such a struggle," she'd say to Greene. To which he answered, "No, it's not. It's a daily renewal."

His message took hold, and Oprah stuck to the program. Three months later she completed the Marine Corps Marathon without walking a

Amby Burfoot's Running Round-Up

Totally by chance, I happened to attend the Marine Corps Marathon that Oprah ran. I wasn't entered or expecting to run, but when I learned that Oprah was going to go the distance, I decided to join her.

I stood near the three-mile mark at the Pentagon, in a pouring rain, and waited to see if I could find Oprah amidst the 15,000 other runners in the field. It wasn't difficult. Before spotting her myself, I heard other spectators yelling, "There she is. There's Oprah."

When she went past, I joined in just behind her. She was running with a friend, while Greene ran just in front of her. The National Enquirer, always on the case, had assigned two quite-fit reporters to go the distance at Oprah's side. I'd estimate I've run more than 70 marathons and written far more than 70 stories about marathons and marathoners, but I feel I've never experienced anything as astounding and inspirational as Oprah, up close and personal, as she ran the marathon distance. Despite the distractions of thousands of spectators and other runners constantly calling out her name or coming up to slap her on the back, she never lost her concentration, her good spirit, or her determination.

She achieved her goal because she had trained hard, and she trained hard because she never stopped believing in herself. If Oprah can run a marathon, anyone can be a successful (and healthy and weight-reducing) runner. All you have to do is believe.

single step. "I'll never forget mile 25 of that race," Greene says. "I turned around to watch her. She was looking great, passing people. She was just so pumped. There were tears in her eyes, and I thought, this is it. This moment symbolizes everything from 222 pounds to where she is now. It was just so moving.

"She could have quit months before the marathon. She certainly had enough legitimate excuses. But she didn't. I like to think her progress and her commitment will show millions of other people that they can improve their lives, too. Maybe they won't run a marathon, but they can run a 5-K. Or they can lose the weight that they've been wanting to get rid of. It's just so inspiring to watch someone transform herself, and that's what Oprah has done.

Chapter 3

Buy the Right Shoes for You

A Guide to Buying Your Most Important Piece of Gear

The great thing about running is that you only need one piece of equipment. The bad thing is that the equipment, your running shoes, is so important that it gets buried under millions of dollars of hype, advertising, and confusing technobabble.

For more than two decades, *Runner's World* magazine has helped consumers decipher and unravel that confusion with semiannual reviews of the best new training shoes. In addition, the magazine publishes simple guides to help readers make the right shoe selections.

A couple of decades ago, the world was a simpler place, and so were running shoes. Today, simple canvas sneakers are as dead as Elvis, which isn't necessarily a bad thing. In just about every way, today's shoes are a whole lot better—more durable, more protective, and more comfortable—than ever before.

The one bad thing: They're also much more complicated. Why? Because running, while it's a simple sport that almost everyone can do, forces your feet and legs through a fairly complex series of movements.

With all the high-tech running shoes available today and all the special features that each shoe claims to have, picking the right pair can be a daunting task. Just follow the advice here, and you'll be able to find the best shoes for you.

STEP 1: LEARN ABOUT PRONATION

Running is a complex biomechanical process in which, generally speaking, you strike the ground first on the outside of your heel. Next, your foot rolls downward and inward slightly as it meets the ground. And lastly, the heel lifts from the ground, and you push off from the ball of the foot to move forward.

The rotation of the foot downward and

inward when you land on the ground is called pronation, and it's a completely natural and normal process. That's worth repeating: Pronation is a natural, normal process. Everyone should pronate to some degree. Pronation is a good thing in that it helps the foot absorb the shock of impact.

Some runners, however, overpronate. That is, their feet roll too far inward. This is a common problem that can lead to injuries, particularly of the lower leg and knee. Some runners supinate (or underpronate); their feet roll inward only a little after contact. These runners are said to have "rigid" feet that don't absorb shock very well. This, too, can lead to injury over time.

STEP 2: FIGURE OUT YOUR FOOT TYPE

Most runners can determine whether they are supinators, overpronators, or normal pronators by checking their arch heights. "The arch determines how your feet and legs will function when you run," explains Joe Ellis, D.P.M., a podiatrist from La Jolla, California, and author of *Running Injury-Free*.

"Our studies show that 50 percent of runners have normal arches, while 25 percent have high arches and the remaining 25 percent have low arches," says John W. Pagliano, D.P.M., a podiatrist in private practice in Long Beach, California.

But how do you figure out your arch height? The easiest way is with the "wet test." Wet the bottom of your bare foot, then make a footprint on a flat, dry surface—a piece of white paper laid on a hard floor works well to show the shape of your foot. If your footprint is very full and wide and

Take the "wet test."

A "wet test" is a quick and easy way of discovering what your footprint tells you about your degree of pronation.

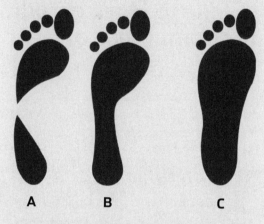

A   B   C

(a) A high-arched foot means you may be a supinator.

(b) A normal foot means you probably are a normal pronator.

(c) A flat foot means you may have a tendency to overpronate.

shows no arch, you have a low arch and a flat foot. If the print shows your entire foot with a moderate curve where the arch rises off the ground, you have a normal arch. And if the footprint is very slight and curved, showing mostly the ball and heel of your foot but very little of the middle of your foot, you have a high arch.

With all the high-tech running shoes available today, picking the right pair can be a daunting task.

STEP 3: GET THE RIGHT SHOE

Your foot type and degree of pronation determine the characteristics that you'll need in a running shoe. One of the most important characteristics to look for is shape. You can see the shape most clearly by looking at the bottom of the shoe.

In general, running shoes come in three shapes—straight, semicurved, and curved—which correspond to the three types of footprints revealed by the wet test. Most experts believe that overpronators should wear a shoe with a straight shape, supinators should wear a shoe with a curved shape, and normal pronators should wear a shoe with a semicurved shape. There are a few other characteristics to consider.

If you have flat feet and overpronate, you need a shoe that will prevent your foot from rolling in too far, that is, a motion-control shoe. These shoes have a straight shape that gives maximum support to your foot. Also look for a firm rather than a soft midsole, a dual-density midsole with the denser material along the inner edge of the shoe to prevent excessive pronation, and a firm heel counter to minimize rear-foot motion.

If you have high-arched feet and supinate, your feet don't absorb shock very well, so you need a cushioned shoe. Also, you want a shoe that allows your feet to roll inward, since this helps absorb shock. "Cushioned shoes tend to be less supportive and work with the foot rather than try to control it," says Dan Norton, a shoe designer who has worked at several of the major running-shoe companies. You want a shoe with a soft, cushioned midsole and a curved or semicurved shape that permits foot motion as you run.

If you have normal arches and pronate normally, you're lucky. You don't need to search out a shoe with special features. You might want to begin by considering shoes that lie somewhere between the motion-control and cushioned types. Manufacturers often refer to such shoes as stability shoes. These shoes, which often have a slightly curved shape, don't control foot motion as much as motion-control shoes.

"Don't worry about the technology. Worry about the fit and the comfort," says Norton

Anatomy of a running shoe

As running shoes have gotten more complicated, so has the terminology used to describe them. The glossary below will help you understand the basic parts of a running shoe.

Upper: The part of the shoe that wraps around and over the top of the foot. It's most of what you see when you look at a running shoe.

Heel counter: A firm cup that is encased in the upper and surrounds the heel. It controls rear-foot motion.

Outsole: The undersurface of the shoe, usually made from carbon rubber.

Midsole: The most important part of a shoe, it is the cushioning layer between the upper and the outsole. It is usually made of ethylene vinyl acetate (EVA), polyurethane (a synthetic rubber that's heavier and longer-lasting than EVA), or a combination of the two. Dual-density midsoles have a firmer material on the inside of the shoe. This helps limit pronation. Many shoe companies also put patented technologies in their midsoles, such as gel and high-tech plastics.

STEP 4: VISIT A SPECIALTY RUNNING STORE

Even if you have followed all the steps outlined here, it pays to go to a specialty running store. The knowledgeable people who work in these stores will be able to tell you if you're a special case who needs extra attention when it comes to shoe selection. Whatever your needs, you'll want help to find the shoe model that works best for you.

STEP 5: MAKE SURE YOUR SHOE FITS

This is the most important step in finding the right shoe. "Don't worry about the technology," says Bob Cook, owner of The Runner's Edge, a running specialty store in Farmingdale, New York. "Worry about the fit and the comfort."

A running shoe that fits will be snug but not tight. Buying running shoes that are too small is a common problem. Your running shoes may need to be a half to a full size larger than your street shoes.

Finding the right shoe for you

Here are some tips for a successful shopping trip.

For best fit, shop in the late afternoon when your feet are at their largest, because your feet will expand during running.

Wear the socks that you'll wear when you run. If you don't have any, buy some before trying on shoes.

Make sure that the salesperson measures both of your feet. Most of us have one foot slightly larger than the other, and you should be fitted for the larger foot.

Before you try on any shoes, the salesperson should talk to you about your running, in order to guide you to appropriate shoe models.

Following are the questions that the salesperson should ask.

How long have you been running?

How much mileage are you running?

Where do you do most of your running?

How much do you weigh?

Are you aware of any foot problems, such as flat feet or overpronation or supination?

The price is right

How much should you pay for running shoes? Any shoe costing $75 or more, no matter who manufactures it, should provide the primary features and protection you need. Step up to $100, and you'll get more durability, more features, and more quality.

Spend the money. A good pair of running shoes should last for 400 to 500 miles and is the only critical purchase you have to make.

Use the following guidelines to determine whether a running shoe fits you properly.

Check for adequate room at the tip of your toe by pressing your thumb into the shoe just above your longest toe. The edge of your thumb should fit between the end of your toe and the front edge of the toe box.

Your heel should fit snugly into the rear of the shoe and should not slide up and down as you walk or run.

The upper (the part of the shoe that wraps around and over the top of the foot) should fit snugly and hold your foot securely, but it should not irritate or press too tightly on any area of your foot.

Take the shoes for a test run. Most specialty running stores allow—even encourage--you to run down the street or around the block so that you can feel the shoes in action.

Use these guidelines in trying out a few different models. Then decide on the pair that fits the best and feels the most comfortable. And if you get them home and find some problems with them as you begin your running program, take them back. "If you have any problems—heel slippage, a burning sensation in the balls of your feet once you

Amby Burfoot's Running Round-Up

With dozens of different companies and models to choose from, and exciting new shoe styles hitting the market every day, selecting your pair of running shoes remains a tough choice. I've found that the process is much simpler if you follow these guidelines.

Stick with proven shoes. New shoes are like new cars and new computers. You should keep away from them for a couple of years until the bugs are all worked out.

Talk to other runners and knowledgeable retail salespeople. Virtually every office and neighborhood in America has experienced runners with a collective knowledge of running shoes. Ask them what shoes they have had good luck with. Evaluate how these runners' needs are similar to or different from your own needs.

When you get your new shoes home, wear them first on short runs. After you're confident that they're broken in and don't cause any blis-

ters or other abrasions, you can use them on longer runs.

Wear your running shoes for running only. They weren't intended for basketball or mowing the lawn, and they'll give you more miles of comfortable, injury-free running if you only use them for running.

Keep your shoes as dry as possible. Whether they're damp with sweat or wringing wet after a workout in a downpour, they'll recover fastest and best if air-dried. (And they won't stink.) Don't put your shoes in the clothes dryer, which is too hot. A small fan does an excellent job of drying out shoes.

Remember that your shoes need replacement after 400 to 500 miles. Even if you don't see much cosmetic deterioration, the shoes' midsoles will have lost their cushioning and resiliency. It's time for a new pair.

start running—bring 'em back," says Dick Haines, owner of Aardvark Sports Shop in Bethlehem, Pennsylvania. He adds, "Remember, there are lots of good shoes out there. We'll find one that's right for you."

And a word for the future: Once you've found a shoe that works for you, stick with it. New models will always tempt you, but keep in mind that the right running shoes help you avoid injury. So, if your shoes fit well and feel good, and you don't have any problems with injuries, stick to a sure thing.

Now, lace up those new running shoes and head out on your path to better fitness.

Chapter 4

Start Right Here

All You Need to Know to Begin Running for the First Time

In the first decade of the new millennium, Americans awakened to a rather strange paradox: We were in the midst of a fatness revolution and a fitness revolution at the same time. Almost every week, headlines screamed out about the rising obesity crisis and the toll it would take on us, both personal—increased diseases among friends and family—and public, in terms of rising medical expenses.

Meanwhile, a fitness revolution was also taking place, though much less noticed. Every year more and more Americans began running, improved their health, and entered races from the 5-K to the marathon.

What does this all mean? Simply that fatness isn't inevitable. It's easy to get in shape; it's just that it takes consistent hard work. In other words, you don't need a lot of expensive equipment or high-priced lessons. You just need the willpower and the dedication to get started and to stick with it.

So you want to start running? You've heard it's inexpensive, great for your health, and the best way to lose weight (and keep it off). You've got friends and coworkers who run, and they're trim, happy, centered, and productive. Running also looks like a straightforward enough sport. There's only one thing that's bothering you: If running is so simple, why do you have so many questions?

You're not alone. Every beginner worries about how to get started and has a lot to ask—about how to get motivated, what to eat, how to avoid injuries, and exactly when and where and how much to run. No problem. We've got the answers—from experts who have been teaching beginning running classes for up to 35 years, and from others who've certainly been around the block. Every runner began with a first step. You can, too.

INSPIRATION

"Help! I need motivation!"

Make all the excuses you want—then get on with it.

You don't have time; you don't have the energy; it's too cold/hot/rainy; the dog ate your shoelaces. Uh-huh. Now go out and run. Online running coach and former educator Dean Hebert has heard so many excuses from his runners that he assembled them into a book, *Coach, I Didn't Run Because . . . Excuses Not to Run and How to Overcome Them.* "These excuses are real to people, and I don't diminish them. I tell my beginning runners to concentrate on the one reason that brought them to running. A clear focus can work magic on your motivation," he says.

Keep track

Keeping a written diary is a highly successful way to stick with an exercise or diet program. It doesn't have to be fancy or sophisticated. Indeed, where you place the diary might be more important than what you write in it. Put a calendar on your fridge or in front of your computer, write down every time you complete a run, and take pride in watching those numbers build up. (Or feel guilty when they don't! That'll get you out.)

Keep at it

Some runners win gold medals and set world records, but no runner has ever done every workout he or she planned. You won't either. Stuff happens, but you can deal as long as you stay focused on the big picture. Shrug off the bad days, get back on the program, and you'll still achieve your goals—losing weight, gaining energy, improving your health, adding distance to your runs, and so on. Remaining persistent is crucial to improved running. "When beginners get discouraged or hit a plateau, I tell them to remember the time and effort invested and the progress they've made," says beginners' coach Jane Serues. "You don't want to slide backward; you want to keep working toward the progress ahead."

Find a fitness friend

Beginning running coaches agree that one of the best ways to stick with your exercise program is to get a training partner. When someone is counting on you as much as you're counting on them, it's much tougher to blow off a workout. But it has to be someone of similar ability who is supportive, not competitive with you. "We emphasize the emotional power of training partners," says Serues, who has introduced 6,000 women to running in the Lehigh Valley of eastern Pennsylvania. "One or two is good. Three or four are even better."

Make the time

Sure, your life is busy enough already. We hear you, but consider the payoffs of just 150 minutes a week of "moderate intensity" exercise, as recommended by the American Heart Association and the American College of Sports Medicine. With five 30-minute run/walk workouts per week, you can expect a reduced risk of chronic illnesses, such as heart disease, stroke, high blood pressure, diabetes, osteoporosis, obesity, colon cancer, breast cancer, anxiety, and depression. In addition, for the first time ever, the two medical-scientific groups acknowledged in 2008 that additional exercise would provide "even greater health benefits."

Don't worry about quitting

New York sports psychologist Ethan Gologor, Ph.D., captain of the New York City Marathon psyching team, points out that we're all quitters in the sense that we have dropped out of some activity at some time. There's nothing wrong with starting again (and again). Says Gologor, author of *Psychodynamic Running: The Complete, Definitive Madman's Guide to Distance Running and the Marathon*. "If you miss one or two workouts, that's not the end of the world. Runners shouldn't 'must' themselves to failure with thoughts like 'I must run every day my plan says to.' You can miss several days and still get back into your routine."

NUTRITION: "I DON'T KNOW WHAT TO EAT!"

Good running and healthy nutrition go hand in hand, from breakfast to late-night snacks.

Pass on the extra carbs

Bread, bagels, pasta, potatoes, and pancakes—you just can't get enough, right? Wrong, says Boston-area sports nutritionist Nancy Clark, R.D., author of the new book *Nancy Clark's Food Guide for New Runners*. Running two or three miles at an easy pace will burn 200 to 300 calories, an amount so

modest that it doesn't demand lumberjack portions of carbs (or anything else) before or after. Clark advocates eating healthy foods throughout the day, and having a small snack an hour or two before you run. "Exercisers shouldn't skip meals early in the day or try to run on fumes," she says. "But you don't require special foods after a workout—just a snack that offers a few carbs and a little protein."

Drink water—but only when you're thirsty

Yes, runners sweat a lot. Yes, they need water, sugar, and electrolytes when they run for 90 minutes or more, particularly in warm weather. But unless you're training for a marathon this summer (which you won't be), you don't need sports drinks and an advanced hydration strategy. Sip a little water before your workout and a little more after. And skip the extra calories in sweetened drinks. "Beginning runners don't need a sports drink, because they're not running far enough," notes Clark.

Eat real food

Runners, even beginners, tend to be driven, results-oriented people. When promised shortcuts, miracle cures, and unbelievable benefits from supplement and "superfood" manufacturers, they're easily swayed. However, eating standard, simple, unprocessed natural foods will give you the same end results. "Every time one of those vitamin or supplement studies produces a negative result, I am reassured that focusing on quality calories is the best advice," says Clark. "I've always believed that the healthiest foods are the real foods—the quality vegetables, fruits, whole grains, low-fat dairy, and lean proteins packed with everything runners need."

If you want to lose weight...

Sorry, but you won't automatically drop five pounds just because you run, says Clark. You also have to reduce your daily food intake. Each mile you run burns roughly 100 calories. Cut out a cookie or two every day, and you can add another 100 calories to your weight-loss effort. "Reducing calorie consumption by just 100 calories a day will theoretically give you a 10-pound weight loss by the end of the year," Clark says. "Hit 200 calories a day, and you'll lose 20 pounds." She suggests cutting calories by eating smaller portions and fewer fried foods.

INJURY PREVENTION: HOW CAN I AVOID INJURY OR WORSE?"

Many runners get minor injuries, but few runners get serious injuries. A few simple steps will keep you on the right path.

Stretch after you run, not before

Runners have long believed that stretching will give them a longer, smoother stride and reduce their risk of injuries. However, in recent years research has failed to prove either point. Budd Coates, four-time Olympic Marathon Trials qualifier, and Jeff Galloway, *Runner's World* columnist and author of *Running: Getting Started*, say they've

never advocated stretching for their beginning runners, and the runners haven't developed injuries. Adds Lewis Maharam, M.D., medical director of the ING New York City Marathon and the Rock 'n' Roll Marathons, as well as a runnersworld.com medical blogger: "A preworkout stretching routine doesn't prevent injuries or improve performance, so there's no reason to do it. The time to do your stretching is after your run, or even later in the evening." Stretch (without straining) your calves, quads, and hamstrings for 10 to 15 minutes.

Beat injuries by going slowly

True, runners get occasional muscle and joint aches, but these should go away quickly. When veteran running coach Galloway began teaching beginners in 1974, he was worried about some of the participants. "But everyone finished the class," he says. "You don't get injured if you follow the 'no huffing, no puffing' rule."

Expect a little tenderness

Sure, runners have to deal with occasional aches and pains. Especially beginners. However, these are temporary complaints that don't lead to long-term damage. In 2008, the *Archives of Internal Medicine* published a study on a group of runners who were first investigated in the mid-1980s when they were 50 years old or older. Twenty-one years later, these runners, now in their mid-70s, were found to have better function and overall health and fewer disabilities than similar individuals who had not been running for two decades. When you experience mild aches and pains, follow the tried-and-true RICE prescription: rest, ice, compression, elevation. Don't overuse pain meds and anti-inflammatories (see "The Pill Problem," page xx). "The over-the-counter meds are not perfectly safe and aren't meant to mask pain," says Dr. Maharam. "Overuse can lead to liver, stomach, and kidney problems."

You're (almost certainly) not going to die

Yes, heart attacks happen, and they make headlines. But these events are extremely rare, averaging about one for every 800,000 half-hour workouts. Meanwhile, it's a well-established medical fact that runners and other highly fit individuals have a 50 percent lower risk of heart attack than nonexercisers. It's more dangerous to sit in front of your TV. The heart is a muscle. If you don't exercise it, it becomes weak and flabby. Still, every runner should know the signs of a heart attack: unusual shortness of breath; chest, arm, or neck tightness (especially on the left side); nausea; and a cold sweat. If you experience these, stop immediately and call your doctor.

Don't fret about the doc

Anyone you ask will say that you should see your physician before beginning a running program, but do you really have to? Maybe not. The American College of Sports Medicine says checkups are necessary only for those with increased risks: men over 40, women over 50, and those with significant medical problems, cardiac risk factors, or a history of heart attack. Even so, it's a good idea, says Dr. Maharam. "You especially need a physical if you haven't seen your doc in a while, and you're just starting to run. Be sure to discuss your plans. Your physician will pay particular attention to certain things during your exam, and you might get an extra test if it's warranted."

GEAR: "DO I NEED FANCY STUFF?"

Running is the simplest, least expensive sport, which is one of its great joys. But choosing good gear can make every mile easier.

Buy the right shoes

You don't absolutely, positively need a new pair of running shoes when you begin running. You can run in your comfortable cross-trainers, sneakers, or walking shoes. But when you're ready, the right pair will make your runs more comfortable while adding extra injury-prevention features. Selecting these shoes, sad to say, can be a complex process. That's why it's smart to go to a specialty running store. The experienced staff will make sure you get shoes that fit right and provide the biomechanical support you need. Expect to pay $85 to $120. "We know how to look at your foot when it hits the road, and that makes a huge difference," says J. D. Denton, senior writer at *Running Times* and owner of a Fleet Feet running store in Davis, California.

Wear polyester

You don't need a lot of expensive gear to run, which is good news in a recession. That said, you'll never regret the dollars you spend on breathable socks, and even shirts and shorts. These garments, made from polyester fabrics, are a world apart from the scratchy material your father ran track in. The best are lightweight, soft, and nonchafing. "They'll prevent blisters and rashes," says Denton, "and they'll actually help keep you cooler in summer and warmer in winter."

Forget about gadgets

Heart-rate monitors, GPS systems on a watch, accelerometers that tell you how fast you're going, cell phones with astonishing tools—none of these glitzy products will help your first efforts. All you really need is a watch with a stopwatch function, available for around $30 at any drugstore, to help you keep track of your walking and running intervals. Don't worry about other fancy gizmos. But if your iPod makes your workouts go better, by all means take it with you—as long as you run in a safe place.

TRAINING: "So how do I do this?"

Having a smart, long-range attitude about your training program is the best way to guarantee your success. Think before you run.

Start slow

Most beginning runners worry that they're not improving fast enough. Don't compare yourself with others. Every runner gets into shape according to his or her own body's schedule. Physiologists have calculated that any and all running paces are fast enough to put you into the moderate-to-vigorous aerobic zone that delivers health benefits. (For more guidance on pacing, see "The Starting Line," page xx.) So take your time and focus on going farther, not faster. "We tell people that they

didn't get out of shape in five weeks, and they're not going to get back in shape in five weeks," says Bob Glover, coauthor of *The Runner's Handbook* and New York Road Runners coach, who taught his first running course in 1973.

And again: Go slow

If you feel out of breath or sick to your stomach, you're running too fast, a mistake made by perhaps 99 percent of beginners. "A lot of people think that they have to go at least a mile at a time, and at a good clip," says Coates. "I always tell my beginning runners to slow down and take more walk breaks." When you slow down and maybe walk more, your breathlessness and nausea will go away. You'll learn that running should be a relaxed activity, and that you should "train, not strain." And, yes, beginning running includes lots of walking. Get over it.

Run tall and relaxed

For the most part, you don't have to worry about your technique. That said, experts agree that you should run tall (not slouched) and straight (not leaning far forward or backward). Don't overstride; that could put extra strain on your knees. "Run with your eyes focused about nine feet ahead," says Serues. "Let your arms relax, down around your waist, and take a natural, comfortable stride."

Whenever and wherever

Is there a best time and place to run? Sure: whenever and wherever are most convenient. Finding ways to fit workouts into your schedule is more important than fretting over the when and where questions. Neighborhood roads, a high school track, a treadmill—all good. Beginners should stick to relatively flat running. Hills dramatically increase the muscular and aerobic strain of a run. Run against traffic, so drivers can see you. After all, you're in this for the long run.

Don't let excuses sidetrack you

Remember the millions of couch-potatoes-turned-runners who came before you. "Beginners all say, 'This seems crazy. Can I do it?'" says Glover. "I tell them, 'Yes, anyone can do this. Runners come in all shapes and all ages. You just have to take your time, and stick with the program.'"

Amby Burfoot's Running Round-Up

If you can walk continuously for 30 minutes, you can transition into a running program by gradually adding running to a couple walks per week. Start running at an easy pace, and stop as soon as you're breathing hard. Walk until you feel recovered. Then run again. If you can run only 10 seconds at a time, that's fine. (And if you can run comfortably for 10 minutes at a time, go for it.)

As you get fitter, gradually run more and walk less. But as soon as you begin breathing hard, slow down. This plan consists of five workouts a week, to accumulate 150 minutes of moderate to vigorous exercise, as advised by leading medical groups.

1ST MONTH: Weeks 1 through 4

Three days per week: Walk 10 minutes. Run/walk 15 minutes. Walk 5 minutes. **Two days per week:** Walk 30 minutes.

2ND MONTH: Weeks 5 through 8

Three days per week: Walk 5 minutes. Run/walk 20 minutes. Walk 5 minutes. **Two days per week:** Walk 30 minutes.

3RD MONTH: Weeks 9 through 12

Three days per week: Walk 2 minutes. Run/walk 25 minutes. Walk 3 minutes. **Two days per week:** Walk 30 minutes.

Americans' health can be viewed as a big triangle, a pyramid of sorts. At the bottom are the many, many people who don't eat very healthfully and virtually never exercise. Near the top are the few who eat wisely and exercise on a regular basis. And way up at the top, at the tippy top, are the runners.

Running isn't morally better than other exercises. A calorie burned is a calorie burned, after all. Running simply burns more calories in less time in more seasons of the year with fewer equipment or gym needs than any other exercise. That's why it's such a great way to get in shape.

When you begin running, the first mile seems impossible. So don't run for a mile. Instead, run for 10 to 15 seconds, walk until you get your breath back, and then run another 15 seconds. You'll probably cover about 50 yards with each run, roughly three percent of a mile.

You see how much easier that is? You don't have to run a mile. You can get there by running three percent of a mile 35 times. And the benefits are exactly the same. So remember: No excuses—get started now.

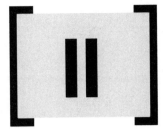

Running and Nutrition

Chapter 5

Eat the Right Foods at the Right Time

Getting Your Pre-Race Nutrition Right Is as Important as Your Taper

Before a big race, runners set aside a period of time, called the taper, that can last from two days to two weeks. The idea is to rest, get strong, and get psyched for the upcoming race. Training wears you down somewhat; the taper allows you to recover and then catapult forward to the high level of performance you hope to achieve on race day.

Tapering involves far more than just reducing your daily training. Another important factor is changing your diet. Indeed, the biggest advances in sports nutrition during the past two decades have been those that have focused on pre-race nutrition.

Nearly everyone has heard about carbohydrate loading, the cornerstone of any pre-event nutrition plan. But a thorough nutritional taper involves much more than just the Ps—pasta, potatoes, and pancakes. There are also the Fs, for example—fats, fiber, and fluids. In this chapter, Liz Applegate, Ph.D., nutrition editor for *Runner's World* magazine, deals with all these topics and many more.

When race day nears, whether it's a 5-K or a marathon, you adjust your training by decreasing your mileage, getting in some extra speedwork, and then tapering the last few days beforehand.

But do you know how to adjust your diet? Improper fueling before a race can result in a lackluster performance. However, by planning a nutritional taper as carefully as you do your training taper, you can stoke up to race your best.

The following guide will tell you when, what, and how much to eat and drink before your next race.

SETTING THE STAGE

Before you taper, estimate your current daily calorie needs by allotting between 17 and 26 calories per pound of body weight, depending on your training intensity. This comes to approximately 2,500 to 4,000 calories for a 150-pound runner.

Carbohydrate intake should be at least 60 percent of your total calories. Keep the fat percentage down to 20 to 25 percent of total calories, with protein at 15 to 20 percent per day.

If you're running a marathon, begin your nutritional plan seven days beforehand. (For shorter races such as 5-Ks and 10-Ks, wait until four days before the race to begin your nutritional taper. See the following section, "Hitting a Stride," for guidance.) Because you'll be tapering your training, do the same with your diet. To avoid gaining weight, you need to bring your calorie intake down about 100 calories for every mile you deduct from your training during your taper. At the same time, you want carbohydrate intake to be sufficient to keep your stores of glycogen (a complex carbohydrate that your body uses for quick energy) full for race day.

Alcohol awareness

The last few days before your race, you'll want to keep away from certain items. Beware of alcohol, especially if you're running a longer race. Alcohol interferes with glycogen and carbohydrate metabolism in the liver, which will shortchange your endurance. It also acts as a diuretic, that is, it accelerates dehydration.

As always—but especially now—go for low-fat, high-carbohydrate foods such as whole-grain cereal, bread, and pasta, along with vegetables and plenty of fruit. Consider taking a multivitamin and mineral supplement that supplies 100 percent of the Daily Value of key vitamins and minerals to ensure adequate intake, particularly if you tend to eat processed or packaged foods that may fall short on good nutrition.

During the sixth and fifth days before a marathon, continue monitoring and adjusting calorie and carbohydrate intake, making sure not to stuff yourself but still eating enough so that you don't feel hungry. It's especially important now to keep your meal times regular and not to miss meals.

HITTING A STRIDE

For shorter races such as 5-Ks and 10-Ks, begin your nutritional taper four days before the race. Cut back slightly on calorie intake as you back off on mileage these few days before the race. Because shorter races (less than an hour) don't tax glycogen stores nearly as much as marathons do, carbohydrate intake is not as crucial. Nevertheless, you'll want to keep carbohydrate intake at about 60 percent of total calories, or roughly 450 grams of carbohydrates per day.

For marathoners, four days before the race is the time to begin increasing your carbohydrate intake to about 65 percent or more of total calories, which amounts to almost 500 grams per day. If you don't have the appetite for that much pasta and potatoes, try liquid sources of carbohydrates, such as fruit juices or sports drinks. And as you boost carbohydrate intake, cut back slightly on fat and protein.

At three days before the race, you've pared down your training, and you may be starting to feel a little sluggish. That's because your body responds to the training taper and the flood of carbohydrates by packing the muscles with more glycogen than usual. And since water gets tucked away with the glycogen in the muscles, you may gain a little weight. Don't worry about it. In the marathon in particular, any water you can store before the race will pay many dividends during the course of those 26.2 miles.

Marathoners should keep in mind that eating 500 grams of carbohydrates a day requires you to be a fat-sleuth, as too much fat will, in effect, crowd out needed carbohydrates.

THE HOMESTRETCH

During the two days before a race, many runners break down nutritionally. Often this happens because they need to travel to a race, which changes their routine, making it hard to stay on a steady eating schedule. Plus, when they do eat, they have less control over what they consume and how it's prepared than they have at home. It's tougher to stay on top of fluid needs as well. (Beware of the dehydrating effects of travel, particularly in airplanes.)

Try to minimize these pitfalls by planning ahead. If you're traveling, find out about restaurants and food stores near your hotel. At home or away, take along nonperishable high-carbohydrate items such as sports bars, granola bars, sports drinks, cereals, and dried fruit. These types of foods are great for augmenting your diet and keeping your carbohydrate consumption up.

Since heavy sweat loss during longer races leads to dehydration, you'll want to "fluid-load" starting two days before you race. Drink plenty of liquids throughout the day, making sure that your urine color is clear or pale yellow, not dark amber. (This is a simple but effective measure of adequate hydration status.) Taking in sports drinks at this time is a good way to get both fluids and carbohydrates.

At this late stage, limiting high-fiber foods such as bran cereals, beans, and some vegetables will help those runners who suffer from bowel problems during running. Stick with foods that agree with you.

On the day before the race, be sure to rest, eat (without overstuffing), and drink plenty of fluids. Provided you have been eating enough and sticking to high-carbohydrate fare that is modest in fat and protein, your glycogen stores will be at their peak by the end of this day. Snack frequently throughout the day and stay with familiar foods. And just to be safe—especially if you're on the road—carry your own water bottle and "go to the well" often to stay hydrated.

Give careful consideration to the meal you eat the night before racing. It should include 800 to 1,000 calories, and—as you know by now—it should be high in carbohydrates and low in fat and protein. Avoid beans, broccoli, and other gas-causing foods, especially if they normally give you problems. Keep alcohol to a strict minimum or skip it altogether. Finally, the night before is not the time to experiment with new foods; the result of the experiment could be diminished performance (or, worse, stomach distress) the next day.

RACE DAY

A good rule of thumb: Eat a light meal the morning of your race, no matter how early it starts. By taking in carbohydrates, particularly before longer races, you'll provide more energy for your muscles. Your pre-race meal should be eaten two to four hours before starting time and should consist of at least 200 grams of carbohydrates, which works out to about 800 calories' worth. In order to speed up your digestion, select foods and beverages that are low in fat and fiber. Don't worry about swings in blood sugar levels, as research shows this doesn't decrease performance.

Bagels, raisins, bananas, sports drinks, pasta, and rice make great pre-race foods. But if the thought of eating in those pre-race morning hours doesn't sit well with your stomach, consider a liquid meal such as a sports drink, a high-carbohydrate beverage, or a nutritional supplement drink.

During the race itself, be sure to stay adequately hydrated. Use those water stops. In longer races, you'll need to replenish with carbohydrates as well. This helps maintain glycogen stores.

On the course, plan to drink from one-half to three-quarters cup every 10 to 20 minutes, depending on weather conditions and your rate of perspiration. As for carbohydrates, consume about 25 grams of carbohydrates per 30 minutes for races that last over an hour. Stick with bananas, orange slices, sports drinks, or other quickly digested sources. With experience, you'll find out what food or drink works best for you.

Drink up

Drink yourself free of dehydration. One study has shown that sprint performance at the end of a 15-K race was improved in runners who consumed a sports drink an hour before race time.

THE POST-RACE PLAN

Post-race refueling won't improve your time, but it's essential for quick recovery. For starters, drink plenty of fluids, about 2 cups for every pound of sweat you lose. Glycogen stores also need rebuilding. And remember, too, that your muscles are most receptive to carbohydrate replenishment during the first hour or so after exercise.

Try to take in between 50 to 100 grams of carbohydrates within the first 15 minutes after your race. Try starting with liquids first; switch to more solid items when your stomach allows you to.

Following a long race, you should aim to consume 600 grams (or 2,400 calories) of carbohydrates in the next 24 hours. Pace yourself at about 50 grams every 2 hours, on average. One study showed that including protein with carbohydrates in those first post-race meals improves the glycogen resynthesis. (According to the study, the optimal ratio was about 3 grams of carbohydrate to 1 gram of protein.) Therefore, a post-race meal of cereal with milk, or maybe some rice with a small portion of chicken, would provide the right carbohydrate and protein combination.

Amby Burfoot's Running Round-Up

You don't have to be a runner for long before you have your first workout that's cut short by stomach distress. The same goes for racing. Start entering races and, far too soon, you'll have one that's ruined by stomach cramps or nausea. This is virtually a universal experience among runners; few escape it.

Fortunately, we do learn. And one of the first and most important things we learn is to stick with simple, tried-and-true foods that we eat almost every day. The night before one of my first Boston Marathons, I was struck by an uncontrollable urge for apple butter. I satisfied the urge that evening but paid a heavy price the next day during the marathon; the apple butter forced me to make several pit stops en route.

You can bet that I have never eaten apple butter again before a race. Instead, I concentrate on foods that are part of my normal diet—pasta, rice, toast, and bagels. These are healthy foods that fuel my muscles rather than knot my stomach. You must certainly have similar foods that you feel comfortable eating every day. These foods, as long as they are carbohydrate-packed, are the ones you should concentrate on for your pre-race meals.

Chapter 6

New Nutrition Truths for Men
How to Maximize Your Running Potential

Thirty years ago, before the first wave of the running boom, men apparently had almost no interest in nutrition. That was something for women to worry about—whether through reading recipes or shopping for the family or preparing meals. Men simply didn't care about these kinds of things.

By coincidence, the running boom coincided with the health and nutrition boom and the rise in feminism. Now men have to care about food, whether they want to or not. They often shop at the grocery store and prepare meals for themselves and their children.

Fortunately, many of today's men, especially runners, care very much about their diets. They understand that men, more than women, are ravaged by heart disease and other illnesses linked to diet as well as other lifestyle factors (like exercise). They also know that diet makes a difference in performance—both how they feel throughout the day and week and how they race on weekends. This chapter addresses many of the nutrition issues that are most important to men and provides tips to help male readers make even better food and cooking decisions.

"I don't worry about my diet," says one high-ranking male triathlete. "I'm sure I get what I need," he continues, "because I eat a lot." But, like so many other men, he may not be adequately fueling his performance and health with this "garbage-disposal" eating method. Men often think that they are free of any special dietary concerns and sometimes don't realize that their diets do make a difference. Diet can affect a man's running and his sexual performance. It can determine the length of his life span and reduce his risk of getting diseases such as prostate cancer. Here are 10 things that every man should do to improve his diet.

1. Eat your way to better sex. Many runners enjoy a better sex life than sedentary folks. Reports suggest that regular exercise improves self-image, which boosts sexual desire and enjoyment.

But an athlete can also tell you that sex is often the last thing on his mind. This can happen because of lower male hormone levels that occur following exhaustive workouts. Training for two hours a day (or, for that matter, training for 40 minutes after a long, stressful day in the office) may not only squelch your desire but it can also lead to weight loss, which can further lower testosterone levels. So check your training mileage, track your sleep and fatigue levels, and make sure that you keep your weight steady by eating frequently—five to six small meals a day, if necessary.

Though no food is a proven aphrodisiac, the mineral zinc, found in oysters, meats, and whole grains, is essential for sperm production and male sexual functioning. (In rare situations, low zinc intake may contribute to impotence.) Adequate vitamin C intake may also contribute to healthy sperm cell production.

2. Take care of your prostate. One in 10 men will get cancer of the prostate—the small gland situated just below the bladder, responsible for producing seminal fluid. Risk factors include family history and race (African-Americans have a 40 percent greater risk than whites do), but accumulating research suggests that diet plays a part, too. Eating a high-fat diet, particularly when the fat comes from animal products, can greatly increase your risk.

Other research shows that certain foods may protect the prostate. Japanese men, for example, have a much lower prostate cancer risk than Europeans. This may be attributable to the popularity in Japan of soybean-based foods such as tofu. Soybeans contain isoflavones, which have been shown to protect against cancer; other beans such as lentils and peas also contain cancer-fighting isoflavones.

3. Knock out stress. A hectic lifestyle means stress, and stress can mean health problems. Studies show that emotional stress can lead to higher levels of artery-clogging low-density lipoprotein (LDL) cholesterol, increasing the risk of heart disease in men. Stress can also aggravate asthma symptoms and a host of digestive problems. Fending off all these ravages of stress requires a comprehensive approach. You need to monitor your sleep patterns and the amount of tension-busting free time you give yourself.

Also, be sure that you get plenty of fiber and keep your alcohol and caffeine intake to a moderate level. (Too little fiber and too much caffeine both can cause digestive problems.) Eating plenty of fresh vegetables, fruits, whole grains, and fiber-filled breakfast cereals will help you get the recommended 25 grams of dietary fiber a day.

Why muscle loss?

Studies have shown that endurance training of about two hours a day breaks down muscle tissue that is then used for energy by working muscles, particularly when stores of glycogen (a complex carbohydrate that your body uses for quick energy) have run low. Because of this, some endurance athletes see a drop in body weight and a loss of muscle over a few months of heavy training.

4. Avoid muscle loss. Okay, so you aren't body-building's Mr. Universe. As a runner, you wouldn't want to be. Yet heavy-duty marathon training can lead to muscle tissue loss, and that isn't good either.

Eating sufficient calories, carbohydrates, and protein daily will help stave off this wasting. You need anywhere from 450 to 600 grams of carbohy-

Eat right, feel right

Studies show that reading comprehension and math computations falter in people who go without eating for four or more hours, whereas eating every three hours or so may enhance cognition by fueling the brain with a steady supply of carbohydrate energy.

drates a day. This means eating more than 12 servings of grains and at least 4 servings each of vegetables and fruits daily. Endurance training pushes protein needs to 25 to 50 percent more than the Daily Value, or 70 to 90 grams total a day. You can meet this requirement with regular servings of fish, beans, cooked grains, poultry, and other lean meats.

5. Re-energize after you run. Whether you run in the morning or squeeze your miles in later, what you eat afterward may determine the quality of your next workout and your energy level for the rest of the day. During training, glycogen stores diminish. Rebuilding these stores soon after exercise is crucial, as that's when muscles are their hungriest.

Munching on a carbohydrate-rich food is a good idea, but studies suggest that a combination of carbohydrates and protein about 30 minutes after hard running can rebuild glycogen stores better than carbohydrates alone. This combo may also speed muscle recovery. Based on these studies, you should consume 80 to 100 grams of carbohydrates and 15 to 40 grams of protein after exercising. This is equivalent to eating either a tuna sandwich with a banana and an apple, or a hefty bowl of breakfast cereal with skim milk and sliced strawberries.

6. Go easy on the booze. You have probably heard that drinking some alcohol is good. That's true. Men who consume modest amounts of alcohol—one or two drinks daily—have a lower risk of heart disease, the leading cause of death in men. The drink of choice is red wine because it contains phenolic substances, which prevent LDL cholesterol from getting stuck on artery walls.

But too much alcohol can interfere with carbohydrate metabolism. Alcohol also adversely affects vitamins (particularly the B vitamins, such as B6 and thiamin) and minerals in the body by accelerating both their breakdown and their rate of loss in the urine. And alcohol, because it's a diuretic (like coffee and tea), can shortchange performance by increasing water loss from the body. Therefore, if you do drink, keep it to one or two drinks per day.

7. Eat steadily throughout the day. With your busy schedule, occasionally skipping breakfast or missing lunch is inevitable. But this will drag your performance down—both at the job and during your workout. Attempting to run on an empty stomach may also squash your performance during long workouts, since going without food for four or more hours begins to eat away at glycogen stores.

Try to eat something every three hours to stay at peak energy levels. Take along easy-to-tote foods such as sports bars, dried fruit, pretzels, and sports drinks for an energizing snack, whether you're at work or motoring down the freeway.

8. Become acquainted with your kitchen. Men often go for take-out food rather than prepare their own meals, but this can bump up fat intake and leave out performance-boosting carbohydrates. Fixing your own meals allows you to choose

Valuable vitamins

Studies of elderly people have shown that immune response improves with vitamin and mineral supplementation. So stay well by eating a variety of fruits, vegetables, whole grains, and lean protein sources. If you don't routinely eat the nutrient-packed foods that you know you should, consider taking a multivitamin and mineral supplement that provides 100 percent of the Daily Value of key vitamins and minerals.

leave you short on the fiber, vitamins, and minerals that are crucial for health and performance. You can expand your nutrient repertoire by trying a new food each week, or by getting in the habit of sampling new grains or pasta dishes at your local gourmet deli. Go for more variety at each meal by, for example, including two steamed vegetables and two grain foods (like rice and whole-grain bread) instead of a single source of each. Having more foods at each meal will also help control portion sizes, which may keep you from overloading on fat or sodium from one particular food.

the ingredients so that you can keep meals low in fat and loaded with vitamins and minerals.

Look for jarred pasta sauces, canned black beans, and frozen, vegetable-filled potpies.

9. Try new foods. Like cross-training, cross-eating adds needed variety to your life—in this case, nutritional variety. Men frequently eat fewer food items than women. Existing on a few dietary staples like bagels, bananas, and sports bars may

10. Strengthen your immunity. Staying healthy means building a strong immune system. Exercise can help boost the number of germ-fighting cells in the body, and eating the right foods helps, too. Adequate intake of protein, zinc, iron, and vitamins C and E, to name a few, is critical for a strong immune system. For example, too little zinc depresses the number of immune cells, which are needed to fight off bacterial infections.

Amby Burfoot's Running Round-Up

Men, here's the bottom line: If we want to live a long, healthy, vibrant life, we have to pay attention to what we eat. And the best way to do this, I believe, is to take advantage of all the foods available to us. Meat and potatoes (heaped with butter) may have worked for the dawn-to-dusk farm workers of a century ago, but they don't make sense any longer, at least not in large quantities.

It makes a lot more sense to graze on four or five modest meals a day than to gorge on two or three. It makes more sense to eat baked or broiled fish or poultry than fat-laden red meats. It makes

more sense to consume a variety of fruits and vegetables than lots of cheeses and sauces. In general, the more different kinds of foods in your diet, the healthier that diet is.

Runners, of course, can never wander too far from the best carbohydrate food groups: grains and cereals. Bread, rice, and pasta are low-fat foods that provide fast energy, fiber, and a host of B vitamins. If you can build a diet around these key foods and supplement it with a wide sampling of fruits and vegetables, you'll have a nutrition foundation that will lead to great health, energy, and longevity.

Chapter 7

Try the Vegetarian Alternative

It's Simple, Healthy, and Power-Packed

In their search for the perfect diet, runners are willing to explore many alternatives, including some considered extreme. One, the vegetarian diet, used to be considered the eating pattern of certain religious fanatics. Today, as it continues to increase in popularity, vegetarianism is seen as an unusually simple, sound, and healthful diet—**and one that many runners find attractive.**

There are many reasons for a strong link between running and vegetarianism. These range from ethics to a concern for the environment to a desire to consume a pure, natural diet that provides plenty of nutrients without a lot of cholesterol and fatty foods.

At the same time, runners are concerned about their performance, which leads them to wonder if a vegetarian diet is sufficient to provide the energy and endurance they need. After all, we tend to imagine vegetarians as emaciated individuals who sit around in the lotus position all day meditating about one thing or another. This may be a great way to achieve personal enlightenment, but what will it do for your 10-K time? The information in this chapter will answer this and similar questions.

If you have ever thought about becoming a vegetarian, you've probably had many doubts. Perhaps you question how you will perform on a vegetarian regimen or how you will take in adequate protein from plant sources alone. Still you must answer the biggest question: Is a vegetarian lifestyle right for you?

To begin with, there are two basic types of vegetarianism. Vegans are vegetarians who eat no meat, chicken, fish, or animal products such as milk, cheese, and eggs. Lacto-ovo vegetarians eat no meat, chicken, or fish but do consume milk, cheese, and eggs. Now for the nutritional questions that haunt many would-be vegetarians.

HOW HEALTHFUL ARE VEGETARIAN DIETS?

Various studies show that most vegetarians are less likely than most meat-eaters to contract a variety of chronic diseases such as heart disease or to become obese. Risk of colon cancer is also lower in vegetarians than in meat-eaters, probably because vegetarian diets tend to be higher in fiber and lower in fat than diets that include meat. And foods such as tofu and other soybean products, which are staples in most vegetarian diets, may have cancer-fighting powers.

Of course, diet isn't the only variable in these studies. Vegetarians, as a whole, tend to take much better care of themselves than meat-eaters. More meat-eaters smoke, abuse alcohol or drugs, or lead sedentary lives than vegetarians and, as a result, tend to experience more chronic illnesses.

But vegetarian diets can be problematic, too. A lacto-ovo vegetarian meal made with high-fat cheeses, for instance, isn't particularly healthful. And a diet that contains some meat (5 to 6 ounces a day) can be as low in fat and high in fiber as many vegetarian diets. Regardless of the eating style you choose, you must watch your fat and fiber intake for optimum health and performance.

HOW DO I COMBINE VEGETARIAN DISHES TO TAKE IN ADEQUATE PROTEIN?

Protein is made up of amino acids, some of which your body requires but cannot manufacture on its own. So meat-eaters and vegetarians alike must take in amino acids through food.

A quick-cooking tip

Those who are curious about eating a vegetarian diet may be put off because they think these kinds of meals take a long time to prepare. Well, the truth is that they don't. Take advantage of frozen vegetarian entrees, canned black beans and refried beans, and quick-cooking pasta and brown rice.

The protein found in beef, chicken, fish, eggs, and milk (animal protein) contains all the amino acids you need, in the right proportion, whereas the protein found in rice and beans (vegetable protein) does not. When grains and beans are combined, however, they provide the perfect mix of amino acids. So vegetarians must pair grains such as wheat, rice, corn, barley, and millet with legumes or beans such as lentils, pinto beans, and soybeans. This guarantees that they are supplying their bodies with the proper amino acid profile. Any combination of grains and beans will do.

To figure serving sizes, consider that a three-ounce serving of meat (about the size of a deck of cards) contains roughly 21 grams of protein. To replace this with a vegetarian source of protein, you must eat a generous cup of cooked beans with a cup of cooked grain. For instance, one cup of cooked lentils served over a large square of corn bread is a great substitute for a three-ounce serving of cooked chicken.

WILL EATING A VEGETARIAN DIET BOOST MY ENDURANCE?

Perhaps. Various studies have shown that training diets that provide at least 600 grams of carbohydrates per day—a quota that's easy to meet with heaping plates of rice and beans—boost endurance. But rice, beans, bread, and pasta, which are all rich in carbohydrates, are also big on volume. As a result, your stomach may fill up well before your muscles do. That could help you lose a few pounds, which might be just what you need in the short term. But over the long term, it could lead to fatigue and breakdown.

WILL I MISS OUT ON ANY KEY NUTRIENTS BY EATING A VEGETARIAN DIET?

In a word, yes. Vitamin B12, for instance, isn't found in plants. Some fermented bean products such as miso and tempeh contain vitamin B12, but they are not reliable sources. So vegetarians must go out of their way to eat foods such as packaged cereal and soy products that are supplemented with the vitamin.

The same is true for iron and zinc. Most plant foods are paltry providers of both minerals, and the iron and zinc they do contain aren't readily absorbed into the body. So vegetarians must take care to consume iron-rich foods, especially since heavy exercise might prompt iron loss. Some good selections are dried fruit, beans, chard greens, and kale, and a multivitamin and mineral supplement

What about protein?

Meeting your protein needs can be challenging on a vegetarian diet. But if you take care to combine grains with cooked beans or add milk, cheese, and eggs to your diet occasionally (once a day for women, several times a week for men), you should have no trouble. Keep in mind, however, that runners need more protein than sedentary people—roughly 25 percent more than the Daily Value or about half a gram of protein for every pound of body weight.

Let's say that you weigh 150 pounds. You would need to take in 75 grams of protein per day, or 10 to 12 servings of grain products (breads, pasta, or rice); 2 cups of cooked beans or bean products such as hummus (which is made from garbanzo beans), tofu (soybean curd), or miso (soybean paste); and a serving or two of nuts such as whole almonds or nut products such as peanut butter. Eating dairy products such as two servings of fat-free or 1 percent milk along with low-fat cottage cheese will help you meet your protein needs, as will adding eggs or egg whites to casseroles, soups, or stir-fried dishes.

that provides 100 percent of the Daily Value for iron and zinc.

As for calcium, vegans have a tough time getting enough. They must substitute soy milk, soy yogurt, or tofu (which is made with calcium carbonate) for dairy products and eat broccoli, bok choy, collard greens, and other leafy greens daily to take in all of the calcium that they can.

WHAT HEALTH RISKS ARE ASSOCIATED WITH EATING A VEGETARIAN DIET?

Some studies suggest that vegetarian diets may lower the levels of sex hormones in female and male athletes. For instance, many amenorrheic women runners (women who don't have regular menstrual cycles) are vegetarians. This has led some scientists to postulate that lower estrogen levels caused by low-fat, high-fiber vegetarian diets are at the root of amenorrhea. Other scientists suspect that the low iron and zinc intakes of many vegetarian runners lead to amenorrhea. Either

Protein Sources

Here are 20 vegetarian foods that provide good ways to get protein.

FOOD	CALORIES	FAT (GRAMS)	PROTEIN (GRAMS)
Black beans, 1 cup cooked	227	1	15
Bread (whole-grain), 2 slices	140	2	6
Brown rice, 1 cup cooked	232	1	5
Corn, 1 cup cooked	178	2	6
Corn bread, 2-inch square	130	4	3
Corn tortilla	67	1	2
Cottage cheese (1%), 1 cup	164	2	28
Egg, 1 large	75	2	6
Egg white, 1 large	16	0	3
Garbanzo beans, 1 cup cooked	285	3	12
Kidney beans, 1 cup cooked	225	1	15
Lentils, 1 cup cooked	231	1	18
Milk (1%), 1 cup	120	2	11
Pasta, 1 cup cooked	200	2	7
Potato, baked with skin	220	1	5
Refried beans, 1 cup cooked	270	3	16
Split peas, 1 cup cooked	231	1	16
Tempeh, ½ cup	165	6	16
Tofu, ½ cup	183	11	20
Yogurt (fat-free), 1 cup	127	0	13

Amby Burfoot's Running Round-Up

During the summer between my sophomore and junior years at college, I decided to become a strict lacto-ovo vegetarian. I told friends that this was an ethical decision—that I was opposed to the needless killing of animals for human consumption. Secretly, I hoped that it would also make me run faster.

It did. My junior year in college was my best ever and led to several outstanding years that followed. It seemed that the vegetarian diet worked for me. Or did it? In truth, there's no way to know. My new successes could have been diet-related or they could have been related to any number of other things, including a harder training schedule. Over the years, I have been asked more questions about vegetarianism than about any other diet topic. I always begin my answers with the above anecdote and end by saying that I don't think anyone should become a vegetarian to improve his race performances. There are too many other excellent arguments for vegetarianism to trivialize the subject with thoughts of faster times.

Have confidence that the vegetarian way of eating is fully compatible with a runner's training and racing needs. And then decide if vegetarianism makes sense for you.

way, estrogen levels sink, and the risk of osteoporosis rises.

A similar situation appears to develop in male athletes. In one study, a group of male endurance athletes (runners, rowers, and cyclists) were divided into two groups, each of which trained similarly. One group, however, ate a lacto-ovo vegetarian diet, while the other ate a diet that supplied the same amount of protein but from animal sources. After six weeks, blood levels of testosterone in the vegetarian athletes had dropped 35 percent. Although dips in testosterone levels pose no health risk, they may depress sexual drive. Whether these levels would return to normal after a period of time on the vegetarian diets wasn't tested.

Chapter 8

15 Superfoods for Runners
Add These Foods to Boost Your Running Performance

Runners believe in superfoods just as they believe in super workouts. They're always looking for that special food—or workout—that will make them stronger and faster. No matter that they know these things are improbable. They keep hoping.

Bee pollen. Algae. Ginseng. All have been promoted at one time or another as ergogenic foods—that is, foods or supplements that can improve performance. And these are just a few among many. Amino acids. Chinese herbs. Chromium picolinate. The list goes on and on.

Reputable sports nutritionists put little stock in these substances, pointing out that anecdote and testimony, even from famous, world-class runners, does not amount to science. Lacking proof from rigorous experiments, these nutritionists tend to disregard the nutritional claims made about self-proclaimed superfoods. That's not to say, however, that nutritionists

don't believe in the power of healthy foods. They do, as this chapter by Liz Applegate, Ph.D., nutrition writer for *Runner's World* magazine, makes clear.

Most runners know that foods such as pasta, bagels, and baby carrots provide good health, top performance, and superior flavor. But they're not the only foods to do so. In fact, there are dozens of lesser-known vegetables, condiments, and entrees that have more nutritional value than you suspect. Some, such as mayonnaise, have been falsely labeled as unhealthy while others, such as cactus, have been pigeonholed as weird. Yet all pack specific nutritional benefits.

Buried Treasures to Boost Your Running

Consider the following foods. Each is tasty, healthful, and, yes, a bit different. Try sampling one or two a week, and you can perk up your meals without sacrificing your health.

1. **Baby lima beans.** One cup of cooked baby limas—delicious in soups, stews, casseroles, and three-bean salads—contains almost 8 grams of fiber (a third of your suggested daily intake), about 30 percent of the Daily Value of iron, 15 percent of the Daily Value for zinc, and about 25 percent of the RDA for magnesium. And that's not all. The same serving size also packs all of your daily requirement of folic acid, an important B vitamin that may prevent birth defects when consumed before and during pregnancy.

2. **Beer.** Be it nonalcoholic or the regular brew, beer is a great source of chromium, a mineral that plays a part in processing carbohydrates for energy. Various studies suggest exercise may increase chromium losses in the urine. And since it's not clear whether chromium in supplement form can boost performance, runners need to look to their diets to supply 50 to 200 micrograms of natural chromium a day. A tall, cold one is a good place to start (and finish): One 12-ounce beer provides about 60 micrograms of chromium.

3. **Blackberry fruit spread.** Blackberries are particularly rich in fiber (just one cup of fresh berries provides more than 6 grams of fiber), but they're a seasonal fruit. Fortunately, you can get blackberry fruit spread anytime. Swirl this tart treat, which is also rich in fiber and vitamin C, into plain low-fat yogurt, or use it as a topping for pancakes, toast, or bagels.

4. **Blackstrap (dark) molasses.** Okay, it looks like sludge, but it packs a powerful nutritional punch. While most sweeteners offer little more than calories (regular table sugar, for instance, provides 46 calories per tablespoon but no essential vitamins or minerals), a table-spoon of blackstrap molasses provides about 20 percent of the Daily Value of iron and 580 milligrams of potassium—about 20 percent of the Daily Value. Pretty good for a sweetener. Use blackstrap molasses to top off a bowl of hot cereal or as a substitute for a portion of the sugar used in baking muffins or cookies. (For instance, if a recipe calls for one cup of sugar, try using $\frac{1}{2}$ cup of sugar with three to four tablespoons of blackstrap molasses.)

5. **Cactus.** Packed with potassium and vitamin C, a one-cup serving of this delicacy provides about 20 percent of the Daily Value for calcium and iron. In addition, one study showed that people with diabetes who eat cooked cactus have improved control over their blood glucose levels and, as a result, are able to minimize health problems such as poor vision and bad circulation that typically occur with the disease. Stick cactus in soups and stir-fry dishes and serve it as an exotic accompaniment to more common main dishes.

6. **Canned chili.** Have you checked out the canned chili aisle in the grocery store? "Lite" chili is in, and it's low in fat and high in performance-boosting protein.

7. **Canned clams.** Most runners eat lots of refined grains and very little meat. As a result, they often fall short of the Daily Value for zinc (15 milligrams), which helps fight infection, repairs wounds, and contributes to the growth of new blood cells and other tissues. To meet your Daily Value for zinc (150 percent of it, to be specific) and pick up 140 percent of the Daily Value for vitamin B12, munch on a three-ounce serving of clams right out of the can. Add clams to marinara sauce and eat them over pasta for a delicious, nutrient-packed meal.

8. **Celery.** Although celery doesn't have a nutrient report card worth writing home about (one stalk contains less than 1 gram of fiber, about 25 percent of the Daily Value for vitamin C, and a smattering of potassium and other nutrients), it does contain a special ingredient called 3-n-butyl phthalide, which may be helpful in lowering blood pressure. Research revealed that 3-n-butyl phthalide lowers blood pressure in lab animals and indicated that it may lower levels of stress hormones that can cause high blood pressure in people. Reach for celery when you need a crunchy snack or a healthful addition to soups, stews, or stir-fried food.

9. **Frozen Chinese pot stickers.** A food that's easy to prepare and low in fat, too, Chinese pot stickers are the perfect accompaniment to steamed rice and vegetables. These tasty chicken and vegetable dumplings contain lots of cancer-fighting cabbage and only about 1 gram of fat each.

10. **Frozen pancakes.** Check this out: Three 4-inch pancakes provide 246 calories (just under 15 percent from fat) and almost 50 grams of carbohydrate. So they're perfect for pre- or post-race carbo loading, especially when you consider their preparation time is only seconds. Garnish a short stack with fresh fruit for added vitamins and minerals.

11. **Mayonnaise.** And we're talking about the real stuff here, too. Regular mayonnaise has much more to offer than calories and fat. Along with 100 calories, a tablespoon of mayonnaise packs more than 50 percent of the Daily Value for vitamin E. That's three to four times the vitamin E found in most oils and margarines.

12. **McDonald's shake.** These low-fat shakes contain less than 5 percent fat calories and a whole lot more. One chocolate shake provides 11 grams of protein (more than a glass of milk), 30 percent of the Daily Value for riboflavin, and 30 percent of the Daily Value for calcium. Plus, 82 percent of its calories come from carbohydrates, so a shake every so often can be considered carbo loading, too.

13. **Pesto.** The olive oil, garlic, basil, and pine nuts that are included in pesto are a winning combination. The olive oil and garlic help depress total blood cholesterol, while basil provides plenty of magnesium and folate (the natural form of the supplement folic acid). And pine nuts pack the essential fats necessary for healthy skin and low blood pressure and may help prevent heart disease and diabetes. Add pesto to pasta, sauces, and soups for great flavor and good nutrition.

14. **Refried beans.** Although they sound fattening, refried beans simply aren't. At 270 calories per cup, canned refried beans contain less than 10 percent fat calories. And this is just the beginning. Each cup provides more than 6 grams of fiber (mostly water-soluble fiber, which helps lower blood cholesterol levels), about 20 percent of the Daily Value for protein, about 25 percent of the Daily Value for magnesium, 23 percent of the Daily Value for zinc, and about 15 percent of the Daily Value for calcium. Plus, fat-free versions are now on the market. Serve refried beans with corn tortillas, rice, or couscous for a high-quality, complex-carbohydrate meal.

15. **Sweet potatoes.** Most people reach for carrots to pack their diets with beta-carotene, but they would benefit more by choosing sweet potatoes, a far better source. One baked sweet potato is virtually fat-free and provides 250 percent of the Daily Value for vitamin A. (In addition to fending off cataracts, cancer, and heart disease, beta-carotene converts to vitamin A once it is inside the body.) However you prepare them—whether they are baked, mashed, or added to stews—sweet potatoes are power spuds.

Amby Burfoot's Running Round-Up

The best way to find your own superfoods is to sample what's available and learn what works best for you. A food that works wonders for one man or woman won't necessarily do the same for another. We are all individuals who react differently to different kinds of foods.

About a dozen years after I had begun running seriously, I sat down one evening to see if I could figure out what foods worked best for me. I was about to begin another serious training build-up, and I wanted to make sure that I was covering my nutritional bases. How could I do this?, I wondered.

It was simple. I wrote down a list of the foods that I ate often, and next to each food I put one to three check marks. Three meant that I always felt strong and energetic after eating this particular food.

I didn't know what to expect when I began this process, but it didn't take long for the results to explode off the paper at me. Rice and bananas. Sounds like a baby food combination, but in fact these were the only two foods to which I assigned three check marks. In the years since, I've added oatmeal to my list of favorite performance-enhancing foods.

Your personal-best foods probably aren't the same as mine, but you'll never know until you make yourself sit down and create a list. It's a deceptively simple process that can yield results. At least it did for me.

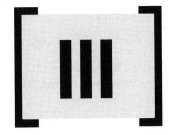

Injury Prevention

Chapter 9

Prevent Five Common Injuries

Avoiding These Injuries Will Keep You Ahead of the Pack

Injuries come in many shapes, sizes, and places, so it's difficult to make generalizations about how to avoid them or recover from them. Each one is unique, especially when you consider that each of us is unique. Still, certain injuries are more common than others. If you can figure out how to avoid these, you're ahead of the game.

When the *Runner's World* editors decided to write about the five most common injuries, we debated them a little. We researched the subject by reviewing the medical literature. We asked each other which injuries we had incurred the most or heard our friends complain about.

But in the end, it wasn't very complicated. Five injuries kept coming up over and over again. So we tackled them head on by asking *Runner's World* writer Dave Kuehls to interview the experts and gather their advice. If you can avoid these five injuries, that's no guarantee that you won't develop others, but it's a big step in the right direction.

Life used to be so much simpler. One day you came home complaining of knee pain. Your mom took a look at your scraped knee, washed it, put an adhesive bandage on it, and sealed the treatment with a kiss. A few days later you forgot that your knee ever hurt.

Today, the pain in your knee is chondromalacia, an insidious wearing away of the cartilage beneath your kneecap. You go to see an orthopedic surgeon who doesn't look at all like Mom. And the prescribed treatment is not something that's over within a minute. It's more likely to take weeks before you're running pain-free again.

Fortunately, many running injuries last only a few weeks. And most are preventable. If you run smart and do all the right things to ensure your running health—things you've heard before, such as strengthening and stretching your leg muscles, wearing proper shoes, and taking easy days or rest days when you're tired—you can avoid most running injuries or at least nip them in the bud.

That is, if you know what you're doing. That's where this guide comes in. Below are the five most common running injuries: Achilles tendinitis, chondromalacia, iliotibial band syndrome, plantar fasciitis, and shinsplints. This guide tells you what they are and how to deal with them—everything from whether or not to run through them, to when it's time to see a doctor. And which doctor or sports-medicine specialist to see.

ACHILLES TENDINITIS

This troublesome heel pain is caused by inflammation of the Achilles tendon. The Achilles is the large tendon connecting the two major calf muscles—the gastrocnemius and soleus—to the back of the heel bone. Under too much stress, the tendon tightens and is forced to work too hard. This causes it to become inflamed (that's tendinitis) and, over time, can produce a covering of scar tissue that is less flexible than the tendon. If the inflamed Achilles continues to be stressed, it can tear or rupture.

Symptoms: Dull or sharp pain anywhere along the back of the tendon, but usually close to the heel. Limited ankle flexibility. Redness or heat over the painful area. A nodule (a lumpy buildup of scar tissue) that can be felt on the tendon. A crackling sound (scar tissue rubbing against the tendon) when the ankle moves.

Causes: Tight or fatigued calf muscles, which transfer too much of the burden of running to the Achilles. This can be brought on by

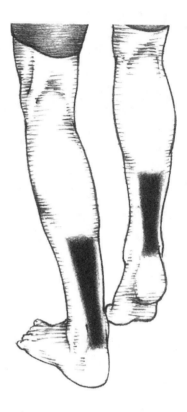

Achilles Tendon

not stretching the calves properly, increasing mileage too quickly, or simply overtraining. Excessive hill running or speedwork, both of which stress the Achilles more than other types of running, can also cause tendinitis. Inflexible running shoes, which force the Achilles to twist, cause some cases. Runners who overpronate (their feet rotate too far inward on impact) are susceptible to Achilles tendinitis.

Self-treatment: Stop running. Take aspirin or ibuprofen, and ice the area for 15 to 20 minutes several times a day until the inflammation subsides.

Self-massage may also help. "I have every therapeutic machine available for the treatment of Achilles tendinitis, and the treatment of choice is massage with a heat-inducing cream or oil," says Marc Chasnov, a physical therapist in Rye Brook, New York. He suggests rubbing semicircles in all directions away from the knotted tissue three times a day.

Once the nodule is gone, stretch the calf muscles. Don't start running again until you can do toe raises without pain. Next, move on to skipping rope, then jumping jacks, and then gradually begin running again. You should be back to easy running in six to eight weeks.

Medical treatment: If your injury does not respond to self-treatment in two weeks, see a physical therapist or orthopedic surgeon. Surgery to scrape scar tissue off the tendon is a last resort and

Feel the stretch

The best stretch for the Achilles is also the simplest. Stand on the balls of your feet on stairs, a curb, or a low rung of a ladder, with your legs straight. Drop both of your heels down and hold for a count of 10. To increase the intensity of the stretch, keep one foot flat and lower the other heel. When done, switch legs.

not very effective. "It usually just stimulates more scar tissue," says Chasnov.

Alternative exercises: cycling in low gear, swimming, and pool running. No weight-bearing exercises.

Preventive measures: Strengthen and stretch the muscles in your feet, calves, and shins. Wear motion-control shoes or orthotics to combat overpronation. Do not run in worn-out shoes. Ease into any running program. Avoid hill work. Incorporate rest into your training schedule.

CHONDROMALACIA

One of the most common knee injuries, chondromalacia is a softening or wearing away and cracking of the cartilage under the kneecap, resulting in pain and inflammation. The cartilage becomes like sandpaper because the kneecap is not riding smoothly over the knees.

Symptoms: Pain beneath or on the side of the kneecap. "It's a soreness, a nagging discomfort," says Dave Apple, M.D., an orthopedic surgeon at Piedmont Hospital in Atlanta. Pain can worsen over a year or so and is most severe after you run hills. Swelling is also present. In severe cases, you can feel—and eventually hear—grinding as the rough cartilage rubs against healthy cartilage when the knee is flexed.

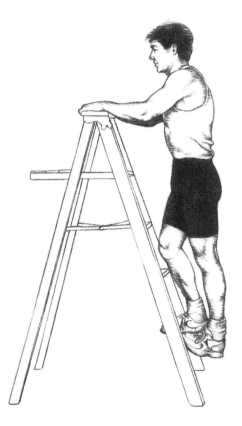

Achilles Stretch

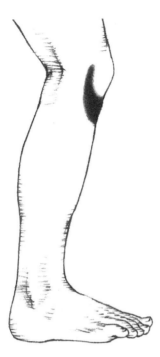

Chondromalacia: A condition whereby a softening or wearing away of the cartilage under the kneecap occurs.

Causes: Overpronation can cause the kneecap to twist sideways. The quadriceps muscles, which normally aid in proper tracking of the kneecap, can prevent the kneecap from tracking smoothly when they are fatigued or weak. A muscle imbalance between weak quads and tighter hamstrings can also pull the kneecap out of its groove. Hill running (especially downhills) can aggravate the condition, as can running on the same side of a cambered road, or, in general, overtraining.

Self-treatment: Stop running. Ice the knee for 15 minutes, two or three times a day. Use a flexible, frozen gel pack that wraps around the knee (or, in a pinch, try a bag of frozen vegetables). Take aspirin three times a day for 12 weeks. "Aspirin has been found to block further breakdown of cartilage," says Dr. Apple. Also try self-massage on the sore spots around the knee.

Once the pain and swelling are gone, do quadriceps strengtheners. Stand on a step or box at least four inches high. Keep your right quadriceps tight while you lower your left leg slowly toward the floor. Then raise the leg back up onto the box and relax. Repeat 40 times with each leg. Continue increasing repetitions in increments of five every two days, all the way up to 60 reps.

Don't forget to stretch your quadriceps and hamstrings. When you start running again, you also might try wearing a rubber sleeve with a hole that fits over the kneecap, which can help the knee track better. You should be back to easy running in four to six weeks.

Medical treatment: If chondromalacia isn't responding to the self-treatment after four weeks, see an orthopedic surgeon. He may prescribe custom-made orthotics to control overpronation. Surgery to scrape away rough edges of cartilage can alleviate some pain. Despite what you may have heard, cortisone injections won't work. "The problem is, you won't feel pain while you're crunching your knee to bits," says Dr. Apple.

Alternative exercises: swimming, pool running, and rowing. Anything that doesn't put pressure on the knee.

Preventive measures: Stretch and strengthen your quadriceps, hamstrings, and calves. If you overpronate, consider switching to motion-control shoes with firm midsoles. You should never run in worn-out shoes. You may need to wear orthotics. Avoid downhill running, and stay off cambered roads. If you can't, try to run on the flattest part of the road. Incorporate rest into your training schedule. Don't overdo it.

ILIOTIBIAL BAND SYNDROME

This condition results in inflammation and pain on the outside of the knee where the iliotibial (IT) band (a ligament that runs along the outside of the thigh) rubs against the femur, the large leg bone.

Symptoms: A dull ache that starts when you're a mile or two into a run, lingers during the run, but disappears soon after you stop. In severe cases, pain can be sharp, and the outside of the knee can be tender or swollen.

Causes: Anything that causes the leg to bend inward, stretching the IT band against the femur, such as bowlegs, overpronation, worn-out running shoes, or workouts on down-

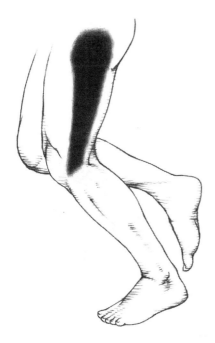

Iliotibial Band Syndrome: In severe cases of iliotibial band syndrome, pain can be sharp and the outside of the knee tender.

Pain: Get rid of IT

The IT band stretch is the most common and effective IT band exercise: Stand with your right leg crossed in back of your left and extend your left arm against a wall, pole, chair, or other stable object. Lean your weight against the object while pushing your right hip to the right. Keep your right foot anchored while allowing your left knee to flex. You should feel the stretch in the iliotibial muscle in your right hip and extending down the outside of your right leg.

hill or indoor, banked surfaces. A tight IT band can contribute to the injury. So can stepping up your training too quickly. It sometimes takes just a single hard workout to cause IT band syndrome.

Self-treatment: "You usually can't run through IT band pain," says Dr. Apple. "But if you do run, back off. Cut back on speedwork, don't run downhill, and make sure to stretch the band a couple of times a day. The main thing you have to do is restore the band's flexibility."

Perform the IT band stretch (see box on page 58). In addition to doing this stretch, ice the knee for around 15 to 20 minutes after running, try some self-massage on the area, and stretch hamstrings and other leg muscles. You should be back to easy running in two to four weeks.

Medical treatment: If you feel your IT band problem isn't responding to self-treatment after four weeks, you need to see an orthopedic surgeon. In severe cases you may need a cortisone injection under the band to alleviate pain.

Alternative exercises: swimming, pool running, cycling, and rowing, but not stairclimbing. "Anything that doesn't put pressure on the outside of the knee is fine," says Dr. Apple.

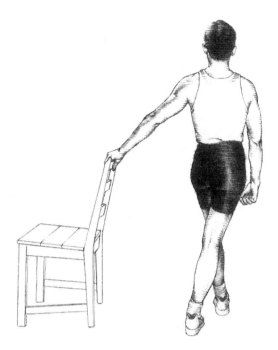

Illiotibial Band Stretch

Preventive measures: Make sure you stretch the IT band (after a workout is the best time). Stretch and strengthen your quadriceps and hamstrings. Warm up well before you run. Avoid hard workouts on cambered roads, down-hill surfaces, or indoor tracks. Ease into any running program.

PLANTAR FASCIITIS

This is an inflammation of the plantar fascia, a thick, fibrous band of tissue in the bottom of the foot, running from the heel to the base of the toes. When placed under too much stress, the fascia stretches too far and tears, which causes inflammation of the fascia and surrounding tissues. The tears are soon covered with scar tissue, which is less flexible than the fascia and only aggravates the problem.

Symptoms: Pain at the base of the heel. "Most people describe it as feeling like a bone bruise or a stone bruise," says Joe Ellis, D.P.M., a sports podiatrist from La Jolla, California, and the author of *Running Injury-Free.* "Plantar fasciitis is most severe in the morning when you get out of bed or at the beginning of a run, because the fascia is tighter at those times. The pain may fade as you walk or run."

Often, a runner will change stride to alleviate pain, but this only provides temporary relief. A bone spur may also develop at the heel, where the fascia has started to tear away.

Causes: Stress, tension, and pulling on the plantar fascia. Runners with tight Achilles tendons

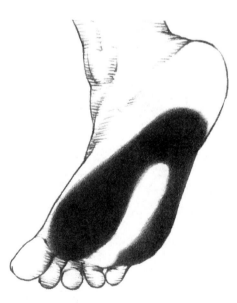

Plantar Fasciitis: The symptom of plantar fasciitis is a pain at the base of the heel similar to a bruising sensation.

The golf ball trick

To help stretch the fascia, you can perform a motion using a golf ball. Start with the golf ball under the base of your big toe and roll the foot laterally over the ball to the base of the second toe and repeat. Do the same motion starting from each toe, always exerting enough pressure so that you feel a little tenderness.

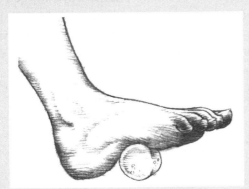

Plantar Fascia Pain Reliever

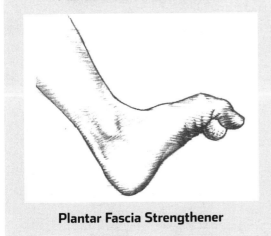

Plantar Fascia Strengthener

which stretch the fasciae, can also make you more susceptible.

Self-treatment: Reduce your running. Take aspirin or ibuprofen daily. Ice the area for 15 to 20 minutes several times a day. Ice-massage the fascia. To do this, fill a paper cup with water and freeze. Peel off the paper, place the ice under your foot, and roll the foot over it, from your heel to the ball of your foot and back again. A frozen-juice can works equally as well.

Medical treatment: If the injury hasn't responded to self-treatment in four weeks, see a podiatrist, who may prescribe orthotics, ultrasound, or friction massage. Surgery to detach the fascia from its insertion into the heel may be recommended if medical treatments don't help after a year. The success rate is 80 percent. Surgery to remove bone spurs usually doesn't work. "The spur isn't the problem," says Dr. Ellis. "It's a reaction to the problem."

Alternative exercises: swimming, pool running, and cycling in low gear. After surgery, only swimming is recommended during rehabilitation.

Preventive measures: Stretch your calf muscles. Strengthen the muscles of the foot by picking up marbles or golf balls with your toes or pulling a towel toward you with your toes. (Grab some of the towel with your toes and pull, then grab some more.)

Do the plantar fascia stretch: While sitting on the floor, with one knee bent and the same ankle flexed toward you, pull the toes back toward the ankle. Hold for a count of 10. Do 10 times. Wear orthotics if you overpronate or have flat feet. Ice the area for 15 to 20 minutes after running. Run on soft surfaces. Don't run in worn-out shoes. Incorporate more rest into your training schedule.

(which put more stress on the fasciae), or high arches and rigid feet, or flat feet that overpronate are most susceptible. Worn-out shoes, which allow feet to overpronate, or shoes that are too stiff,

SHINSPLINTS

A very common and nagging injury, shinsplints are an inflammation of the tendons on the inside of the front of the lower leg. (Sports-medicine specialists don't like to use the term "shinsplints" because it commonly refers to several lower-leg injuries. This section uses it anyway but focuses on the specific problem that is the most common: tendinitis of the lower leg.)

Symptoms: An aching, throbbing, or tenderness along the inside of the shin (though it can radiate to the outside also) about halfway down, or all along the shin from the ankle to the knee. Pain when you press on the inflamed area. Pain is most severe at the start of a run, but it can go away during a run once the muscles are loosened up (unlike a stress fracture of the shinbone, which hurts all the time). With tendinitis, pain resumes after the run.

Causes: Tired or inflexible calf muscles put too much stress on tendons, which become strained and torn. Overpronation aggravates this problem, as does running on hard surfaces such as concrete sidewalks.

Beginning runners are the most susceptible to shinsplints for a variety of reasons, but the most common is that they're using leg muscles that haven't been stressed in the same way before. Another common cause of shinsplints among beginners is poor choice of running shoes or running in something other than running shoes. Runners who have started running after a long layoff are also prone to shinsplints because they often increase their mileage too quickly.

Self-treatment: Many runners experience mild shin soreness, which usually can be tolerated. "If shinsplints hit you at the beginning of a season, a certain amount of running through it will help the body adapt," says David O'Brian, D.P.M., a podiatrist in private practice in Roselle, Illinois. "But if it's a persistent problem, you shouldn't run through it."

If it does persist, ice the inflamed area for 15 minutes, three times a day, and take aspirin or ibuprofen. Ice immediately after running. To hasten recovery, cut down on running or stop altogether. Recovery time: two to four weeks.

Medical treatment: If the injury doesn't respond to self-treatment and rest in two to four weeks, see a podiatrist, who may prescribe custom-

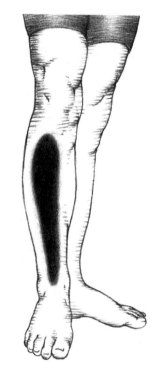

Shinsplints: Shinsplints are an inflammation of the tendons on the inside of the front of the lower leg.

"The best injury-prevention advice I know is also the most boring: rest."

made orthotics to control overpronation. Ultrasound and anti-inflammatories may also be prescribed. Surgery is rarely required.

Alternative exercises: Nonimpact exercises such as swimming, pool running, walking, and cycling in low gear.

Preventive measures: You should exercise the tendons and muscles in the front of the leg (see box, right). You can also strengthen the lower leg with band exercises. Anchor one end of an exercise band to a heavy object, such as the leg of a sofa. Stretch the band, then loop the free end around your forefoot. Move the foot up and down and side to side against the band's resistance to exercise different muscle groups. The band can be ordered from a doctor or bought at some sporting goods stores. Ask for "tension tubing."

Finally, make sure to wear motion-control shoes—and orthotics if your doctor says you need them. Don't run in worn-out shoes. Warm up well, and run on soft surfaces. Avoid overstriding, which puts more stress on shins.

Shinsplint solutions

To stretch and strengthen the tendons and muscles in the front of the leg, sit on a table or chair and loop an ankle weight around your foot. Without bending your knee, move your foot up and down from the ankle. Or have a partner grasp the foot to provide resistance.

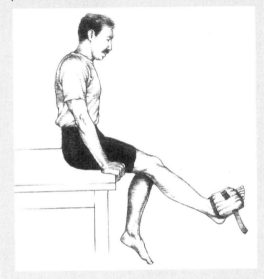

Amby Burfoot's Running Round-Up

The best injury-prevention advice I know is also the most boring: rest. What's more, it leads to zany conclusions like, "If I never ran at all, I would never get injured, so maybe I should head for the couch instead of the roads."

I suppose that I've been guilty of similar black-and-white thought patterns myself. The thought that I had when I was younger and hungrier was: "If I don't run 20 miles today, someone else will, and that person will beat me in the next race." I won lots of races in those days. I was also injured a lot.

And, looking back, I wonder if I might not have won even more races by tempering my training a bit and avoiding those injuries (one of which thwarted my only real chance at the Olympic Games).

Today, I know that resting one day just makes me (and probably you) more enthusiastic about running the next day. And I understand better what judicious rest can do. It can help you recover from injuries. It can help prevent injuries. It can help you train and race better. All in all, that's a compelling package.

Chapter 10

Train Right to Beat Running Injuries

A Foot Doctor Tells You How to Stay on Your Feet

The runner's doctor is the sports podiatrist. Running philosopher George Sheehan, M.D., was the first to discover this, just as he was the first to discover many things from the medical and philosophical sides of running. And during his life he did much to promote the ways a podiatrist could help injured runners.

This isn't to say that podiatrists are the only medically trained professionals who can help or that other physicians (especially orthopedic specialists) aren't better suited to analyze and treat certain injuries. What's more, many runners swear by their favorite chiropractor, physical therapist, or massage therapist. Still, podiatrists generally fare best in treating the many foot and lower-leg maladies that occasionally trouble runners.

At *Runner's World* magazine we learned this long ago and immediately began contacting podiatrists who are also serious runners (there are many) to help us prepare articles. One of the first and best was Joe Ellis, D.P.M.—an enthusiastic

runner, a great podiatrist, and a frequent contributor to *Runner's World*. In this chapter, Dr. Ellis outlines a simple but effective program that can help keep you injury-free.

Most runners know injuries. They're almost part of the game. Run long enough or hard enough, and you'll probably come down with an ache that will temporarily sideline you. Fortunately, most running injuries are short term. After a few days or weeks of rest, you can return to your regular routine. Still, there is a better way: Don't get injured in the first place.

Impossible, you say? Not at all. If you adopt the principles outlined on these pages, you'll have a reasonable chance of running in good health indefinitely. Ignore them, and . . . well, you know. You sow what you reap.

RUN RIGHT

Carefully choose where you run. The best surfaces for running are firm but not too hard, relatively flat (without camber), and smooth (without ruts or holes). Generally, roads make fine running surfaces, but keep in mind that most are canted so that water will run off the center of the road. As you run down the road against traffic, the slant causes your right foot to pronate (roll inward) and your left foot to supinate (roll outward). So map out your routes over the flattest streets that you can find. Here's a look at other possible running venues.

Cinder paths: A packed cinder path can be an ideal running surface—provided it is well-maintained, not lumpy or rutted. And not wet. On rainy days a cinder trail can become muddy and slippery. Many towns and cities have fitness trails in their parks and recreation areas. Seek out one near your home.

Lawns and other grassy areas: Because they're soft, you might think that golf courses or cross-country courses would be good places to run. But the unevenness of these surfaces forces the muscles and tendons in your feet and legs to work harder than they would on a flat course and increases the possibility of injury. When you consider that more than half the population has some biomechanical abnormality, you begin to see the risks of cross-country running. It can be downright treacherous if you head out over terrain where ruts and holes lie hidden in the grass. Most runners' ankle sprains occur on cross-coun-

try courses. You're better off running on dirt trails, because you can see the rough spots and avoid them.

Sidewalks: Stay away from sidewalks unless you are running in heavy traffic and need to get off the street. Concrete is significantly harder than asphalt, and because sidewalks aren't continuous, you have to jump off and on at every corner. Furthermore, many sidewalks are cracked and uneven. If you catch your toe on a raised chunk of walk, next thing you know you'll be nose-down against the pavement.

Tracks: Tracks offer an even surface that's firm but not too hard. The one disadvantage is that they force you to turn frequently and can strain your muscles unevenly. But if you change direction every two or three laps, you'll lessen the chances of injury. Also, run in the far outside lanes, especially during warmups and cooldowns. The angle of the curve is less there, so it generates reduced forces on your legs.

Beaches: Most beaches are poor places to run. Generally, the sand is too soft and causes uneven footing, which strains and stresses your leg muscles. Also, the beach is slanted, and just as on a crowned road, your legs are forced to work unevenly—one pronating too much and the other supinating. If you can't resist a seaside jaunt, run at low tide when you can get onto packed sand and a flatter stretch of beach. Also, don't run too far in one direction; turn around to reverse the stresses on your legs.

WAKE UP AND WARM UP

Be sure to warm up and cool down. When you first get up in the morning, your muscles and soft tissues are tight. In fact, at that time your muscles are generally about 10 percent shorter than their normal resting length. When you start to exercise, your muscles stretch, reaching up to 10 percent longer than resting length. This means you have a 20 percent change in muscle length from the time you get out of bed until your muscles are well warmed up.

According to basic laws of physics, muscles work more efficiently when they are longer; they can exert more force with less effort. This means, too, that longer muscles are much less prone to injury.

Make it a practice to warm up before a run or race. Pedal for a few minutes indoors on a stationary bike, or jump rope for a few turns before you head down the road. If you would rather warm up on the run, begin with a walk or a slow jog and gradually move into your training pace.

Cooling down can also help you avoid injury. An easy jog after a hard workout or race has been shown to speed recovery by helping remove any lactic acid that may have accumulated. It also gently brings your muscles back to a resting state.

REACH FOR THE STARS

Stretch those muscles. Without flexibility, you are an injury waiting to happen. Tight muscles cannot go through their full range of motion. Lack of flexibility is probably the biggest cause of Achilles tendinitis and is a major factor in plantar fasciitis and shinsplints.

Although muscles in the back of your upper legs (the hamstrings) tend to be the workhorses, don't forget to stretch the muscles in the front of your legs as well. They're busy, too.

Stretching is not the same as warming up.

Take to the track

Outdoor tracks are almost always better than indoor tracks because they are larger and unbanked.

Indoor tracks often have a steep camber, which is murder on the knees. Also, most indoor tracks are smaller and require you to run more laps per mile—meaning more turns per mile.

Trying to stretch a tight muscle may cause injury. The best time to stretch is after a run, when your muscles are warm and elongated. Make stretching part of your routine every day.

When you stretch, move slowly and gradually into each position and hold it for just two seconds before relaxing again. Repeat each stretch 8 to 12 times. Never stretch a muscle to the point of pain. Pain indicates that you are stretching too hard or that some injury needs attention.

REST IS BEST

Schedule rest in your program. If you train hard every day, you'll wear your body down rather than build it up. You need to recover after a tough

Reward your muscles

A good warmup and cooldown are especially important before and after a hard workout such as intervals or a race in which you push your muscles to their limits. The extra time you spend warming up your muscles before a training run or race and cooling down afterward is worth the effort in improved efficiency and decreased likelihood of getting injured.

workout or a race, giving your muscles a chance to mend and stock up on glycogen for your next hard effort.

Just as some people need more sleep than others, some people need more recovery. You may discover that your body performs best when you rest for two days after a hard workout. Or you may even need three easy days. Experiment with various combinations of hard and easy days and compare the merits of easy running versus rest or cross-training.

EXPLORE OTHER AVENUES

Open up to cross-training. Runners once took a run-or-nothing approach to their sport, and many still do, believing that other sports cannot benefit their running and may in fact hurt it. The wiser runner now explores other options, both to supplement running during periods of good health and to substitute for running during injury phases. It's a rare runner today who doesn't employ some cross-training.

Participating in another sport a couple of times a week gives your feet and legs a welcome respite from the constant pounding of running and strengthens muscles that running does not

exercise. In both of these ways, cross-training can help protect you from injury.

Replace an easy run or rest day with a cross-training workout. After all, often it isn't total rest that your body needs, merely a break from the overspecialized action of running.

The more muscles you can involve in your training program, the less likely you are to sustain an overuse injury. Additionally, by working more of your major muscle groups, you improve your overall state of fitness.

If you do become injured through running and have been cross-training regularly, you will have an activity to turn to that will keep you fit while you recover. Overuse symptoms such as soreness, or injuries caused by too much shock or jarring, can often be relieved through swimming or cycling. By using a stair-climber, rowing machine, or cross-country ski machine, you can take the stress off an injured area and still get an excellent cardiovascular workout.

RECOVERY IS KEY

Recover properly after races. Racing pushes the limits of your speed and endurance, and too much racing can push you beyond your ability to avoid injury. Racing is hard on your body, so you must give yourself plenty of time to recover after each event.

Occasionally, you may read or hear about someone who runs an incredible number of races—a runner who runs a marathon every week for a year, for example. It's difficult to believe anyone can do that without getting injured, but there are always some people who can beat the odds. A few people can smoke three packs of cigarettes a day and live to be 100. But that doesn't mean that

Hard/easy training

Most experts recommend that you never schedule hard workouts two days in a row. Give yourself at least one day of easy running or rest between hard efforts. If you run fast one day, train slowly the next. If you run long one day, go short the following day. This is the "hard/easy" method of training.

you can play the odds without suffering the usual painful consequences.

LOG YOUR RUNS

Keeping a training log of your daily runs may seem compulsive or boring, but charting your distance, pace, course, the weather, and how you felt can give you an important perspective. With a running log, you can trace your progress and detect errors accurately and objectively. You can see if you have been training too little or too much.

Review your log weekly with a critical eye. Pretend it's someone else's training program and that you're checking how effective and safe it is. You may be amazed at the training errors you find. Correct these errors, and you'll become a better runner—and one more likely to stay injury-free.

REBOUNDING FROM INJURIES

If you do get injured, come back slowly . . . much more slowly than you might think.

After a layoff or an injury, your feet and legs need time to get reaccustomed to the effort of running. They have become somewhat soft and lazy, and it takes time to build them to the point where they can once again absorb the forces of running.

Furthermore, it's possible that your injury hasn't healed completely. Even though you may not feel any symptoms, the area you hurt will be weaker than it was before your injury—and more susceptible to reinjury. If you stress your body too much too soon, the same symptoms are likely to reappear.

Depending on how long your layoff was and

Top training tips

Let your training schedule be your guide, but never your prison guard. One of the surest ways to become injured is to train hard on a day when you're fatigued or feeling the soreness of an injury about to happen. Even if you're following all the rules—running on a good surface, warming up, stretching, using a hard/easy pattern—other factors of your lifestyle figure into your physical well-being and level of fatigue. Stress or lack of sleep can take a toll as well.

If you feel fatigued or overly sluggish or if you notice twinges of muscular pain, ease up on your training. If you have planned speedwork, run easy instead or take a day off altogether. You will not lose fitness over a day, or even a few days, of rest. Unfortunately, most runners have a hard time following this advice.

Let's say that you are training for a certain race and your schedule calls for a 10 percent increase in mileage this week, yet you're feeling a little twinge in your hamstrings. How do you respond? Do you go ahead and follow the schedule, or do you alter it?

You know the right answer. Yet many runners insist on adhering to the printed training schedule as if it were gospel. They refuse to deviate by a single mile from that program, since they believe that any modification will ruin their chances of running a good race. In fact, the reverse is true. They would benefit more by giving their body a chance to recover.

Training schedules are built on the assumption that you aren't experiencing any unusual pains before, during, or after the run. If pain or fatigue does strike, don't hesitate to modify your workouts.

whether or not you were able to do any cross-training to maintain fitness, you might need to return to your running program with a walk/jog regimen. Although you would rather eat asphalt

Amby Burfoot's Running Round-Up

The question of running surfaces, which Dr. Ellis covers at the beginning of this chapter, has long fascinated me. What really is the best surface to run on? If the answer were simple, then we would all take a big step forward in the battle against running injuries.

Of course, the answer isn't simple, as he explains. Every surface seems to have its pros and cons. Confusing, yes, but this situation nonetheless leads me to a tentative conclusion: Run on all surfaces. All the time. Deliberately. As part of your injury-prevention program.

The way I figure it, running on just one surface adds fuel to the overuse syndrome. Say you run on the roads every day. Every footfall is almost exactly like the one before it. The same muscles, tendons, and bones get stressed in the same way over and over again.

Whereas if you vary surfaces, the stresses vary. Now you have to be careful. New stress, such as that which comes from running on a beach, for example, can be a powerful injury mechanism. So be sure that your first beach run is a short and easy one. Don't do a hard 10-mile run.

Changing surfaces in an intelligent manner is a little like cross-training. It helps you prevent injuries by giving certain muscles and joints a rest while strengthening other muscles and joints.

---

than be caught walking, do it anyway. You'll still be exercising your muscles but without the hard pounding of running.

If you try to take shortcuts or cheat your body's natural timetable, you're asking for trouble. You simply cannot rush your recovery. As you become stronger, increase your weekly distance by no more than 10 percent per week. This rule applies when you're healthy, too.

Finally, be sure to eat well. During a layoff, many runners cut back on their diets to prevent weight gain. This isn't necessary. You need extra nutrients to help your body mend the injured area and fuel your training once you renew your running program. If you do gain a few pounds during your recovery period, they'll just melt away when you begin running again.

So eat. And train wisely. There's no reason why you can't continue running healthy year after year.

Chapter 11

Self-Treatments That Work

Here's a Low-Cost Insurance Plan for Your Running Problems

Many runners are lousy patients. They go to a doctor to get advice and then ignore it. Tell a runner to quit running for two to three weeks to rest an injury, and many will last just two to three days. After that, they figure that they can jog just a little to see how the injury feels. If it's okay, why not run a bit more tomorrow and more still the day after tomorrow?

Runners are too active to take the break they need. But here's a good alternative: Engage runners in their own therapy and recovery. That's an active role. Besides, runners are generally quite smart and quite analytical. They enjoy trying to understand an injury and trying out ways to help it heal.

That's the philosophy of this chapter: Help runners be their own doctors. This can't always work, obviously. A serious injury requires serious medical attention. But many running injuries aren't serious, and they can be cleared up better by the athlete who's finely attuned to his body than by anyone else. Runner, heal thyself.

Injuries happen. And when they do, you can call your doctor, make an appointment for some-

time next week, and hope the problem doesn't worsen in the meantime. Or you can treat it yourself at home, immediately, with the help of this guide.

"With a home remedy, you can cure most problems in a week or less," says Warren A. Scott, M.D., chief of sports medicine at Kaiser Permanente Medical Center in Santa Clara, California. "Left untreated, an injury can hang on for several months or up to a year or more."

This guide covers everything you need to know, from black toenails to exercise-induced asthma. And the remedies come from Dr. Scott and the medical experts who have worked with *Runner's World* magazine for many years.

Granted, not all injuries can be handled

at home. If your symptoms are severe and your injury is at an advanced stage, or if self-treatment doesn't seem to be working, see a sports-oriented physician.

ASTHMA, EXERCISE-INDUCED

A contraction of the muscles surrounding the air passages, which narrows these passages and causes wheezing, shortness of breath, and heaviness in the chest. Cold temperatures, dry air, and high altitude aggravate the condition, which is suffered by 10 to 15 percent of the population.

Remedies: Before a run or race, warm up for about 10 minutes. Then start running hard, which may cause the asthmatic response, triggering the release of adrenaline, which then dilates the bronchial tubes. When you're able to, run hard for five minutes, then slow for five minutes; repeat several times, then walk. Stretch and walk a little more. Perform this routine 15 to 30 minutes before you race or run. The intensity of this warmup results in a refractory period of 60 to 90 minutes during

Keeping injury at bay

Of course, the best advice is not to get injured in the first place. You can help prevent injuries by following these smart training principles: Wear good running shoes that fit well and replace them before their midsole cushioning wears out; increase mileage by no more than 10 percent a week; follow hard training days with easy days or days off; stretch and strength-train regularly; and when something starts to hurt, back off or stop running until the pain is gone.

When asthma strikes

If you can't run for long without an asthma attack no matter what you do, try running at intervals of three to five minutes with two to three minutes' rest in between. Eventually, you should build up some endurance and be able to run longer. The bottom line is that exercise is excellent for asthma.

which you should be able to exercise without an asthma attack.

Since cold, dry air can trigger asthma attacks, wear a surgical mask (which you can purchase at a pharmacy or drugstore) or wrap a scarf over your mouth when running in cold weather. If you have allergies and notice more frequent asthma attacks during the spring and late summer, wearing a mask may help then as well. Always inhale through your nose. Also, beware of air pollution and remember that you will have more trouble breathing at high altitudes.

Anxiety can exacerbate an asthma attack. Some experts recommend 30-minute relaxation or meditation sessions several times a week to teach you to relax readily at times of stress. Home remedies may not be enough. Consult a sports-oriented physician about taking one of several safe, effective asthma medications now available.

ATHLETE'S FOOT

A fungal infection that causes itchy or painful scaling, redness, and blisters between the toes and on the soles of the feet.

Remedies: Apply a fungicide such as Desenex, Tinactin, Lotrimin, or Lamisil. Use these products two or three times a day for two to four weeks, and continue to use them for one to two weeks after symptoms are gone. The fungus remains even after the irritation disappears.

To relieve itching, apply an astringent solution, such as Domeboro, or soak your feet in baking soda mixed with water. Remove dead skin with a pumice stone, or rub fine sandpaper along the bottoms of your feet and discard the sandpaper.

Athlete's foot fungus is ubiquitous and thrives in dark, moist places. You may get reinfected. If you do, alternate the fungicides you use so that the fungus does not build a tolerance to one brand.

BACK PAIN

A source of pain or aching in the back, which may have any of several causes.

Remedies: Should you run with back pain? If running doesn't make it worse, go ahead. "Sitting puts more stress on your back than running does," says Dr. Scott. "In fact, exercise rather than rest is recommended for most patients with back problems." If running isn't comfortable, swim, go cycling, or try some other activity. Walking is excellent.

For pain relief, use ice (see "Three of the Best Cures for Running Injuries" on page 75). But rather than wrap the ice against your back, place it on your bed and lie on it (you may have to bolster your back a bit with pillows if you're too uncomfortable). Some people favor a hot/cold regimen from the start. Alternate 20 minutes of ice with 20 minutes of heat.

Some back problems lie deep in the muscles, where icing won't have an effect. If pushing the site of the injury with your thumb does not cause pain, the injury probably lies too deep.

People with chronic back problems should do stretching and strengthening exercises regularly. Try back extensions, lower-back stretches, pelvic tilts, bent-leg crunches, and trunk twists. Warm up beforehand. When running, stick to soft surfaces and avoid hills, irregular surfaces, and small running tracks with tight turns. When you sleep, put a pillow between your knees when lying on your side; put two pillows under your knees when lying on your back.

If your back pain radiates into your legs, or if rest and home treatments don't bring relief, you need to see a sports-oriented physician.

BLACK TOENAILS

A pooling of blood under the toenail, caused by the toe rubbing or hitting the top of your shoe. Often the toe will throb with the pressure of the blood.

Remedies: To relieve the pressure, you need to make a hole in the nail and drain the blood. Either heat the tip of a small, straightened paper clip and use it to burn through the nail until a drop of blood comes out, or sterilize the tip of a $1/16$-inch drill bit with heat or alcohol and, by spinning the instrument between your finger and thumb, drill a hole in the nail. Stick your foot in a pan of water until all the blood comes out. (If you're squeamish about doing this, see a sports-oriented physician.) Apply an antibacterial cream. Relieve inflammation with ice and anti-inflammatories.

If your black toenail isn't painful, you don't have to drain the blood. Lubricate with antifungal cream and cover it with a bandage. But monitor the nail, as it will probably loosen and fall off over the next few months. When it gets loose, carefully pull it off and continue to apply the antifungal cream. In the meantime, buy a pair of running shoes with more room in the toe box.

BLISTERS

Fluid accumulation between the skin's inner and outer layers because of excess friction.

Remedies: When possible, leave the blister alone for 24 hours to allow it to heal itself. If the fluid isn't reabsorbed, lance the blister as follows: Sterilize a needle by heating it in a flame or boiling water or by soaking it in alcohol. Swab the blister with a disinfectant such as alcohol. Prick two holes on opposite sides of the blister and press it gently with sterile gauze to push out the fluid. Don't remove the loose skin. Smear the blister with 1% hydrocortisone cream, such as Preparation H, and cover it with a sterile gauze pad. If the blister refills, lance again and then soak it in Epsom salts or an astringent solution, such as Domeboro. Before putting on shoes, make a doughnut shape out of molefoam and place it around the blister, then put another layer on top to cover the whole area. For recurring blisters, eliminate the cause: Wear running shoes that are the right size and shape. Also wear synthetic-blend socks. Before you run, apply petroleum jelly or talcum powder to reduce friction.

CALF STRAIN

Pain in the calf, as well as swelling, tenderness, and muscle tightness, resulting from sudden over-loading of the muscles during speedwork, hill running, or running on uneven trails.

Remedies: Treat with ice and anti-inflammatories. Wrap your calf with a four-inch elastic bandage. It should be tight enough to provide relief but not so tight that it cuts off circulation. Wear this all day long and during running for a couple of days.

Stretch your calf 5 to 10 times a day. Try adding ¼-inch cork heel lifts to your shoes, and be sure to wear street shoes with a heel height that reduces stress on the muscles; running shoes are often a good choice. Avoid walking barefoot.

People with recurring calf problems should look for shoes that are thicker in the rear foot and have sturdy heel counters.

CALLUSES

Areas of thickened skin caused by repetitive friction (such as that of running in ill-fitting shoes) or by abnormalities of the bony structure of the foot. Usually painless, calluses are a natural protective reaction of the skin over pressure sites.

Remedies: When a callus first develops, file it with an emery board, sandpaper, or a pumice stone after bathing, and apply petroleum jelly, lanolin, or other moisturizers to the skin. If a thicker callus has formed, use a peeling and softening agent such as Ultra Mide 25 lotion. Don't let calluses get too big; they can crack and become infected.

Very thick, painful calluses should be treated by a sports-oriented physician. To reduce friction when you run, wear thicker socks. Watch for blisters that may occur next to thick calluses, and treat them as described earlier.

FLAT FEET

An inherited condition in which there is little or no arch to the bottom of the foot. (Note: Running cannot cause flat feet.)

Remedies: Flat feet in themselves are not a problem. Many runners with flat feet overpronate, however, and overpronation can cause problems in your feet, shins, and knees. If running is giving you aches and pains, first check your shoes; a motion-control shoe with a straight "last" is best. (The last is the shape the shoe is based upon. You can see this shape by turning a shoe upside down.) Over-the-counter arch supports or orthotics can provide additional support. If none of these help, see a sports-oriented physician for custom-made orthotics.

HAMSTRING PAIN

Pain in the muscles at the back of the thigh, occurring during sprinting or speedwork.

Remedies: Treat with ice and anti-inflammatories, and stretch the hamstring several times a day. Wrap your thigh with a six-inch elastic bandage. The muscle should be squeezed but comfortable.

Do leg curls to strengthen the hamstrings. When doing them, lift with one leg at a time so that a strong leg cannot compensate for a weaker one, and make sure that you feel the work just in the hamstring, not the buttocks and calf.

HEAT EXHAUSTION AND HEATSTROKE

These are similar problems, but they are not the same. Heat exhaustion refers to overheating of the body from excessive loss of water or, in rare cases, salt depletion. Symptoms include thirst, headache, pallor, dizziness, and possibly nausea or vomiting. In severe cases, your heart may race, and you may feel disoriented.

Heatstroke occurs when the body's thermoregulatory system stops working. Many of the symptoms are the same as for heat exhaustion. Cessation of sweating, difficulty walking, disorientation, and fainting or unconsciousness, however, indicate heatstroke. Runners suffering heatstroke will be too disoriented to help themselves. Learn to recognize the symptoms and treat the problem in someone else.

Remedies: For heat exhaustion, stop running and get out of the sun, preferably into an air-conditioned building. Drink water or, better still, a sports beverage, taking it slowly rather than gulping it down. If you don't feel better within 30 minutes, go to a hospital emergency room.

Heat exhaustion is not fatal, but heatstroke can be. The key symptom to look for is disorientation. A person who is functioning well mentally isn't in danger. Someone who's becoming "jelly brained" is in trouble. Pack ice around the runner's neck, armpits, and groin, splash water on the skin, and fan the runner. Elevate the legs. If the person is conscious, give plenty of fluids—one to two quarts—preferably a sports beverage, but water is fine. The person will probably be nauseated and may not want to drink anything, but fluids are essential.

If you get heatstroke once, you may be likely

to get it again. All runners should take care to dress appropriately for the heat. Make sure you wear synthetics, not cotton. Wear a light cap, sunglasses, and sunscreen (which actually helps cool your skin), and drink, drink, drink. Try to schedule your runs during the cooler hours of the day—morning or early evening.

HYPOTHERMIA

Low body temperature—96°F or lower—which can be fatal if left untreated. Symptoms include shivering, slow pulse, lethargy, and a decrease in alertness. In severe cases, muscles become rigid, and the victim can lose consciousness. Dehydration makes you more prone to hypothermia.

Remedies: Keep moving to generate heat. Get to a warm place, wrap yourself in blankets, and drink warm liquids. Snuggle up to the Saint Bernard for his body heat, but refuse the whiskey around his neck—alcoholic beverages do not warm you. In fact, they cause more heat loss and promote fluid loss.

Runners most at risk are those who run in rural areas and on trails. Run with a partner, and dress appropriately—in layers, all synthetics. Cotton doesn't wick away your sweat, and wet skin loses 25 times more heat than dry skin. Wear a polypropylene hat and gloves. Carry a fanny pack, and take along one to two quarts of a sports beverage.

LEG-LENGTH DISCREPANCY

A difference in the length of the legs. This alters the alignment of the spine and makes it more vul-nerable to the shock forces generated by running. A leg-length discrepancy isn't painful in itself, but it can cause other problems and injuries. If you experience regular bouts of iliotibial band syndrome or have sciatica-like pain that radiates from your buttocks down into your legs, you may have a leg-length discrepancy.

Remedies: Here's a home test for determining if you have a leg-length discrepancy: In your underwear, stand with good posture in front of a full-length mirror. Look to see if your shoulders are level (if you have played a lot of throwing sports, your dominant shoulder will hang lower and may not be an indication of leg-length discrepancy). Look at your pelvis, then let your body sag and look again. Put your fingers on the bony areas at the front of the hip and look to see if they are level. If they're not, place magazines under the foot of the shorter leg, building up until both sides are even.

If the difference amounts to more than ½ inch and you have suffered from foot, ankle, knee, thigh, hip, or back pain, see a sports-oriented physician. If the difference is about ¼ inch, try a ¼-inch cork heel lift in all your shoes to relieve the problem.

MUSCLE SORENESS

Muscle pain and inflammation following a race, speedwork, downhill running, or other hard workouts.

Remedies: At the end of a hard run, race, or marathon, walk rather than stop completely. Then cool your legs off with cold water poured over the entire leg. Take anti-inflammatories, stretch often, and, if possible, get a massage. After a marathon, take three days off from running and go cycling instead. Pick up running again on the fourth day if you want.

Three of the Best Cures for Running Injuries

Ice, anti-inflammatories, and stretching are common treatments for many running injuries. Here are the best ways to implement them.

How To Ice An Injury

Cover the skin with two layers of plastic wrap. Put ice on top and compress with an elastic bandage or tight-fitting clothing such as spandex or Lycra. Ice for 20 minutes, stop for 10 minutes. Ice again for 20 minutes, stop for 10. Ice for 20, stop for 10. "If you can do this three times a day for three days in a row, you'll get a tremendous anti-inflammatory effect," says Dr. Scott. If you don't have the time for this regimen, do what you can. Crushed ice, 1- to 2-pound bags of frozen peas, and gel packs work well.

"Heat does not have the anti-inflammatory effect that ice does," says Dr. Scott, "but hot tubs and heating pads can be very relaxing to your muscles and your mind. Go ahead and use them if you want." Rubs and balms applied to the skin have no healing effect. They create a mild stinging sensation in the skin to trick the brain and distract you from your pain, Dr. Scott adds.

Using Anti-Inflammatory Medicines

Inflammation, common in running injuries, is characterized by pain, swelling, redness, and warmth and is treated with anti-inflammatory medications. Ibuprofen and naproxen sodium are the best, but aspirin is okay, too.

Follow the instructions on the bottle, and take these medicines for one to two weeks. Always take them with food.

If you have chronic aches and pains that you can't get rid of, such as those associated with osteoarthritis, and you've been to the doctor to have them checked out, use acetaminophen to relieve pain. It's very safe and works well.

A Few Words On Stretching

When stretching, make sure that you feel the tension in the muscle you are stretching, which isn't necessarily the site of the injury. Do not bounce. Hold the stretch until you feel the muscles relax, usually between 15 and 30 seconds.

It's best to stretch warm muscles, but it's okay to stretch gently when you haven't warmed up. Where stretching is indicated as part of the treatment for an injury, it's a good idea to stretch several times a day.

To help prevent muscle soreness, add some downhill running to your training, every two to three weeks, especially when you're preparing for a downhill race. Your quadriceps will thank you.

OVERPRONATION

Excessive inward roll of the foot after landing, such that the foot continues to roll when it should be pushing off. This twists the foot, shin, and knee and can cause pain in all those areas. If you are an overpronator, you'll find excessive wear on the inner side of your running shoes, and they'll tilt inward if you place them on a flat surface. Flat feet contribute to overpronation.

Remedies: Wear shoes with straight or semicurved lasts. Motion-control or stability shoes with firm, multidensity midsoles and external control features that limit pronation are best.

Over-the-counter orthotics or arch supports can help, too. You know you are making improvements when the wear pattern on your shoes becomes more normal. Overpronation causes extra stress on and tightness in the muscles, so do a little extra stretching.

OVERTRAINING

Fatigue, stale training, poor race performance, irritability, and loss of enthusiasm for running, caused by excessive mileage or too many hard workouts. Serious overtraining can cause sleep disturbances, hampered immune function, poor appetite, and in women, the cessation of menstrual periods.

Remedies: Cut back on your running for a minimum of two weeks. Experiment with cutting back on mileage, adding rest days,

To run or not to run?

Should you run with an injury? "It's okay as long as you run at a level below the threshold of pain," says Warren A. Scott, M.D. When an injury occurs, cut back your mileage and intensity until you can run without pain (but don't ever take medications or ice an injury before testing whether or not you can run). If it hurts no matter what, stop running, and cross-train. Walking, cycling, swimming, pool running, rowing, stair-climbing, and cross-country skiing all work with most running injuries.

If you need to stop running, take a week off, and then try a walk/run. If that feels okay, you can begin to return to running. If it doesn't feel good, take another week off, and test your legs again. Always reintroduce yourself to running through a walk/run regimen that eventually progresses to regular, steady running.

and substituting cross-training to see what works best.

If you suspect serious overtraining, cut your running back to only two or three days a week, 30 to 45 minutes at an easy-to-moderate effort. You can supplement this with more stretching and some cross-training on other days of the week, but no more than an hour at an easy-to-moderate effort.

When you're feeling better and you're ready to increase your running, look at your training over the coming year, and plan periods when you'll train hard and race; follow these with periods of easier running and lower mileage.

RUNNER'S KNEE

Pain all around and under the kneecap, and stiffness of the knee joint. In severe cases, flexing the knee may produce a painful grinding sensation. Runner's knee results from running too much or too hard, too soon.

Remedies: Poke around the knee. If you find a sore spot, ice it; if you don't, ice won't help. Take anti-inflammatories. If the knee swells, ice it, and see a sports-oriented physician. Swelling indicates a major problem, and it may take three to four months for the knee to heal.

Runner's knee can occur when hamstrings are tight, when quadriceps are much stronger than hamstrings, or, in the case of new runners, when quadriceps are weak. All runners should stretch and strengthen their quadriceps and hamstrings regularly.

If you can run through this injury, avoid downhills; flat running and uphills are easier. Wear shoes with adequate sole padding and good motion-control properties. Consider wearing a rubber sleeve with a hole that fits over the kneecap to reduce pain caused by too much flexing.

SCIATICA

Sciatica is a pain in the butt, literally. Caused by an irritation of the sciatic nerve, this pain can radiate down the back of the leg and all the way to the foot. It feels like burning, pins and needles, or an electrical sensation. It has many causes, including tight hamstrings, tight buttocks, biomechanical problems, leg-length discrepancy, back sprain, or a herniated disk.

Remedies: Do not ice, but do take anti-inflammatories. Lots of muscles will get tight; stretch the back, buttocks, hamstrings, iliotibial band, gluteal muscles, and calves. Consider cross-training, and when the pain diminishes, try a walk/run. Sitting can aggravate sciatica. Make sure that your sitting posture is good (especially in the car) and use pillows, if needed, to adjust your back and buttocks into a more comfortable position.

Sciatica is secondary to an underlying problem. A leg-length discrepancy is often the culprit. If home treatments don't relieve the pain or if your condition gets worse, see a sports-oriented doctor. (Note: Don't ignore sciatica pain. It will follow you to your grave if you don't deal with it.)

SIDE STITCHES

A sharp pain usually felt just below the rib cage (though sometimes farther up the torso), caused by a cramp in the diaphragm, gas in the intestines, or food in the stomach. Stitches nor-mally come on during hard workouts or races.

Remedies: If you get a stitch on your right side (which is more common), slow down for 30 seconds or so and exhale forcefully each time your left foot hits the ground. If the stitch is on the left, exhale hard when your right foot lands. Continue until the pain recedes. If this doesn't help, try slow, deep "belly breathing" (your abdomen should go in and out with each breath). Or run with your hands on top of your head and your elbows back while you breathe deeply from your belly.

Another remedy is to take your fist and dig it under your rib cage. Push the fist in with your other arm and bend your torso over almost to 90 degrees. Run like this for 10 steps. This stretches the diaphragm (most stitches are caused by a spasm of the diaphragm). If none of these techniques work, stop and walk until the pain subsides.

And here's a no-brainer: To prevent stitches caused by food in the stomach, don't eat before you run.

SUPINATION (OR UNDERPRONATION)

Insufficient inward roll of the foot after landing. This places extra stress on the foot and can

Supinator symptoms

Runners with high arches and tight Achilles tendons tend to be supinators. Shoes will wear on the entire outside edge, and the side of the shoe becomes overstretched. If you place shoes on a flat surface, they tilt outward.

Amby Burfoot's Running Round-Up

The hardest lesson that I had to learn as a runner was the importance of rest—total rest—when recovering from an injury. On more occasions than I'd like to admit, I prolonged my injury problems by failing to let them heal completely before running again.

One year, having developed a stress fracture in my foot, I went to a doctor who said I was fine—I just needed to take six weeks off from running. I took two days off, but then started running again. Just a little at first, and then a little more, and then a little more. After three weeks I was almost back to my usual training program. Until I took a hard run one day and fractured the foot bone all over again. The result, of course, was that I lost three months of training instead of six weeks. I've made similar, less serious mistakes with injuries, and I have known hundreds of other runners who have done the same. Now I am wiser (I hope), and I see things more clearly.

I know the truth about injuries: Rest cures them. Usually in remarkably little time. When you have a nagging ache or pain, take a couple of days off. If it doesn't get better right away, take a week off, two weeks if you need to. It seems like a lot of time when you're not running, but it's nothing compared to the amount of time you'll lose if you're chronically injured.

So get healthy first. Totally healthy. Then ease your way back into running.

result in iliotibial band syndrome and Achilles tendinitis.

Remedies: Wear shoes with curved lasts to allow pronation. Lightweight trainers are often best, as they allow more foot motion. Also, check for flexibility on the inner side of the shoe. Supinators should do extra stretching for the calves, hamstrings, quadriceps, and iliotibial band.

Chapter 12

You Can Run, But You Can't Hide . . . from the Heat

When the weather turns hot, you need to change your running habits

Running is a high calorie-burn activity, and most of the time you appreciate this effect. After all, it's what makes running such a great weight-loss tool. In summer, however, there are times when you might not feel so positive about that calorie burn.

Like on the hottest, most humid days. That's when you begin to realize that the calorie is a measure of energy release. As such, it's bound to raise your body temperature at a time when you'd rather encounter a cooling breeze.

But even one-hundred-degree days don't have to stop you. Runners from the hottest cities in the United States have learned to adjust their training and racing strategies to match the conditions. Here, writer John Hanc visits some of those places to learn how the local runners adapt.

Shortly after I arrived in Phoenix and checked in at my hotel, Mike Sheedy of the Arizona Road Runners contacted me. "We have a 14-mile run planned for tomorrow, and we heard you'd like to join us." Yes, definitely! "We run on trails in South Mountain Park. It's beautiful." Sounds great! "And we can pick you up at your hotel." Works for me! "Good, we'll be there at 3:30." Hmmm. "Three thirty?" I finally asked. "In the morning?" There was a chuckle on the other end of the line. "We try to start around 4 o'clock. That's the only time we can run out here. It's best to finish before 7 because it can be almost 100 degrees by 8 o'clock.

Our 4 a.m., 14-mile run through the desert was memorable not just because of the beauty of the desert at dawn but because of how well we were able to run. The key to success? Preparation and attentiveness.

Everybody wore a hat, everybody carried fluids—and everybody shared them. It seemed like I couldn't run more than a quarter-mile without a bottle of water or flask of sports drink being pushed in front of my face. "Take a sip," ordered one of the veterans, when I declined his initial offer. "You can't fool around out here."

There was something else the Phoenix runners demonstrated that I didn't notice in my group runs back home in New York: a sense of responsibility. They all kept an eye on each other, especially newcomers. "You can get into trouble real quick in this heat," said John Conant, a Tempe runner who had seen someone collapse at a local 8-K just a few weeks earlier. "It was hot, the guy hadn't been hydrating during the week, and he didn't drink during the race." In other words, if you don't use your head in the heat, you may find yourself falling on it.

GO SLOW: BATON ROUGE

The heat of Baton Rouge, Louisiana, bears little resemblance to the dry, desert heat of Phoenix. "Down here, it's hot and sticky," says longtime resident Kenny Dunaway. From mid-May through the end of October, the weather is "oppressively tropical," he says. "It's as close to jungle running as you can get in North America." The average daily heat and humidity in Baton Rouge in July (91 degrees, 74 percent humidity) are comparable to midsummer in Nigeria. Dunaway has been running in these American tropics since high school. And although the climate is far different from the Valley of the Sun, the attitude among Bayou runners

toward the heat is similar. "We take it seriously," he says.

Preparations for Sunday long runs start on Saturday, when, Dunaway says, "I eat light and drink heavy"—as in water, not Lone Star Beer, which he saves for the night after the run, along with all the spicy Cajun food that he forgoes the night before. "Your body has to digest all that, and in the really intense heat, that's tough on your stomach," says Dunaway. The night before summer long runs, he sticks with salads and fruits, which are not only light but also have a high water content to assist with hydration.

The hot, moist conditions Dunaway and his running partners face in Louisiana demand extra caution. Humidity on top of heat drastically decreases the body's ability to cool itself. "Sweating doesn't cool the body; it's the evaporation of the sweat that makes you feel cooler," says Lisa Bliss, M.D., ultrarunner and medical director of the Badwater Ultramarathon. "When it's humid, it's harder for the sweat to evaporate." The most effective way to deal with the oppressive combination of high humidity and heat? "Let your body self-select the pace," says Dr. Bliss.

In other words, when it's hot, slow down. "If it ain't happening, it ain't happening," says Dunaway. "What we say here is 'Don't be a hero in the heat.'"

RUN, DON'T HIDE: MIAMI

All the heat vets agree that you need to keep your pace easy when the temps and humidity climb, but none of them, including Steve Brookner, president of the Miami-based Bikila Athletic Club, suggest hiding from the heat. "The good thing about Miami is that we can train outdoors year-round," says Brookner. "The bad thing is that there are days when you open your door, even at 5 a.m., and you're hit with hot, sticky air. You think, This run is going to suck, but it doesn't if you're prepared." The Bikila club members carefully plan their running routes to pass by water fountains and stashes of fluids that they put out beforehand. That way, everyone has ample opportunity to drink up.

Brookner advises newcomers to the Miami running scene to simply get used to the heat through limited exposure. He tells newbies to go out during the hottest part of the day and do a very slow, short walk or run a few easy miles a couple of times a week for their first few weeks.

Medical experts agree. "Spending all your time in air-conditioning and then expecting to run well outdoors in the heat is not going to cut it," says William Roberts, M.D., medical director of the Twin Cities Marathon. If you want to train in the heat, you have to learn to live in it first. Gradually exposing yourself to the hot weather—for as little as 30 minutes a day—helps induce changes that make the body more tolerant of heat stress.

Here are the hot-weather tips Brookner gives new members of his club:

Train at 5 a.m. "The world is so full of promise when viewed at sunrise," Brookner says. True, but equally important, it's a little cooler. Put in your miles before the sun is high.

Cross-train indoors. Build your cardio base while taking a break from the heat and humidity by swapping an outdoor bike ride for an inside spin class.

Do speedwork on a treadmill. Intensity of exercise is a major factor in heat distress—the harder you run, the higher your risk. Plus, when you try to run fast in extreme heat, Brookner points out, "your perceived effort almost always exceeds your actual effort." To make your intervals safer and more productive, stay in and run as fast as you like in air-conditioned comfort.

Ease into the heat. Do a slow, two- to three-mile walk or very easy run at the hottest part of the day, two times per week for three or four weeks, to acclimate to the heat. "It makes the morning run feel cool," says Brookner.

Have a hydration plan before you start. Know where your water stops are, either by plotting your runs in areas that have water fountains or by stashing bottles at strategic points along your route ahead of time. Also get in touch with local running clubs and training groups to find out where they might put out jugs, so you can share.

Don't just drink the water. A combo run-and-swim workout is perfect on really hot days. One of Brookner's favorites is a three-mile run from the Cocoplum traffic circle to Matheson-Hammock Park in Coral Gables. There, he and his buddies dive into the cool, clear waters of the nearby lagoon, swim for 15 to 30 minutes, get out, and run back. You can re-create this duathlon anywhere there's a body of water, or even a local pool.

Plan to race in cool temperatures. For Brookner, registering for a fall marathon "up north," such as Marine Corps or New York, basically guarantees relief from the heat. "When I show up in New York for the marathon in November and it's in the 70s, the New Yorkers are all like 'ugh,' and I'm saying, 'Bring it on!'"

WATER: HOW MUCH SHOULD YOU DRINK?

Drink too little, you worry about dehydration. Drink too much, you worry about hyponatremia (low blood-sodium levels). Dr Bliss has personally experienced the effects of both.

In 2004, Dr. Bliss ran Badwater and, in the 125-degree heat of Death Valley, became hyponatremic. "You're sweating so much and everyone's telling you to drink," says Dr. Bliss. "I kept drinking, and when I finally hopped on a scale, I'd gained nine pounds. I was dizzy and disoriented." Fortunately, the solution for Dr. Bliss was simple. "All I had to do was stop drinking," she says. She kept running, and the symptoms went away as her body shed the excess water through sweating and urination—allowing her to finish in 15th place overall.

Weighing in during the course of an event helps ensure you aren't gaining weight (a sign of overhydrating) or losing too much weight (dehydrating). Of course, we're not suggesting you train with a scale. But weighing yourself before and after runs is the best way to find out if you are taking in the right amount of fluids, which is different for everyone. To estimate your fluid needs, weigh yourself naked before and after a hard one-hour run. Convert the amount of weight lost to ounces to figure out your sweat rate per hour—so a loss of one pound means you sweated about 16 ounces of fluid. In this case, going forward you would try to replenish fluids at a rate of about 16 ounces per hour.

If figuring out your sweat rate is too much work, the most recent American College of Sports Medicine guidelines suggest drinking anywhere from about 14 to 27 ounces per hour, with the higher end of the range applying to "faster, heavier individuals competing in warm environments and the lower rates for the slower, lighter persons competing in cooler environments." When you're out for more than 30 minutes, choose sports drinks over water, since the carbs and electrolytes they contain help you stay energized and better hydrated during longer runs.

ARE YOU READY TO RUN IN THE HEAT?

According to Dr. Roberts, ambient temperature is only a small factor in predicting heat stress. "At Twin Cities, we've had cases of heatstroke at 50 degrees," he says. "And there have been marathons in Rio de Janeiro without any problems. So much depends on your acclimation levels." Dr. Roberts has researched cases of fatal heatstroke among athletes and found that the runner's general health and use of medications were contributing factors, just as important as dehydration and weather conditions. He offers this checklist to determine if you're ready to run in the heat. If you answer "no" to any of questions 1 through 6 or "yes" to question 7, Dr. Roberts advises either exercising indoors or keeping your run very short and very easy.

1. Are you acclimated—have you been in similar temperatures during the past two weeks?

2. Are you well rested (having gotten at least seven hours of sleep last night), and have you been in cooled or air-conditioned environments for some part of the last 24 hours?

3. Are you hydrated? (If you are hydrated, your urine will be pale yellow in color. If it is dark like apple juice, you're dehydrated.)

4. Are you healthy—no recent illnesses?

5. Are you well nourished?

6. Have you avoided alcohol in the past 24 hours?

7. Are you taking medications with ephedrine or other prescription medicines that might interfere with your thermal regulation (information you can find in the literature that comes with the medication or get from a pharmacist)?

DRESSING TO STAY SAFE UNDER THE SUN

Shirt: Wear a loose-fitting, long-sleeve running top that is light in color (to reflect the sun) and made of a wicking technical fiber. Flowing, longer shirts can keep you feeling cooler than tanks because they offer more protection from the sun's heat.

Shorts: Opt for longer, loose-fitting running shorts, which will protect more of your legs from the sun and offer more ventilation to keep you cooler. Shorts should be light in color and made of a lightweight technical fiber. But choose apparel without significant mesh panels, since mesh offers minimal sun protection.

Hat: Choose a hat with a substantial brim and made of technical fibers (like Coolmax) to help wick sweat. Caps with a "sun skirt" (some of which are removable) offer additional protection for your ears, back of head, and neck. Or try a "cold cap." Soak an old baseball cap in water and put it in the fridge for at least 30 minutes or overnight before a morning run.

Sunglasses: Select lightweight models designed for sports activities that offer good coverage. The American Optometric Association recommends lenses that block out 99 to 100 percent of both UVA and UVB rays for optimal eye protection.

Fuel belt: Look for a fuel belt that is capable of carrying multiple mini-bottles or gel flasks so that you can customize your fueling strategy—replacing both carbs and electrolytes on the run—depending on the length of your workout.

Neck wrap: Lay a bandanna out in a diamond shape. Place a row of ice cubes in a horizontal line, just below one tip of the bandanna. Then roll it up like a burrito, and tie it around your neck.

Water: Depending on the length of your run, consider carrying one or two ergonomically shaped, handheld bottles with foam strap handles (each bottle typically holds about 20 ounces), or wear a hydration pack that can carry 50 to 70 ounces of fluids.

THE MOST IMPORTANT ITEM TO WEAR: SUNSCREEN

"Start taking it seriously," says 2004 Olympic bronze medalist Deena Kastor about sun protection. Kastor knows. She's been diagnosed three times with malignant melanoma, the most serious form of skin cancer. Fortunately, each time it was caught early and removed. Kastor now gets checkups every three months.

"In high school, I wasn't such a stickler about putting on sunscreen and protecting myself," she says. "I'm paying the price right now."

Chances are, many of us haven't been sticklers, either. A recent, widely publicized study found more abnormal moles and lesions in marathoners than nonmarathoners and also reported that only 56 percent of the runners said they put on sunscreen regularly. "The study is not a reason to stop running outdoors," says Peter O'Neill, M.D., a dermatologist and marathoner from Garden City, New York. "But it is a reason to start taking sun protection seriously."

Hot summer weather should never be taken lightly by runners. I have seen Olympic athletes stumble off a track when they ran themselves into heatstroke, and have written feature stories about teenage runners who died after a training run in soupy heat. High heat and high-intensity running can be a dangerous combination.

That doesn't mean that you can't run healthfully in the heat. You can. Very easily. By observing all the tips presented in this article(most important: to run slow and easy on the hottest days)and by always running with someone on hot days. That way, if you or your training partner start to feel light-headed, you've got a friend right at your side.

Drinking fluids before and after running can help keep your body temperature under control, but you have to be certain not to drink too much. A few years back, we figured that runners sweat so much it was impossible to over-drink. Now we know about hyponatremia, described above. The science of running is always gaining new insights. But to be the healthiest runner you can be, you have to follow the new advances. So be sure to drink without over-drinking

—Deena Kastor

Dr. O'Neill recommends using a sunscreen that's waterproof, has an SPF of 30, and offers "broad spectrum" protection, which means it protects against both UVA and UVB rays. "Some sunscreens only protect against B," he says. "But it's the A, the longer wave of ultraviolet light, that penetrates the skin more deeply."

Slather on a good sunscreen at least 20 minutes before you head out so that your skin has time to absorb the lotion. Dr. O'Neill is also a fan of protective clothing. "It's nice to run in just a tank top and shorts," he says, "but you're better off dressing like those guys in the desert who wear the long-sleeve, lightweight fabrics." Kastor wears them during her training runs in California. "The long-sleeve shirts are really thin and light, they have added SPF in the fabric, and they feel fine," she says.

While all the precautions Kastor is now taking haven't been enough yet to overcome either her genetic predisposition or her youthful sun transgressions, she's approaching the situation with a healthy attitude. "That's what this sport is all about," she says. "We run because it's a healthy thing to do."

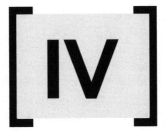

Women's Running

Chapter 13

Run Smart and Informed to Save Your Life

Being Aware Is Only Part of Running Safely

The safety question is the most troubling issue that women runners face. On the one hand, simply raising it restricts women runners. Instead of thinking of their workouts as a time of freedom and release when they can expand their horizons, they see limitations—the kind of shackles that women have long had to fight against. On the other hand, not to consider the safety question is sheer insanity.

At *Runner's World* magazine, we encourage women to run by pointing out all the positive things about running. And we do this often and easily. After all, our women readers are constantly telling us about the many benefits that they have received. We get testimonials in the mail nearly every day.

But we can't stop there. Women have also been attacked, raped, and murdered while running. Writers and editors can't stop violence against women, but we can tell women how to be vigilant and how to protect themselves. That's the purpose of this chapter: to inform women runners while still liberating them.

Every 22 seconds someone becomes a victim of violent crime. Every minute in America, 1.3 adult women are raped. If you think that your runner's speed and fitness will protect you against assault, you are giving someone out there a huge opportunity to hurt you. To protect yourself, you must first get rid of that it-could-never-happen-to-me attitude, and then take the precautions that are necessary to protect yourself from violent crime.

To find out how you can run safely, J. J. Bittenbinder, formerly with the Chicago Police Department, now an inspector and lecturer assigned to the Cook County Sheriff's Department in Illinois, offers some tips. After more than two decades of working with more than a thousand offenders, witnesses, and victims of violent street crime, Bittenbinder has seen it all. And he has come up with some tough strategies to keep you safe on the streets. Indeed, what he has to say could save your life.

Q: Do women runners need to be constantly aware that they are potential victims?

A: I'd hate for women to run scared every step of the way. You have to realize that bad stuff can happen to anybody, anyplace, anytime. But if you have a plan of action, you won't have to concentrate on the fear. Every bad guy is different, but you have to be trained to do certain things and use certain skills if a bad situation comes up. Then your attitude changes—instead of being afraid, you say to yourself, "This stuff can happen, but I know how to prevent it." You'll be more self-assured, and believe me, that comes through in how you look and behave toward potential bad guys.

Q: Is there anything that a woman can carry with her while she's running that she can use if someone threatens her?

A: Yes. You can try a self-defense spray, such as pepper spray (but make sure it's legal to use where you run), or a personal alarm. And not only will these things help you get out of a threatening situation, but just carrying them will make you feel tougher. And if you feel tough, you'll look tough. And the bad guys will be more likely to leave you alone.

Q: How harmful are they?

A: Self-defense sprays cause enough pain in an attacker's eyes to stop that person instantly, but they won't cause permanent blindness. I recommend the varieties that contain a

mix of ultraviolet dye, tear gas, and pepper juice. They act immediately.

Q: How do you use a spray, and is there any danger of it going off accidentally while you run?

A: No, it won't go off accidentally. Carry it in your hand or clip it on your waistband. It weighs only a few ounces, so you won't be bothered by it. I recommend that women carry it so that others can see it. Like an animal baring its teeth, you are displaying your weapon of aggression. To use, pump it like you would any other spray.

But before you go out on your next run with a product like this, I recommend that you test it at home. Spray a small amount on a paper napkin, dab your finger in it, and rub it lightly an inch or so below your eye— make sure you don't rub it in your eye. If it's effective, you should feel a slight burning. Then, take the spray out in your backyard to see how far it squirts. If it goes 10 feet, then you know to use it when somebody comes within that distance. And if somebody should come up at you from behind, squirt it over your shoulder.

Q: Where can you purchase sprays and alarms?

A: Sporting goods stores should carry them. Many are available through mail order.

Q: Should runners carry money or identification?

A: Carry some coins in case you want to run to a phone booth and call for help. And sure, carrying identification (your name and an emergency phone number) is a good idea.

Q: We tell runners not to wear headphones. Do you agree with this viewpoint?

A: Get rid of them. I really don't like those things. They're a bit like wearing sunglasses in the dark. I appreciate that lots of people love them. In fact, I've had many women come up to me and say, "But I feel so confident when I'm listening to my own music." Well, that's because you are blocking out reality. You are in never-never land. When you wear those things, you may not have that extra 3- to 4-yard head start to break away at pace, and that factor could be the difference between making it or not—all because you couldn't hear the bad guy approaching.

Q: What time of day should women run?

A: Early-morning hours are the best because the bad guys are still in bed. We get a lot of reports of sexual assaults in the early evening, around 6 o'clock.

Q: What if a stranger is approaching a woman—should she ignore him or acknowledge him?

A: When a man and woman approach each other, there comes a point when the woman looks away. And the reason she looks away is because, if she doesn't, she may encourage a comment from this guy that she doesn't especially want to hear. So she looks away—most often down.

But that's like saying, "I'm weak," or "I don't want to be here." I suggest that you wave your eyes across him one time, but don't look down when you are done. Look to the other side or over his head. Remember,

What to wear?

As a woman you have the right to wear whatever you want when you run. But if two women are running side by side, with one wearing baggy sweats and the other flashy skin-fitting tights, for example, the second woman will not feel as confident because she is revealing more of her body. She may look away when people approach. Or she may look down at her feet—a sign the bad guys look for when they are evaluating how vulnerable someone is.

If you want to wear sexier clothes, it's up to you to be alert to what's going on around you. You will attract attention—some good and some bad—so you have to look tough to discourage the attention that you don't want. By the way, I have a T-shirt with Northside Homicide on the front—I guarantee you, with a T-shirt like that, no one is going to mess with you.

it's the one who looks the toughest who won't get picked as a victim. Meeting someone's gaze adds to a strong self-image, which is exactly what you want to project.

Q: Do you advise that women run with dogs?

A: Yes. A dog is an unknown thing to a bad guy. He doesn't know what the dog is capable of, and he doesn't know about the intensity of the bond between dog and master. Just don't call your dog Muffin or something like that when a suspicious character is around. I like Fang or Bandit a lot better.

Q: Is there a profile of a bad guy?

A: No. Because they look like you and me and your father and uncles and brothers and neighbors. Because that's who they are. Don't assume that a guy dressed like a runner won't pose a threat, either.

A safe place to run

Where should women run? Are country roads safer than city streets? The boonies are not the place to be. If the bad guy looks both ways on a country road and it's empty, he knows there will be nobody to interrupt him. But a deserted city street doesn't make things as easy—there could always be somebody looking out a window or driving around a corner. Run where there are people and activities around you. And vary your routes and the time you exercise so that someone who notices you won't be able to track your whereabouts by the minute.

Q: So what do you do if a runner comes up alongside you and begins running with you?

A: It's all right to talk to him and run with him, if you want. Just don't leave your regular running route. If he suggests going somewhere else, refuse. On the other hand, if you feel scared right away because this guy is staring at your chest or making crude remarks, you say, "Don't talk like that. Leave me alone." If he moves too close, use your spray or personal alarm.

Q: What if you are being followed—should you confront the person and say, "Are you following me?"

A: No. Don't ask questions. If you are suspicious, forget your normal route and take off for an area where there is more traffic or people. Never, ever ignore your instincts. When you feel the hair rise on the back of your neck, that's a few million years' worth of evolution at work. Don't ignore it—ever.

Q: What if somebody is trailing you in a car or stops to ask directions?

A: If anybody ever stops to ask, "Do you know . . . ?" or "Have you got . . . ?" or "Can you spare . . . ?" just say, "No." Don't enter into a conversation. If he keeps it up, you should yell "No" again and "Leave me alone. Get out of here." And believe me, you will be inspired to run away, even if you are at the end of your workout.

Q: What if someone grabs you? What can you do?

A: Flee if you can, but use the spray if you can't get away. If for some reason you have dropped it and he is trying to grab you, you have to use your legs to fight off the attack. Women don't have the upper-body strength necessary to keep a man's body off them. But you—especially runners—have the strength in your legs. If you get knocked down, start kicking hard.

Meanwhile, yell, but don't yell for help. Too many people tune that out. You have to yell, "Fire! Fire! Fire!" And keep on kicking, yelling, and using the spray or the alarm if you're able to. Don't ever get on your knees during this struggle because he could get you in a choke hold, and then it's all over.

Q: Let's make the scenario more threatening. What if the bad guy is trying to force you into his car, and he has a gun? How should you react?

A: First of all, remember this: You must never get into a car.

When you do, it's over. Ted Bundy

picked up his victims in a car; Dahmer used a car; Gacy used a car. They all used cars. And all those women whose bodies were found in forest reserves—they weren't out there hiking in the woods when they were attacked. They were taken there in a car.

You must resist quickly. You must run away. If he gets a hold of your jacket or shirt, you rip it off or pull it over your head and break away. Remember: The first few seconds of contact between a victim and offender are crucial—the offender has the least amount of control at that time because he's not sure how you are going to react. The more time you spend with him, the more he's got control.

Q: But what about the gun—won't you risk being shot?

A: So what? It's better than getting in the car. Believe me, if you get in the car, you're dead. Just run. Let's look at the chances of your getting shot and killed. If you break and run, you'll have a 50 percent chance of being hit. And if you're hit, you'll have another 50 percent chance of being seriously wounded and then another 50 percent chance of being killed. Well, that's only a 12.5 percent chance of being killed. Pretty good odds compared to the car. Furthermore, the Department of Justice reports that the real figure is less than 5 percent.

Q: Have you ever interviewed a runner who has been the victim of an attack?

A: No. But recently a Chicago woman who was running on the lakefront at dusk was attacked. Two young guys slashed her. They weren't trying to rob her because she had no money with her. They wanted to rape her, but she resisted, and they ran away. A cab driver passing by saw her lying on the ground and took her to the hospital. She survived because she fought back.

Q: Unfortunately, rapes occur. What does the victim need to know about reporting the crime?

A: The first thing you'll want to do is go to the hospital. And I realize that this may be extremely difficult, but you must not bathe or clean yourself in any way. I know it's the first thing a woman instinctively believes she must do, but the fluids retrieved during the physical exam are what enable police to positively identify the offender through DNA analysis. And he will go to jail.

Q: How would you describe the woman runner who presents herself as a tough target?

A: She looks self-assured. Her head is up, and she looks straight ahead instead of down at her feet. She doesn't wear headphones. She carries a spray or alarm in her hand to help her fight off an attack, and she pays attention to everybody and everything, even cars that are traveling around her. If she hears somebody come up from behind, she makes a point of turning around to look at who it is. And if she is the least bit suspicious, she makes sure that the guy sees the spray or alarm in her hand so that he knows she could make things difficult for him.

Amby Burfoot's Running Round-Up

In addition to following the good advice in the preceding pages, women runners can do one more simple thing: They can run with a group. There's strength in numbers, after all, not to mention it's a lot of fun.

All across the country, small (and sometimes large) groups of women get together for regularly scheduled runs. They meet in the early morning before daybreak and in the evening after the sun has set. They run together because it adds to their motivation (it's hard to skip a workout if others are waiting for you), because it becomes a social time, because it's easier to train hard with teammates, and for dozens of other reasons unique to every group. Often, safety is the least of their concerns but an important payoff nonetheless.

If you can't find a women's running group, look to run with a male friend. It only takes one, and many women can run as fast as the guys, so it's no problem keeping up. If you can't keep up with the fast guys, then run with them on their easy days when they run slowly. Check for running partners at work, with your running club, or in the neighborhood. If you have just one or two days a week when you have to run in the dark or in an area where you don't feel secure, you may be able to schedule escorted runs on those days.

A final (and regrettable) word about trail running. As trail running becomes more and more popular, increasing numbers of women find themselves drawn to it. And why not? It's hard to beat a relaxed run in a scenic, natural environment. Unfortunately, trail running raises a number of safety concerns, so don't go it alone. Get together with a friend or friends to enjoy trail running as a group activity.

Chapter 14

38 Ways to Improve Your Running

You'll Be a Better Runner with This Primer

The *Runner's World* editors have spent years discussing and debating the differences between men and women. No, we're not dense. We've simply been trying to figure out the most intelligent way to write about women's running.

When women first began running in sizable numbers in the mid-1970s, we searched for the obvious topics: pregnancy, menstrual periods, running bras, and so forth. In our rush to provide women-specific stories, we concentrated too much on the physical differences between men and women. We ignored all the ways women runners might be like men runners and focused instead on the ways they were different.

Convinced later that we had stereotyped women in this manner, we plunged headlong in the opposite direction in the 1980s. We even dropped our monthly "Women's Running" column from the magazine. Women didn't need special treatment, we decided. They could learn everything they needed to know about running by reading the same articles as our male readers.

We've made many changes since then, and I hope we have things right now. While we acknowledge the many similarities between men's and women's running, we also see differences. Differences that are not just physiological but also social and emotional. This chapter examines many of the key issues for women runners.

Knowledge is power—in running as in any other pursuit. The more you know about training, nutrition, and health, the better you'll be at getting the most from your running, whether that means fitness, weight loss, great race performances, or just plain fun. Below, you'll find lots of useful information from experts around the country to help you reach your goals.

Some of these facts and tips apply to all runners, but many address the specific needs of women. You may well recognize things that you already know, but you're bound to discover many new ideas that can help you become the runner you want to be.

1. Running is a state of mind. The only thing that determines your success, or lack of success, is the way you think about your running. If it works for you—if it relieves stress, burns calories, gives you time to yourself, enhances your self-esteem—then it doesn't matter what any other person or any stopwatch says about your running.

2. Exploring your competitive side offers benefits beyond running. Racing helps you tap into your goal-setting, assertive, self-disciplined side. Channeled correctly, these attributes can boost your success in other parts of your life, such as in the workplace.

3. You don't have to be the competitive type to enter a race every now and then. You'll find that lots of other racers aren't overly competitive, either. They're out there because it's fun and social and it motivates them to keep on running.

4. A woman runner should consider herself an athlete, whether she's fast or slow, tall or short, small or large.

5. In the United States, heart disease kills 10 times more women than breast cancer does each year. One of the best weapons for fighting heart disease is exercise. Exercise lowers your blood pressure and resting heart rate, raises your good high-density lipoprotein (HDL) cholesterol levels, and helps you maintain a healthy weight.

6. A survey of thousands of U.S. women found that while 44 percent of the respon- **dents actually were overweight, fully 73 percent thought they were.** So women who run for weight control, like all women, may lose perspective on what is an appropriate body size.

7. Trying to lose fat by eating less and running more and more doesn't work. The more you exercise and the less you eat, the more likely your body is to hibernate. That is, you'll conserve calories and thwart your efforts to lose fat. The better bet is to exercise reasonably and to increase your food intake early in the day to fuel your training. Eat breakfast, lunch, and an afternoon snack. Then eat lightly for dinner and afterward.

8. The two minerals that women runners need to pay the most attention to are calcium and iron. (Iron is especially important for women who are menstruating.) Your Daily Value for calcium is 1,000 milligrams; good sources are dairy products, dark green leafy vegetables, broccoli, canned sardines, and salmon. Your Daily Value for iron is 18 milligrams; foods high in iron include liver, fortified dry cereals, beef, and spinach.

9. Taking antioxidant supplements may substantially reduce muscle damage and inflammation. A research study that measured levels of malondialdehyde (a barometer of muscle tissue oxidation) in 25 women, before and after 30 minutes on the treadmill, found that post-exercise levels increased by 32 percent in women who did not take antioxidants, but decreased by 28 percent in those who had taken 400 international units of vitamin E daily for three months.

10. For female runners, controlled anaerobic training—intervals, hill repeats—may lead to gains in strength and speed similar to those produced by steroids but without the noxious side effects. Why? High-intensity anaerobic running is one of the most potent stimulators of natural human growth hormones—those that contribute to stronger muscles and, ultimately, enhanced performance.

11. Fast running burns more calories, but slow running burns more calories than just about any other activity. In short, nothing will help you lose weight and keep it off the way running does. Besides, it's inexpensive, it's accessible, and, if necessary, it can be done while pushing a stroller.

12. Speedwork allows you to explore the boundaries of your ability and can add an exciting element to your regular running. Though you may have taken up running just for fitness, after a while it can be fun to see just how fast you can go.

Start with short "pickups" (bursts of speed) sprinkled throughout a regular run and move up to formal, once-a-week interval sessions on a track (for example, running four to six fast 400s with 200-meter recovery jogs in between). You'll be delighted with the results.

13. One of the smartest things that a woman runner can do is to include strength training in her weekly regimen. Lifting weights can help prevent injuries by correcting the muscle imbalances caused by running. It has also been proven to enhance bone health and elevate moods.

Testing times

Women runners who train intensively, have been pregnant in the past two years, or consume fewer than 2,500 calories a day should get a more comprehensive blood test than the routine one for iron status, since these test only for anemia, the final stage of iron deficiency. Instead, request more revealing tests, including those for serum ferritin, transferrin saturation, and total iron-building capacity.

14. We all have our strengths and weaknesses. One important study of running injuries shows that women are much more likely than men to suffer ankle sprains, shinsplints, stress fractures, and hip problems. (Having said this, women are much less susceptible to Achilles tendinitis, plantar fasciitis, and quadriceps injuries.) To help you avoid injuries, make cross-training—such as pool running, bicycling, and weight training—part of your program.

15. Just because you're married and have young children and a job doesn't mean that you don't have time to run. Running is time-efficient and the best stress reducer on the market. You need this time. Taking it for yourself (by, say, letting your husband babysit while you run) will benefit the whole family.

16. Morning is the best time for women to run, for lots of reasons. One, it's the safest time; statistics show that women are more likely to be attacked late in the day. Two, studies have shown that morning exercisers are more likely to stick with it, because what you do first thing in the day gets done—not so with "maybe later on." Three, it saves you a round of dressing, undressing, and showering at lunchtime or later. Four, it gives you a feeling of accomplishment, which is a great mental and physical start for the day.

17. Running while wearing headphones outdoors is a safety hazard in more ways than one. You won't be able to hear cars, cyclists, or someone approaching who intends to do you harm. And attackers will always pick a victim who looks vulnerable. When you have headphones on, that means you.

18. Women who run alone should take precautions. Leave a note at home stating when you left, where you'll be running, and when you expect to return. Carry a personal alarm or self-defense spray (but make sure it's legal to use where you run). Stick to well-populated areas and don't always run the same predictable route. Avoid running at night. Don't wear jewelry or headphones. Pay attention to your surroundings. Carry identification but include only your name and an emergency phone number.

19. Running with another woman or with a group of women on a regular basis will help keep you motivated and ensure your safety. Plus, it's a lot more fun than running alone. Women runners become more than training partners; they're confidantes and counselors, too.

20. Like women, men are a good source of many things for running, from camaraderie to information to safety to inspiration. Running is the perfect melting-pot sport for the sexes.

21. Running with a dog provides the best of both worlds—you get to run alone but with a friend. A dog is both a faithful companion who will go anywhere, anytime, and a loyal guardian who will discourage anyone from harming you. The optimal running dog is medium-sized with a bloodline bred for endurance. An easy rule of thumb: Hunting breeds make the best runners.

22. It may not be much consolation, but men are sometimes verbally harassed and occasionally threatened on the run, just as women are. Run smart, but don't let insignificant taunting limit your freedom.

23. A run is a wonderful first date. It's relaxed and casual, yet you get a chance to show off your body, your stamina, and your style. It can mean as much or as little as you and your date wish it to mean. Conversation is rarely a problem, thanks to all those mood-lifting endorphins. If things go well, you can move on to a post-run meal.

24. Statistically, women run approximately 10 percent slower than men at all distances (based on the average difference between men's and women's world records). And although a University of California analysis showed that elite women have been improving twice as fast as elite men over the past three decades (14 meters a minute per decade versus 7 for men), women are not going to catch up with men.

This improvement in women's running can be traced to, among other things, dramatic increases in the number of females competing,

Women to Remember

Women runners should know about the history of their sport. Here is a list of the most significant dates in women's distance running. Study them. Quiz your training partners. Quiz the guys. They should know these things, too.

April 19, 1967: Kathrine Switzer runs the "men-only" Boston Marathon, and Jock Semple tries to rip her number off. The resulting photo puts women's running on the map.

June 2, 1972: The first women-only road race, the Crazy Legs 10-K, is held in New York City's Central Park. (It later becomes the L'eggs Mini Marathon. Today it's the New York Mini Marathon.)

October 22, 1978: Grete Waitz wins her first of nine New York City Marathons in a world record 2:32:30.

August 5, 1984: In Los Angeles, Joan Benoit Samuelson wins the first women's Olympic Marathon.

April 21, 1985: Ingrid Kristiansen sets the women's world record in the marathon, running 2:21:06 in London.

November 1, 1987: At age 42, Priscilla Welch wins the women's race at the New York City Marathon.

September 17, 1989: Ann Trason wins outright the USA 24-Hour Championships in Queens, New York. She outdistances the second-place (male) finisher by 3½ miles.

March 21, 1992: Lynn Jennings wins her third-straight World Cross-Country Championships in Boston.

September 8-12, 1993: Chinese women rewrite the distance-running record books, setting world records for 1500 meters, 3000 meters, and 10,000 meters.

July 18, 1994: Yekaterina Podkopayeva, 42, becomes the first masters woman to break 4 minutes for 1500 meters with a 3:59.78 in Nice, France.

April 19, 1998: The Kenyan Tegla Loroupe smashes Ingrid Kristiansen's 13-year women's marathon world record in Rotterdam, shattering the 2:21 barrier with a time of 2:20:47.

October 13, 2002: In Chicago, Great Britain's Paula Radcliffe demolishes the previous women's marathon world record by 1 minute 29 seconds. Her time of 2:17:18 beat her own personal best—set just six months earlier in London—by 1 minute 38 seconds.

April 13, 2003: Paula Radcliffe destroys her own world record by slashing 1 minute 53 seconds off it in the London Marathon. She clocks in at 2:15:25.

opportunities to compete, and better coaching. Of course, certain individual women can far outpace most men. Paula Radcliffe's marathon world record of 2:15:25 is faster than what 99.9 percent of the world's men are capable of achieving.

25. Women sweat less than men. Contrary to popular belief, however, women dissipate heat as well as men. The reason for this is that women are smaller and have a higher body-surface-to-volume ratio, which means that although their vaporative cooling is less efficient, they need less of it to achieve the same result. Nonetheless, drink plenty of water (until your urine runs clear) to offset the effects of sweating and prevent dehydration.

26. Women generally have narrower feet than men, so when you're buying running

The female factor

While no one has ever proven the old theory that women are better marathoners than men (because they have more body fat to burn), you never hear anyone argue the opposite. Men tend to use their strength to push ahead in short races, but this can backfire in the marathon. Women seem perfectly content to find a comfort zone and stay there. This makes them ideally suited for the marathon—the ultimate keep-your-cool and keep-your-pace distance. So set your sights on a marathon.

shoes, your best bet will probably be a pair designed especially for women. But everybody's different; if your feet are wide, you may actually feel more comfortable in shoes designed for men. The bottom line is to buy the shoe that fits your feet. If there is any question—or if you suffer blisters or injuries because of ill-fitting shoes—consult a podiatrist who specializes in treating runners.

27. No matter what your breast size, it's a good idea to wear a sports bra when you run. By controlling breast motion, a sports bra will make you feel more comfortable. Look for one that stretches horizontally but not vertically. And, most important, try it on before you buy. A sports bra should fit snugly, yet not feel too constrictive. Run or jump in place to see if it gives you the support you need.

28. Running doesn't make your breasts sag or make your uterus collapse, but these old myths resurface from time to time. In fact, running tightens and firms all the muscles it uses,

so it will help prevent sagging rather than cause it. There are no recorded cases of running resulting in a fallen uterus (or any other organ, for that matter). Where this idea got started is a mystery.

29. A Harvard University study found that running women produce a less potent form of estrogen than their sedentary counterparts. As a result, women runners cut by half their risks of developing breast and uterine cancers and by two-thirds their risk of contracting the form of diabetes that most commonly plagues women.

30. Running can help produce healthy skin. According to dermatologists, running stimulates blood circulation, transports nutrients, and flushes out waste products. All of this leads to a reduction in subcutaneous fat, which will make your skin clearer and your facial features more distinct.

31. "That time of the month" (or even the few days preceding it) is not the time when women run their worst. The hardest time for women to run fast is about a week before menstruation begins (a week after ovulation). That's when women's levels of the key hormone progesterone peak, inducing a much-higher-than-normal breathing rate during exercise. The excess ventilation tends to make running feel more difficult than usual.

32. There's no need to pass up a run or a race just because you're having your period. If you're suffering from cramps, running will often alleviate the pain, because of the release during exercise of pain-relieving chemicals called endorphins. Speedwork or a hill session can be especially effective, according to researcher Jody Weitzman of Women's Health and Support Services in Maryland. To guard against the risk of leakage, you should try using two tampons (side by side) for extra protection. Just be sure to remove them after your run.

33. If you run so much that your periods become light or nonexistent, then you may be endangering your bones. Amenorrhea (lack of a monthly period) means that little or no estrogen is circulating in your body. Estrogen is essential for the replacement of bone minerals. Amenorrheic women can stop—but not reverse—the damage by taking estrogen and getting plenty of calcium. Any woman with infrequent periods or no periods should consult her gynecologist, preferably one sensitive to the needs of runners.

34. Medical wisdom upholds that moderate exercise during a normal pregnancy is completely safe for the baby. The most important precaution: Avoid getting overheated (a core body temperature above 101 degrees could increase the risk of birth defects). Early in your pregnancy, take your temperature rectally, immediately after a run. As long as your temperature is below 101 degrees, you can maintain that same level of effort throughout your pregnancy. If you increase your intensity or duration, check your temperature again. Also, skip the post-run hot tub.

35. If you were a regular runner before you became pregnant, you might have a bigger baby—good news, since larger infants tend to be stronger and weather physical adversity better. Researchers at Columbia University in New York City found that women who burned up to 1,000 calories a week through exercise gave birth to infants weighing 5 percent more than offspring of inactive moms. Those who burned 2,000 calories per week delivered babies weighing 10 percent more.

36. If you ran early in your pregnancy, you might want to try switching to a lower-impact exercise during the latter stages and after delivery. Because of the release of the hormone relaxin during pregnancy, some ligaments and tendons might soften, making you more vulnerable to injury. Walking, swimming, stationary bicycling, and pool running (you'll be even more buoyant than usual) are good choices.

37. Phooey! If your nursing baby gags and spits your breast milk back at you, it may be because babies dislike the taste of post-exercise breast milk, which is high in lactic acid and imparts a sour flavor. A study at Indiana University in Bloomington found that nursing moms who logged 35 minutes on the treadmill faced off with grimacing, reluctant infants if they nursed soon afterward. Researchers recommend that you either collect milk for later feeding or breast-feed before running.

38. Older female runners can be very positive role models for girls learning about the sport. Any show of support can be helpful. This could perhaps be something as simple as attending a high school cross-country meet and cheering for the girl down the street.

Amby Burfoot's Running Round-Up

I have long argued that women are better suited to running than men. The reason? Reread point number one on page 94, and you have it: Running is a state of mind. Or, as I would explain it at greater length: Women are better runners than men because they have fewer state-of-mind obstacles to overcome.

The biggest obstacle men face is their typical notion of competition in sports. Men think that sports are about beating the other guy. That may be true in boxing, but it's not true in running. Runners must learn to compete with themselves and not against anyone else. If they race against others, they will soon give up, because they will find so many others who are faster than they are.

Women seem to find it easier to understand that running is its own reward. It's not a question of your win/loss record, your batting average, your strokes per round, or any other sports statistic. It's not a matter of what you can do to an opponent; it's a matter of what running does for you.

If it makes you feel better, if it helps you control your weight, if it gives you 30 minutes of quiet time every day, then that's enough. Women accept this and learn to run with great success even if they never succeed at beating anyone.

Chapter 15

The Answers You Need to Know

Answers to Some Important Questions from Women Runners

Since many women runners don't have a long history of sports participation, every new step they take on the way to becoming a runner and an athlete is filled with questions. Questions about nutrition, technique, and, most important, their changing bodies.

No doubt about it. When you begin running, your body changes, and never in ways you expected. You may gain pounds at first, when you had expected to lose weight. Your muscles will get sore, when you only wanted them to get firmer. You'll need to drink more; you'll have strange, new food cravings; and you may notice differences at the most basic level of your female physiology—your periods, for example.

Because all of this is new and different, it will make you nervous. At one time or another, you'll think that something is surely wrong with you. You'll wonder about the answers to questions that you don't dare ask.

Here are two thoughts: It's unlikely that there's anything wrong with you, and ask anyway. Decades of research have shown that running

changes people in many ways that are almost all positive. Where not positive, the changes are generally not negative either. They're just different.

But ask your questions anyway. The answers will reassure you. For starters, here's a sampling of questions that women runners often ask.

Most women are a bit sheepish about asking certain health questions. You know the ones. Questions about your period and your breasts and bladder control that are next to impossible to blurt out when you're looking a physician straight in the eye. Too bad that these questions are often easier to leave unspoken. You hope that you'll come across the answers somewhere else.

Welcome to somewhere else. Six ticklish questions below have been answered by the experts. Their answers aren't scary, and you'll learn a lot from them. It is our hope that these answers will encourage you to talk more directly with your physician next time. Remember that there's no such thing as a stupid question.

RUNNING AND YOUR BREASTS

Q: I've been running for years but only recently began experiencing discomfort in my breasts. Should I wear a sports bra when I run? Will running for 15 years without wearing a special bra contribute to sagging breasts as I get older?

A: Wearing a sports bra is a good idea. Why? Because sports bras are designed specifically to minimize breast discomfort and stretching that may occur during exercise. But just because you have been running without one doesn't mean that your breasts will automatically sag as you age. Four factors contribute to sagging breasts: breast size, body weight, history of pregnancy, and genetic makeup. In combination, they determine whether your breasts will sag or not.

Many women experience breast discomfort on a monthly basis, often just before their periods. Most discomfort occurs as the breast bounces upward and then drops back down. So a sports bra, which is designed to reduce breast motion, may alleviate some pain.

But one type of bra won't work for every woman. You have to let your body be your guide. Keep in mind that bras are made either to bind and compress or to divide and conquer. Women with small breasts and no

unusual feelings of tenderness often favor the compression style.

But if you wear a size C cup or larger or experience cyclical changes in your breasts, you may do better with a bra that encapsulates each breast. I recommend wearing a style with seamless cups to prevent nipple burn, and a wide nonelastic band under the breasts to help prevent the bra from riding up as you run. The straps and cup support should be nonelastic as well, and the bra should have covered metal attachments that hook in the back. Styles that connect in the front allow more breast motion.

As for sagging, most of it results from pregnancy and lactation, not running. Breasts are composed primarily of glandular tissue and fat. If your breast size increases while you are nursing or as a consequence of a gain in weight, no ligaments exist to support the extra tissue. Stretching and sagging are the unwelcome results.

RUNNING DURING PREGNANCY

Q: I'm confused about how much exercise a well-conditioned pregnant woman can perform safely. I'd like to continue doing speedwork and long runs, yet many physicians recommend limiting exercise intensity to no more than 140 heartbeats per minute. That's not much of a workout for me. Are there other guidelines to follow?

A: Many obstetricians use 140 beats per minute as an exercise guideline for pregnant runners, despite the fact that there is no scientific evidence to back it up. Because 140 ends up being too high for sedentary women and too low for women like you, I tell my patients to pay strict attention to their perceived level of exertion and to run more conservatively.

I advise you to continue running at a speed that feels easy to you, slowing or even stopping if you begin cramping, gasping for breath, or feeling dizzy. Skip the speedwork, don't attempt to improve your times or build distance during the next nine months, and limit your workouts to no more than 30 minutes.

Why? Because after 30 minutes, core body temperature begins to rise, and elevated core temperatures can cause birth defects. Besides, no one knows exactly how long the flow of blood can be diverted from the uterus (as happens during exercise) before the fetus is compromised. For this reason, reserve a few minutes at the end of your workout to cool down slowly. Blood won't circulate back to the fetus if you stop abruptly, so end your run with a walk.

WHEN YOU DON'T GET YOUR PERIOD

Q: I haven't had my period for nearly a year now, but I'm keen to start a family. I assume my amenorrhea is caused by strenuous training. How should I go about decreasing my mileage in order to conceive in four to six months?

A: Menstrual dysfunction isn't always caused by intense training. Perhaps your percentage of body fat is too low to prompt your period.

Slowing things down

Many women runners shoot for the perfect pregnancy and the perfect child. And that's okay. But to achieve that goal, you may have to decrease some very important numbers in your life. For instance, if you're accustomed to training at an eight-minute pace, you may have to slow down a bit. And you may have to decrease your mileage as well.

Maybe you have a thyroid problem or even premature menopause. (You don't have to be middle-aged to experience menopause; it's not age but an egg deficit in the ovaries that causes menopause.)

I suggest that you see your family physician or gynecologist for a checkup that includes a pelvic examination, a hormonal evaluation, and a discussion or careful measurement of how much you are eating.

Because I avoid advising runners to alter their running schedules, I generally recommend drug therapy, such as clomiphene (Clomid) or other hormonal stimulants, to induce ovulation. Many women who have an aversion to drugs may opt on their own to cut back on their training. And if diet is a contributing factor, they may also choose to consume more food. Some even do both—run slightly less and eat more.

Although I realize that your first priority is conception, you must keep in mind that when you don't menstruate, your body probably doesn't produce enough estrogen. Low levels of estrogen lead to osteoporosis, which predisposes you to breaking bones now and as you age.

So it's essential that you supply your

Further Resources on Women's Health Issues

Want more information on women's health issues? Try one or more of the organizations listed below which provide publications created especially for women involved in sports and fitness activities.

Melpomene Institute for Women's Health Research, 550 Rice Street, Suite 104, St. Paul, MN 55103 (651) 789-0140

melpomene.org

Named for the plucky Greek woman who sneaked into the first Olympic Marathon in 1896, Melpomene was founded in 1981 as a unique research and resource center for active women. The institute provides a wide array of publications, including numerous brochures, books, the *Melpomene Journal*, and informational packets on subjects ranging from body image and PMS to breast care, eating disorders, and osteoporosis.

National Women's Health Network, 1413 K Street NW, 4th floor, Washington, DC 20005 (202) 682-2640

womenshealthnetwork.org

This network answers specific questions on all women's health issues, provides referrals to clinics and organizations in your area, and publishes more than 50 different packets on a wide variety of health subjects including AIDS, infertility, breast cancer, hysterectomy, and menopause.

Women's Sports Foundation, 1899 Hempstead Turnpike, Suite 400, NY 11554 (800) 227-3988

womenssportsfoundation.org

Call the foundation to receive brochures on women's health concerns and sporting activities. The foundation also offers 15 informational packets on topics such as nutrition and weight control, pregnancy and exercise, and the psychology of sport.

body with the hormones it has stopped manufacturing. Although running does counteract the effects of low estrogen, it also puts additional stress on your bones. Unless your hormonal balance is restored, you may find yourself nursing a broken bone before an infant.

EFFECTS OF BIRTH CONTROL PILLS

Q: I read somewhere that birth control pills reduce aerobic capacity. Is this true? Will they impair my ability to run competitively?

A: For contraceptive protection, the Pill is your best bet. That much is certain. But even in this day and age, scientists still know very little about the Pill's effect on overall health and athletic performance. Opinions vary, but since you asked for mine, here goes.

If you want to perform at your best, I advise against taking the Pill. As a naturalist, I believe the Pill throws off your body's natural balance. Studies published several years ago indicate that maximal oxygen capacity (max VO2), which measures the greatest volume of oxygen that can be dispatched to your muscles during exercise, falls significantly in active women who use oral contraceptives. And other studies have demonstrated that women on the Pill lose some endurance and isometric strength.

Furthermore, many women say that they feel tired and sluggish once they start taking oral contraceptives. Although weight gain may be the culprit, I suspect the changes in blood cholesterol and triglycerides (a form of fat in the bloodstream) are more at fault.

Pill users have elevated levels of triglycerides, which are readily available for the body to use as fuel when you run. But the metabolism of one gram of triglyceride requires more oxygen than the metabolism of one gram of carbohydrate (glucose), so triglycerides are considered a less-efficient fuel. This may be why women on the Pill find running more difficult: Their bodies are using triglycerides instead of carbohydrate as fuel. Perhaps this is also why max VO2 drops in Pill users.

I suggest that you talk to a gynecologist—a sports gynecologist if possible—for more information on oral contraceptives and athletic performance. And then weigh your options.

EATING RIGHT

Q: I eat a low-fat, high-carbohydrate diet, but I'm not sure whether I take in enough protein. As a woman runner, do I need more protein than other people? Are there any signs of protein deficiency that I should be aware of?

A: Many women squeeze the protein right out of their diets simply by skimping on calories. If you average only 1,500 to 1,800 calories a day and make a point of eating lots of carbohydrates, it's very difficult to meet your protein, vitamin, and mineral needs.

A breakfast of fruit and a bagel, for instance, is high in carbohydrates and low in fat but doesn't contain the quality protein you need to replace what you use during hard training. Perhaps you fall into the same trap by avoiding meat for health reasons.

Vegetarians lower their fat intake and the amount of protein they take in unless they include vegetables such as black beans, kidney beans, and lentils in combination with grain products in their diets.

What happens if you don't get enough protein? You may experience more injuries, fatigue, and mood swings or frequent bouts of illness (such as nagging colds or chronic respiratory infections). You may experience menstrual irregularities or cease having your period altogether. And the quality of your training and racing will suffer for sure.

Because the body uses protein for fuel during endurance exercise, all runners should boost their protein intake to 50 percent more than the Daily Value. For your own personal guideline, multiply your body weight in pounds by 0.54. Say that you weigh 130 pounds: 130 times 0.54 is 70.2. So you would need no fewer than 70 grams of

A pro-protein menu

This is a sample diet that supplies 80 grams of quality protein within an 1,800- calorie diet.

Breakfast: 1 cup plain low-fat yogurt topped with fresh peaches and nectarines, whole-wheat bagel with low-sugar jam, herbal tea

Lunch: 2 ounces tuna tossed with fresh greens, olive oil, and vinegar; pita bread; fresh fruit compote with kiwifruit, oranges, and strawberries

Snacks (to be eaten throughout the day): Soft pretzel, sports bar, 2 cups air-popped popcorn

Dinner: Baked potato with 3/4 cup low-fat cottage cheese, 1 cup steamed broccoli, two oatmeal cookies

protein a day—and a menu to get you started (see box below).

GAINING CONTROL OF YOUR BLADDER

Q: My running partner is just starting to train again after the birth of her daughter, and she's having a difficult time. She must perform Kegel exercises to strengthen her pelvic muscles, wear a diaphragm to stop urinary leakage, and use a pad to absorb the leaks she does have while running. Is the same fate in store for me when I get pregnant? And what about my bladder? Can it actually drop as a result of running too much?

A: Your running partner has stress incontinence, a problem many women experience in some form or another after labor. In fact, about 22 percent of all adult women are incontinent. Many report their first episodes after childbirth or pelvic surgery, which sometimes displaces pelvic organs and weakens muscles along the pelvic floor.

In your friend's case, the tube connecting the bladder and urethra (the bladder neck) has dropped out of normal position. So whenever she does anything that creates intra-abdominal pressure or stress, such as coughing, sneezing, laughing, or running, leakage occurs.

Stress incontinence after childbirth usually doesn't last for more than three months. In the meantime, your friend should dispense with her diaphragm (it will not help, although a tampon may), continue her Kegel exercises, and consult a specialist who may prescribe drugs, a biofeedback program, or weighted vaginal cones, which are

Amby Burfoot's Running Round-Up

In searching for a health-care provider, women runners face two central issues. First, finding a physician they feel confident in and comfortable with, whether that physician is male or female. Second, finding a doctor who understands sports medicine and the special needs, physical and mental, of women who regularly exercise.

No one but you can decide when you feel right about a primary-care physician—your first line of defense in any health-care situation. You have to talk with the individual, evaluate the way he or she interacts with you and answers your questions, and then make the most intelligent choice you can. With some luck, you'll find a doctor who at least understands that exercise is important to you.

At times, this will be absolutely essential to your care and treatment. A physician who doesn't keep up with exercise physiology may actually miss certain diagnoses among women runners—for example, false anemia, which isn't anemia at all but is the increased blood volume common to regular runners. Just as important, a doctor who doesn't understand the psychological benefits of running will often tell you to quit running when in fact you may be able to continue at a more moderate level or at least switch to a cross-training regimen.

So when you're interviewing physicians, don't hesitate to ask questions about their experience with exercise and sports medicine. You need a doctor who can treat you as a whole person, including you, the runner. Don't settle for one who sees only your parts but not the way they fit together.

inserted like tampons and tend to slip out unless the wearer contracts the appropriate muscles. (By contracting the proper muscles, many women can control incontinence.) She should consider surgery, which isn't always successful, only as a last resort.

There's no way to predict whether you, too, will experience stress incontinence after childbirth. Your best defense, however, is a regular training program of correctly executed Kegels. The first step is to identify the muscles involved in the exercise. While you're on the toilet, tighten your muscles to stop the flow of urine. These are the muscles you need to contract during a Kegel. Many women mistakenly isolate abdominal, thigh, or buttock muscles instead.

To begin, do 3 sets of Kegels a day. Do 5 contractions in each set, holding each contraction for 3 seconds. Gradually increase the time to 5 and then 10 seconds. Work up to 10 contractions of 10 seconds each, and do them 3 to 5 times a day. Be sure to schedule a few sets while you're running. By the way, running may jiggle your pelvic organs a bit but will not cause your bladder to drop.

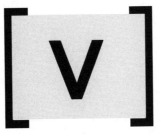

Building Strength, Endurance, and Speed

Chapter 16

25 Best Training Tips

Run Better, Stronger, and Faster

When *Runner's World* celebrated its 25th anniversary in the early 1990s, we asked the magazine's first editor, Joe Henderson, to write a special article for us. Even after he left his full-time, day-to-day responsibilities with the magazine, Joe continued his active role in the running community, publishing a newsletter, speaking at many races, and serving as a sort of elder spokesman for the sport. We figured that this made him the perfect person to write about the most important advances in training knowledge and technique that he had observed over the years.

Joe's article hits them all. You can't find a better big-picture snapshot of training developments in recent decades than this one.

Best of all, many of these guidelines remain as true as when they were discovered, whether that was yesterday or 20 years ago. As you read this chapter, ask yourself this simple question: Does my training program violate one of these principles? If it does, you should seriously consider making a change.

In January 1966 New Zealander Arthur Lydiard's revolutionary training methods had just arrived in the United States, imported chiefly by University of Oregon and U.S. Olympic coach Bill Bowerman. At the same time, Ken Cooper, M.D., was testing his running-as-exercise training plan on Air Force personnel in Texas and preparing to write a revolutionary fitness book called *Aerobics*.

These separate forces of change would soon meet and merge on the roads, where people of all ability levels began running. The number of runners increased steadily through the 1960s, 1970s, 1980s, and 1990s. As the sport grew, so did an interest in finding the best ways to train. Coaches, researchers, and runners tried various methods and techniques in their search to improve performance and to make running an enjoyable, healthful, long-lasting activity. Here are the 25 most important training advances of the past 30 years.

1. Training without straining. Effective training, said famed New Zealand coach Arthur Lydiard, traces a fine line between hard enough and too hard. This principle grew from the theories of Hans Selye, the endocrinologist credited with describing how stress works on the human body, who found that repeated exposure to a mild stress stimulates adaptation. In other words, through running, which is a stress, the body learns to adapt to the demands of running and eventually performs better. Selye also pointed out, however, that too much stress overwhelms the body's ability to cope. Thus, if you run too hard, your body will not be able to adapt. This philosophy formed the cornerstone of Lydiard's system, which encouraged runners to train hard without straining.

2. Aerobic training. Dr. Cooper, the president and founder of the Cooper Aerobics Center in Dallas, plucked the term aerobics from physiology jargon and made it an international phenomenon. His research concluded that prolonged low-intensity exercise improved physical endurance better than brief, explosive workouts. Training aerobically meant choosing a running pace that allowed you to talk and that kept the heart rate at about three-quarters of maximum. The result was an easier, yet still effective, training effort.

3. Specificity in training. This philosophy states that you will reap in races what you sow in training. Long, slow runs prepare you to race slowly, whereas short, fast runs only train you to race short distances. Jeff Galloway applied this rule of adaptation to his now-popular marathon-training program, which requires a long run of 26 miles.

4. Long runs. The long run was Lydiard's most lasting gift to training. Few runners still do his 100-mile weeks, but almost everyone—from a miler to a marathoner—runs longer than his norm at least once a week. The long run builds endurance, and it provides a great opportunity to spend time with friends.

5. Surviving the marathon. Speaking of long runs, about 15 years ago a new breed of runner

Get the tempo right

Jack Daniels, Ph.D., assistant professor of physical education and an exercise physiologist at the State University of New York in Cortland, has followed the principle of specificity in training (see point 3, above). Daniels applied this philosophy when using tempo runs (runs that start easy, build up to a steady speed, and then finish at an easy pace), at about a 10-K race pace, to lift slow runners out of their training ruts. The typical distance runner's training schedule now includes some of both: Long runs are used to increase strength; short, fast workouts are used to build speed. The final mix and mileage depend on the type of race you're preparing for.

came to dominate marathons—at least numerically. These athletes treated the event not as a race for time or place but as a survival test to be passed just by finishing. In the 1970s Jack Scaff, M.D., of the Honolulu Marathon Clinic, developed a program to prepare runners to reach the marathon starting line in good health and able to complete the distance. His program downplayed high levels of weekly mileage and speedwork and emphasized the long training run.

6. Hill training. Hill work, another staple of the Lydiard system, was overlooked early on in the rush to 100-mile weeks. Lydiard's runners used hills in two ways. Regularly, they would do their long runs on extremely hilly courses. Also, prior to the sharpening phase of their training, which emphasized speedwork, they would do hill repeats. We now know that hills are speedwork in disguise. Uphill running strengthens the upper leg muscles, which produce speed, and downhills force runners to go faster.

7. Speed training. Runners once shunned speedwork because it meant circling the track endlessly in an exhausting race against the stopwatch. It meant enduring boredom and pain. Not anymore. Jack Daniels provided more humane, but no less effective, choices: tempo runs, done at a steady pace but lasting only about 20 minutes; and cruise intervals, run at tempo pace but broken into three to six repeats with brief rest periods between them.

8. Races as training. Four-time Olympian George Young, now a successful college coach in Arizona, pointed out that the most effective speed training occurs where it is most exciting to do: in races. Now, with races on the schedule almost every weekend in most areas, many runners take their speedwork this way, which helps explain why the 5-K and 8-K are the fastest-growing race distances. Similarly, runners looking to do a long training run with a group help flesh out the fields for half-marathons and longer races.

9. Recovering from races. As the road-racing schedule grew to fill the year and to crowd each weekend, so, too, did the temptation to overrace. New Zealander Jack Foster, who held the masters marathon record for 16 years, came up with a valuable rule of thumb: He followed his races with a recovery period totaling one day for each mile of racing. He didn't stop running during that recovery period; he simply wouldn't race or train hard again until the appropriate time had passed.

10. Hard and easy days. Coaches and runners learned that recovery from hard training is also important. Long runs, hills, and speedwork all place the runner on training's edge. Bill Bowerman produced as many top runners as any college coach ever has. Tests on his young, strong athletes showed that none thrived on more than three hard training days in a row, and most did best by alternating a hard day with an easy one.

11. Recovering from hard days. Long, slow distance (LSD) provides the means to recover from hard workouts. LSD—a product of the 1960s—was originally misunderstood as an invitation to run too long and slowly. A better term would have been gentle running. As originally practiced, long, slow distance meant

Why easy days pay off

One of coach Bill Bowerman's athletes, Kenny Moore, became a two-time Olympic marathoner. He would train hard one day and easily the next two. The importance of easy days was confirmed by exercise physiologist David L. Costill, Ph.D., director of the Human Performance Laboratory at Ball State University in Muncie, Indiana, whose research showed that most runners need 48 to 72 hours to recover fully from even a moderately hard effort.

running slower miles between more difficult workouts. It fits perfectly into the hard/easy training plan, and this remains its best use.

12. Days off. LSD goes one step further and becomes rest. In other words, take a day off. The word "rest" was once a dirty word among runners. Real runners ran every day. It took advice from some of the sport's heaviest hitters and most respected physiologists to convince runners that resting could sometimes be as valuable as training—especially for older runners with slower recovery rates. Rest days, of course, mesh with Bowerman's hard/easy plan and Dr. Cooper's five-day schedule for fitness running (see point 25 on page xx). Two more converts to this philosophy, the late George Sheehan, M.D., and Galloway, switched to practicing and then preaching every-other-day training.

13. Tapering before races. Gentle running became important in preparation for racing, too. Runners training for marathons used to take their last long run—and often the longest one—a

week before their race. The smart ones now space these efforts three weeks apart to restore full life to their legs. Research done by Dr. Costill indicates that runners need to cut back on their mileage level for three days to three weeks prior to a race, depending on the degree of training that they have been doing and the length and seriousness of the race.

14. Running cycles. If you take Bowerman's hard/easy system and extend it beyond days to seasons or even years, you have peaking. Lydiard maintained that no one could race and train at their highest level year-round. He recommended scheduling alternate seasons of peak training and relaxed training. Lydiard's runners, winners of five Olympic medals, were masters of peaking. The all-time best athlete to use this training principle was four-time Olympic winner Lasse Viren, whom Lydiard influenced.

15. Training by time. Digital watches put an accurate measure of performance on every runner's wrist. They provided race splits and final times instantly. But another important value was more subtle. The digitals also let runners adopt another of Lydiard's recommendations: Train by periods of time instead of distance. This freed runners from measuring road courses and trying to run those courses faster with each workout. Thus, it helped prevent runners from working too hard during an average training run.

16. Preventing overuse injuries. The purpose of training is to improve, to get stronger and faster. So it is easy to get caught in an ever-increasing schedule that has you constantly building on speed, distance, and hills on the theory that more work and a harder effort will continue to improve your performance. But runners soon learned that they were overdoing it. They trained too long, too fast, and too often, and found their breaking points. Podiatrists treated growing numbers of injuries over the years, until runners began to realize that sometimes less is more.

17. Listen to your body. Dr. Sheehan taught this valuable lesson. He told runners that they didn't need to follow complex training formulas, monitor their pulses, or even try to run a certain pace. All that a runner needed to do in distance training, said Dr. Sheehan, was "set the inner dial to 'comfortable,' neither too hard nor too easy. The pace that feels right is right." He endorsed Gunnar Borg's scale of perceived exertion, which measured feelings instead of heartbeats or minutes per mile. Heart-rate monitors arrived later to do the same type of listening electronically.

18. Stretching. Runners needed to learn to listen to their bodies not only to determine what level of training exertion was right for them but also to detect minor problems and correct them before they became injuries. Dr. Sheehan wrote, "Three things happen when you run, and two of them are bad." The good one is that you become a more efficient runner. The first bad one is that runners—especially those who run the same slow pace all the time—lose flexibility. Their muscles grow tighter and more susceptible to injury. To prevent this, runners were encouraged to do slow, gentle, yogalike stretches.

19. Strengthening. The second bad thing that happens to runners, wrote Dr. Sheehan, is that they develop strength imbalances. Muscles at the back of the legs overpower those in front, a setup for injury. In addition, the muscles of the upper body lag in strength behind those of the lower body, which get all the exercise. Dr. Sheehan advised that runners should supplement their miles with exercises that restore strength balances and make fitness more complete.

20. Carbo loading. Beyond taking care of their muscles, runners learned about the important effects of diet. They began to shun meat in favor of low-fat proteins and high-energy carbohydrates. The technique of carbo loading before races was first tested by Swedish physiologists, and British marathoner Ron Hill proved its value. Dr. Costill found that carbo reloading after races and hard training was equally valuable.

21. Hydration. Dr. Costill pointed out the folly of not drinking enough water before, during, and after long runs. He showed that as the dehydrating body's temperature rose, performance declined, and the risk of heat injury increased. Runners started to drink more water, and then more than water. They began downing sweetened and electrolyte-laden solutions. Florida researchers invented Gatorade, and soon many other replacement fluids flooded the market.

22. Cross-training. Also known as alternative or supplemental training, cross-training received its greatest push from the triathlon boom that began in the mid-1980s. Triathletes sent runners the message that total fitness requires more than running and gave them the okay to switch activities on days when extra miles seemed unwise or unappealing. Swimming and bicycling are but two among dozens of activities that runners can mix and match for a complete fitness program.

23. Water training. Running in a pool while wearing a flotation vest or belt may be the single most valuable variation on land running. Injured runners can continue normal training efforts and stay running-fit without aggravating the problem that put them in deep water. Oft-injured Mary Slaney gave water work credence when she trained this way for six weeks following a mishap at the 1984 Olympic Trials. A few days after returning to the track, she broke the world record for 2000 meters.

24. Walking. The word *walk* used to make runners turn away in disgust. They wouldn't think of stopping to walk during a run and certainly not in a race. Tom Osler, who successfully mixed walking breaks into his own ultra-marathons, started changing this thinking. He wrote that runners could greatly increase the length of their longest run by inserting brief walks at regular intervals. Marathoners whose only goal is to finish will purposely take walking breaks. Galloway even found that some marathoners could improve their times by taking a one-minute walking break every mile. Also, runners coming back from injuries or illness, and new runners building their endurance, can mix walking with running in an effort to increase distances.

25. Fitness training. Dr. Cooper once ran for sport, but he came to see a wider role for the activity. He took his running-for-fitness message to nonathletes who would never have thought of training to enter a race. That's fine, said Dr. Cooper. It's not necessary. Instead, he proposed a

Amby Burfoot's Running Round-Up

Our knowledge of training changes—but slowly. The process is far more evolutionary than revolutionary. If I were coaching a would-be Olympian today, I would tell him to review the principles in this chapter carefully and to make them the foundation of any training program. Because these are the basics, and no runner can advance very far without observing them.

Strengthening, hill training, and cross-training are still very popular. Runners, and in particular runners past age 40, have come to recognize the importance of strength training; one important component of strength training is hill work. The growth of cross-training is everywhere, and even though the physiologists continue to make the "specificity" argument—that the only thing that makes you a better runner is running—thousands of runners have found that cross-training makes them stronger, healthier, and more injury-resistant. And these three combined will certainly make anyone a better runner.

running program of two to three miles, three to five times a week. As health studies in the mid-1990s showed more and more Americans becoming overweight, Dr. Cooper's philosophy encouraged many of these formerly sedentary people to begin running for weight control and health improvement.

Chapter 17

The Need for Speed

Spice Up Your Speedwork with Variety

As a young runner, I was lucky. My coach, a runner himself, believed that the sport was meant to be enjoyed for many intrinsic reasons: the beauty of movement, the beauty of nature, the beauty of an activity that combined the two. He thought that running should be fun and taught us to enjoy its varied splendors. We prospered.

But we never learned how to do speedwork. I think— in fact, I'm quite sure—this was because my coach himself had had an unpleasant experience with a college coach bent on subjecting him to torturous track workouts. He resolved that, as a coach, he would never do the same to his young charges.

On the whole, I'm glad he didn't. He taught us the aesthetics of running—far more important than the mechanics. Still, I think I could have run faster and gained a deeper appreciation of the sport if we had done more speedwork of the type Olympian Jeff Galloway describes. And, as Galloway is quick to point out, this kind of running can and should be fun. You only have to approach it correctly.

Most runners burn out on speedwork because they don't allow themselves to have fun—the workouts are too hard and repetitive. Most of us

perform our speedwork according to that worn-out adage, "No pain, no gain." The result? Often, it's little or no gain.

But if you start doing workouts that are fun, you'll want to do more of them. And that alone will help you improve, to race better. Yes, I said fun, even when it comes to speedwork, the type of training many runners dread most. Speedwork can and should be fun. It simply has to be tailored to your particular ability and needs.

Speedwork helps you run faster and stronger in three ways: It improves running form, eases your adaptation to oxygen debt, and helps you push through the mental barriers of discomfort and doubt. Hard work, of course. But it doesn't have to be those dreadful interval repeats on the track with short rests.

The Speed Doctor

Speedwork is great for improving your form, your ability to handle oxygen debt, and your skill at overcoming mental barriers, but it can also fix specific problems with your running. Here are some common problems and how speedwork can cure them.

You lose steam at the end of races. Try longer speed workouts. Instead of 10 repeats of 440s as your longest workout before a 10-K race, increase the number of repetitions over eight weekly workouts to 20 repeats of 440s, running each five to seven seconds faster than your goal race pace. Try to run the last four of each workout two to three seconds faster than the other 440s (but never run all out).

Just past midrace, you gradually slow down. For the 10-K, build your speedwork gradually until the hard repetitions equal 14 to 16 repeats of 440s (at seven to eight seconds faster than goal pace). Run each of the middle four to five repeats of 440s at two seconds faster than the others.

You always run a slow first mile. For the 10-K, run a maximum of 12 repeats of 440s at 8 to 10 seconds faster than goal pace, then hang on through the rest of the workout, running six to eight seconds faster than goal pace.

Hills wipe you out. Study the course that you plan to run. Run a hill workout once a week, gradually increasing to three to four more hills of the same size and grade as those on the course. You may also run the same number of hills, but make each one longer and/or steeper than those on the race course. Be sure to work on efficient downhill running to balance your skills.

Oxygen debt prevents you from running your best. Cut down the rest between repetitions during your interval workouts. For the 10-K, gradually build to 20 repeats of 440s at three to five seconds faster than race pace. Take the shortest rest interval (jogging) that you can tolerate and finish the workout in the time assigned.

In fact, the best—and fastest—way to build strength and speed is by combining hill, fartlek, and interval sessions into one. If you approach the following workouts with a little imagination and inspiration, you can enjoy some moments of real joy and satisfaction.

THE UPSIDE OF HILL RUNNING

Running hills increases strength and drive from the legs and also helps prepare you for taxing interval workouts. It may be the best type of speedwork.

A few years ago, I was concerned that a talented high school sophomore would burn out by running too much track work. So, during track season, he and I ran four to nine 400-meter hills (on a moderate five percent grade). With no other speedwork, and after just eight of these weekly sessions, he lowered his mile personal record from 4:32 to 4:18.

Many coaches and strength experts believe that hills provide better leg strength for running than weights or machines. Pushing up the incline builds the lower leg muscles.

Weight lifting strengthens those same muscles but won't train them for the demands of running. The large and small muscles in the legs must work together perfectly to produce a smooth stride. Hill running does that by building strength and coordination at the same time.

That added leg strength also improves running posture. An efficiently moving body saves energy. Additionally, good running posture reduces wear and tear on easily injured parts of the body.

What's more, hill training forces you to develop quick push-off and faster leg turnover.

Unlike the explosive strength that high jumpers and long jumpers rely on, distance-running strength is measured in quick little pushes. Given the number of steps you take per mile, even a small increase in efficiency will pay off in a 10-K, and even more so in a marathon.

You only need to do hill work once a week. Pick a hill with a moderate grade, five to eight percent. Start with three to four repetitions, and gradually increase to a maximum of eight to a dozen. Your goal is to build strength, not oxygen debt, so take plenty of rest between each hill. Remember: Short, steep hills develop quick, dynamic strength, while long, sustained hills build stamina.

FEEL GOOD ABOUT FARTLEKS

You have probably run fartlek workouts—even if you were too embarrassed to pronounce the word in public. It's the simplest form of speedwork: You just accelerate when you feel good, then jog easily until you recover.

Popularized in Europe, fartlek (the Swedish word for "speed play") prepares you for the turbulence of racing. Many runners feel that they get a better workout when they do fartlek than when they do track work because the random nature of the running helps them push beyond artificial physiological and psychological barriers.

Let's assume that you tell yourself you'll end an acceleration at a street corner. Even though you're tired and in need of a rest, you push past the corner. You have entered the "worry zone" of races when most runners question themselves and then slow down. By pushing through fatigue, you'll learn to run past your doubts and keep moving toward your goal.

Head for the hills

Maintaining the correct running form is an important part of hill training. Keep a short stride with your feet directly underneath you. Once you find the perfect stride, you'll feel lighter and smoother. If you overstride during hill work, you'll miss out on some of the possible form improvements, and your recovery will slow.

WAYS IN WHICH FARTLEK REWARDS YOU

Fartlek can help improve your running in many ways. For example, if you have trouble surging or staying with someone who surges, then work on this in fartlek sessions. When tired, push the pace for 50 to 60 yards, then come back to your basic pace instead of just jogging to recover.

If you slow down in the middle of races, then work extra hard in the middle of each fartlek workout. You can train yourself to perform at top capacity at the end of races by saving the roughest part of your workout for last and trying to overcome fatigue.

A useful fartlek tip

Remember to increase the distance of your fartlek workouts according to the distance of your goal race. To prepare for a 10-K, try running the hard parts slightly faster than race pace for a total workout of three to four miles. If you're training for a marathon, you can increase the length of your fartlek bursts, run them slower, and log four to six miles of fartlek running in the middle of an eight- to ten-mile workout.

Keeping Your Speed Safe

According to some studies, speedwork ranks among the leading causes of running injuries. Fortunately, you can reduce your chance of injury by being prepared for speed, inserting strategic rest before you need it, and running under control. Here are some basic tips.

Start slowly. To prepare for speed, pick up your pace gradually. Instead of jumping into track work after months of slow running, begin with a series of four to eight weeks of once-a-week hill workouts. These will give you a strength-building transition zone. Run the first two hill workouts conservatively, then gradually increase the intensity of subsequent hill sessions.

Warm up well. To get your leg muscles ready for speedwork, warm up with 10 to 20 minutes of slow running and walking. Speedwork demands top performance from the body, and so it's also important to take four to eight light accelerations (100 to 200 yards). Starting at a slow pace, gradually pick up speed until you are running about the pace you'll run in the workout, then decelerate. Jog slowly or walk between accelerations. Afterward, walk or jog for three to five minutes.

Don't forget about rest. When you add speedwork to your program, you put extra stress on the muscles. This produces more microtears in the muscles and tendons. Unless you build some quality rest into your program, the microtears will accumulate and result in an injury.

Most six- to seven-day-a-week runners can improve performance by dropping to five days a week (three running days, one day off, two running days, one day off). Keep the same mileage per week, but add swimming or biking on the easy days. Schedule your hard days before an easy day and after a day off. Never run two hard days back to back.

Stick to it. Start a year-round program of light acceleration work—a few repetitions with maximum rest between. You can use them as warm-ups (as above) or to keep sharp during easy days or the off-season. After an easy five- to ten-minute warmup, pick up the pace for 100 yards or so at random places around the track. Or choose specific parts of the track where you'll start and finish. Run on trails or roads if you like, but wherever you run, stay relaxed throughout each repetition. Don't time them, don't run all-out, and don't feel too tired during this workout. Run hard enough to feel invigorated, not fatigued.

Fartlek is easier and more fun with a partner. By sharing the hard running, both of you get a better workout, reduce stress, and simulate race situations.

THE IMPORTANCE OF INTERVAL TRAINING

Interval training does two things better than other types of speed training: It improves your running mechanics and provides direct feedback on pace. While repetitions may be boring, they allow you to develop a fast running rhythm in a controlled environment, which helps improve running form. Your time for each lap tells you exactly how you're performing and teaches pace judgment. Scientifically designed interval workouts can gradually help you tolerate oxygen debt. When muscles are overloaded, they cannot process enough oxygen to burn fuel efficiently, hence the term "oxygen debt." As you add one or two repetitions to a workout each week, you can increase your body's capacity to handle this oxygen debt.

Interval sessions also help you peak for races. By reducing the rest interval between the hard repetitions, you'll find that your body gets more prepared for the intensity of a hard race.

To compensate for individual problems, such as midrace letdown, run interval workouts like fartlek sessions. Try surging in the midst of hard repetitions or going out fast and hanging on. This psychological war with yourself will push you into and past the worry zone.

HOW TO MAKE IT FUN

It's the little things that make you feel good about your workout, and that makes it easier. To add a little spice to running hills, for example, break them up mentally: Relax for the first third, run the second third hard, and hold the pace over the top.

The most powerful motivator may be the chemistry of your running partners. Of course, everyone needs to have a cooperative attitude and to avoid goading each other to be "the workout winner." With the right group, you'll establish respect and gain irreplaceable friendships.

Alone or with others, play games. Imagine that a fierce competitor is just ahead of you. As you near the end of the hill or repetition, visualize

Mixing and matching

You'll find you can reach a high level of conditioning by properly mixing your speedwork components— hills for strength, fartlek for mental toughness, and intervals for peaking. In addition, light accelerations will keep you in good form throughout the year. Each stage develops strengths and capabilities that you'll need during the next phase of training.

yourself gaining and then cruising by at the finish. Many runners prefer world-class fantasies.

Billy Mills did. On practically every run for three years, this mediocre college runner imagined that the world-record holder (Ron Clarke of Australia at that time) was just ahead. Finishing each run in a blaze of glory, Mills would visualize himself lunging for the tape in quest of the gold medal.

Mills's fantasy became reality. This almost unknown runner rounded the final straightaway of the 1964 Olympic 10,000 meter final a distant third. When he saw the finish tape, he didn't have to think. His mind and body were exhausted, but they did what they had been doing for the past 1,000 days. He didn't even have to lunge for the tape to take the gold medal.

Amby Burfoot's Running Round-Up

The loneliness of the long-distance runner. The camaraderie of the long-distance runner. Which one will it be?

Both, no doubt. Each in its proper place. And the place for camaraderie, in my mind, is when doing speedwork. As long as I have been running, I have always performed my best and had the most fun when I was part of a regular speedwork training group in college with a tight group of buddies in my late twenties, or with my colleagues at work now.

Running hard and fast at least once a week in the company of friends has long been among my greatest running pleasures. As Jeff Galloway says, there's a chemistry that develops among training partners.

The chemistry changes depending upon the runners, of course, but two things remain constant: Running hard and fast with a group is fun, and this kind of speedwork makes you faster. You would be hard-pressed to find a better training combination than this.

Chapter 18

The FIRST Way to Train

A group of runners and scientists at Furman University have devised a scientific, highly time-efficient way to get in great shape

Train Less, Run Faster"—you've heard the refrain before. It's a longtime favorite of snake-oil coaches with credentials from Charlatan University. Of course, everyone knows that to get faster, you have to log more miles and run intervals until your rear end is dragging on the track behind you. Not this time. The "Train Less, Run Faster" claim is backed by the experiences of real runners who followed a daring new marathon-training program from scientist-runners with advanced degrees in physical education and exercise physiology at Furman University in Greenville, South Carolina—and got results.

It's daring because it defies conventional wisdom by limiting participants to just three running workouts a week. And daring, in the extreme, because it tells runners they'll get faster on fewer workouts. You should give the program a try. It just might work for you.

The Furman Institute of Running and Scientific Training (FIRST) marathon program was born, in a sense, when Bill Pierce and Scott Murr decided to enter a few triathlons way back in the mid-1980s. Just one problem: They hit the wall when they added biking and swimming to their running. The demands of three-sport training were too much, so they cut back their running from six days a week to four.

To their surprise, they didn't slow down in local road races. So they cut back to three days of running. "Lo and behold, our 10-K, half-marathon, and marathon times didn't suffer at all," says Pierce. "The more we discussed this—and we discussed it a lot—the more we became convinced that a three-day program, with some cross-training, was enough to maintain our running fitness."

Pierce, chair of Furman's Health and Exercise Science department, has run 31 marathons, with a best of 2:44:50. At 55, he still manages to knock out a 3:10 every fall by practicing what he preaches: running three workouts a week. While Pierce has retired from triathlons, Murr, 42, with a doctorate in exercise physiology, still wants to complete another Hawaii Ironman, having already done five. He has run a 2:46 marathon, also on three training runs a week.

Pierce's and Murr's discussions, and personal successes, amounted to little more than that until early 2003 when Pierce got university permission to form FIRST. "It helped," he notes with a smile, "that I didn't ask for any funding." By that time, he had assembled a team of four FIRST cofounders, including Murr, Furman exercise physiologist Ray Moss, Ph.D., and former Greenville Track Club president Mickey McCauley.

In the fall of 2003, FIRST launched its training program. Applicants were told they would have to undergo pre- and post-program physiological testing in Furman's Human Performance Lab, and run three very specific running workouts each week. There were no restrictions on additional running or cross-training workouts, and there was no "final exam" test race.

The post-program lab tests showed that subjects had improved their running economy by 2 percent, their maximal oxygen uptake by 4.8 percent, and their lactate-threshold running pace by 4.4 percent. In other words, the three workouts had led to better fitness and race potential. FIRST was off and running.

Fast forward to summer 2004. FIRST advertised a free marathon-training program that would last 16 weeks and culminate with the Kiawah Island Marathon on December 11. To enter the program, you had to be able to run 10 miles. All participants also had to agree to lab testing, and promise not to run more than three days a week. In other words, this time the program came with a clear running restriction. Partially as a counterbalance, participants were encouraged to do two additional days of cross-training, such as bicycling, strength training, rowing, or elliptical training.

From about 50 applicants, FIRST selected 25 subjects (17 with past marathon experience, eight first-timers), including engineers, accountants, managers, administrators, sales representatives, teachers, a nurse, an attorney, and a physician. They began training in August with individualized workouts that Pierce calculated from the lab testing and a questionnaire. Each participant ran just three days a week, doing one long run, one tempo run, and one speed workout. They trained on their own, in their own neighborhoods, according to their own daily and weekly schedules.

In December, 23 of the original 25 ran at Kiawah. One had dropped out of the program because her house flooded, and one because of injury. "I had expected that we would lose at least five runners to injuries," says Pierce, "so I was very happy with this outcome. It seemed to prove that our workouts, which were harder than most of the runners were accustomed to, didn't lead to a rash of injuries."

Two participants dropped down to the half-marathon, because they had developed minor injuries during training but recovered in time to attempt the shorter distance. Both finished the half-marathon with good performances.

That left 21 FIRST marathoners on the starting line. How did they do? All 21 finished, with 15 setting personal bests. Four of the six who didn't set PRs ran faster than their most recent marathon.

"It was so exhilarating to watch them come in, and it was quite a relief, too," says Pierce. "When you're responsible for 21 people who cut back their marathon training because you told them to, well, that can make you a little nervous."

What's more, as post-race lab testing showed, the FIRST participants had improved their maximal oxygen uptake by an average of 4.2 percent and their lactate threshold running speed by 2.3 percent. Bonus: They also reduced their body fat by an average of 8.7 percent. "We think the results show that our program was a big success," says Pierce. "Our people didn't get hurt, and most ran their best-ever marathon. I think we showed that you can teach people to train more efficiently."

BE A FIRST-TIMER

Official participants in Furman's marathon program undergo lab testing, attend monthly meetings, and receive individualized advice, and sometimes even daily e-mails. But anyone can adapt and use the program's basic principles. Just follow the eight rules below, and the 16-week FIRST training plan at the end of this chapter. For more information, check out furman.edu/FIRST.

1. Run Efficiently, Run for Life

Bill Pierce is a tough, performance-oriented guy, but he insists on explaining the FIRST program from a fitness and philosophical perspective. He believes that a three-day running week will make running easier and more accessible to many potential runners and marathoners. It will also limit overtraining and burnout. Finally, with several

days of cross-training, it should cut your injury risk substantially. This may lead to faster race times. More importantly to Pierce, it adds up to a program that many time-stressed people can follow healthfully for years. "Our most important objective is to help runners develop and maintain lifelong participation in running," says Pierce. "Our second goal is to help them achieve as much as possible on a minimum of run training."

2. Run Three Times a Week . . . And No More

This is the centerpiece of the entire FIRST program. FIRST runners do only three running workouts a week. This decreases the overall time commitment of the program, and the risk of injuries—important considerations to many runners. Each of the three workouts has a specific goal. That's something few runners have considered. "With most runners, when I ask them what they're hoping to accomplish on a given run, they look back at me with a blank stare," says Pierce. "I don't think they've ever thought about this question before. We have." The three FIRST workouts—a long run, a tempo run, and a speed workout—are designed to improve your endurance, lactate-threshold running pace, and leg speed.

3. Build Your Long Run to 20 Miles

The FIRST marathon training program builds up to two 20-mile workouts, the second one taking place three weeks before your marathon race date. But covering 20 miles is the easy part of the FIRST program. The harder part is the pace—

60 to 75 seconds slower per mile than your 10-K race pace. Many other marathon programs allow you to run slower than this, by as much as 30 to 40 seconds per mile. "It's true that our long runs won't let you admire the scenery as much," says Pierce. "But they aren't painful, either. They just push you a little beyond the comfort zone. If you're going to race a marathon, you have to do some hard long runs to get the toughness and focus you'll need on race day."

4. Run Three Different Kinds of Tempo Runs

The tempo run has become a mainstay of many training programs, but the FIRST program carries the concept a little farther than most, adding more variety and nuance. FIRST runners do three different kinds of tempo runs—short tempos (three to four miles), mid tempos (five to seven miles), and long tempos (eight to ten miles). Each of these is run at a different pace. "We've found that the long tempo run is particularly helpful," says Pierce. "You're basically running at your marathon goal pace, so you're getting maximum specificity of training, and improving your efficiency at the pace you want to run in your marathon."

5. Run the Right Pace for You

The paces in the FIRST plan are somewhat faster than those recommended by other training plans. Of course, with just three running days a week, you should be well rested for each workout. Here are the paces you'll need to run, each expressed relative to your current 10-K race pace. For the repeat workouts, take a 400-meter jog between each one.

Pierce has a rule for speed training: Start modestly, but after a month, try to get the total distance of all the fast repeats to equal about three miles or 5000 meters (i.e., running 5 x 1000 meters, or 12 to 13 x 400 meters).

6. Cross-Train Twice a Week . . . Hard

During the first year of the program, the FIRST coaches asked their subjects to cross-train twice a week, but they didn't provide any additional instruction. Now they do because they think too many of the runners lollygagged through the cross-training. This caused them to miss out on some potential training benefits. "We believe that if you

LONG RUN	10-K RACE PACE + 60 TO 75 SECONDS/MILE
Long Tempo	10-K + 30 to 35 seconds
Mid Tempo	10-K + 15 to 20 seconds
Short Tempo	10-K pace
1600 mm Repeats	10-K -35 to 40 seconds
1200 mm Repeats	10-K -40 to 45 seconds
800 mm Repeats	10-K -45 to 50 seconds
400 mm Repeats	10-K -55 to 60 seconds

cross-train correctly, you can use it to increase your overall training intensity, without increasing your injury risk," says Pierce. "At the same time, you can still go out and run hard the next day." But the point is this: Even though the original test group didn't cross-train as hard as they could have or should have, they still set a slew of PRs.

7. Don't Try to Make Up for Lost Time

Stuff happens. During a 16-week marathon program, lots of stuff happens. You get sick; you sprain your ankle; you have to go on a last-minute business trip. And so on. Result: You miss some key workouts, maybe even several weeks of workouts. Then what? "You can't make up what you missed," says Pierce, "and you certainly shouldn't double up on your workouts to catch up with your program. Often, if you had a slight cold or too much travel, you can recover and get back where you want to be relatively quickly. But if you have foot pain or ITB syndrome or something like that, you've got to take care of your injury first, and get healthy again." This can take weeks, and it's really tough if you've been looking forward to a big race. You have to accept it, though, and oftentimes you get better and can run an accompanying half-marathon. But you shouldn't try the marathon until you're fully prepared for it. Reschedule another in a few months' time.

8. Follow a Three-Week Taper

The FIRST program builds for 13 weeks, with the second 20-mile long run coming at the end of the

Amby Burfoot's Running Round-Up

In the early 2000s I made several trips to Greenville, South Carolina, to get to know the people behind the FIRST program. It was an eye-opening experience. First of all, I was struck by their resolve to help serious but quite average runners get better on less training. Their success rate was also impressive, at least to judge by the many "thank you" letters and e-mails they received from happy runners.

But the real education came in the several workouts I did with Bill Pierce, Scott Murr, and their noontime training partners. On the first day we ran 5 x 800 meters really hard. I was in good shape and managed to finish the repeats a stride or two ahead of Pierce, who's several years younger than me. I felt like thumping myself on the chest.

Two days later, it was a different story, however. Pierce had played tennis on the intervening day, while I had done nothing. I felt recovered from our 800-meter repeats two days earlier, and I expected to match Pierce stride for stride on our tempo run. It didn't happen that way. He pulled away from me in the first mile, and eventually finished the 4-mile tempo effort about 45 seconds ahead of me.

Those two workouts taught me that the FIRST program is a tough program, even if it does focus on just three running workouts a week. Pierce had obviously conditioned himself to run hard three times a week. I wasn't ready yet, and quickly learned that the FIRST program requires a solid adaptation period. The good news is that you only have to run hard three times a week. The bad news is that you have to run quite hard on those days. Of course, that's the whole point. And once you adapt to the FIRST way of training, which takes a couple of weeks, it pays great dividends.

thirteenth week. After that, the program begins to taper off, with 15- and 10-mile long runs during weeks 14 and 15. The speedwork and tempo runs taper down just a little, with a final eight-mile tempo run at marathon goal pace coming 10 days before the marathon. "The marathon taper has tripled in length during my career," Pierce notes. "When I first started out in the 1970s, we only did a six-day taper for our marathons. Now the conventional wisdom is three weeks, and that makes sense to me. It seems about the right amount of time to make sure you've got the maximum spring back in your step." If you feel sluggish doing just the easy running in the final week (this is very common, by the way), do five or six 100-meter strides or pickups after the Tuesday and Thursday workouts. Get in some extra stretching afterward as well.

The FIRST Training Plan

The FIRST marathon program includes three running workouts per week—a speed workout, a tempo run, and a long run. Here's the full, 16-week marathon training program. (To tailor it for you, see tip number 5: "Run the Right Pace for You" on page xx.) Participants are also encouraged to cross-train for 40 to 45 minutes on two other days per week.

WEEK	TUESDAY–SPEED (METERS)	THURSDAY–TEMPO (MILES)	SATURDAY–LONG (MILES)
1	8 X 400	3	10
2	4 X 1200	5	12
3	4 X 1200	7	13
4	4 X 1200	3	10
5	10 X 400	5	14
6	10 X 400	5	15
7	7 X 800	8	17
8	3 X 1600	10	13
9	12 X 400	3	18
10	8 X 800	5	15
11	4 X 1600	8	20
12	12 X 400	5	15
13	6 X 1200	5	20
14	7 X 800	4	15
15	3 X 1600	8	10
16	30 min easy	20 min easy	

Chapter 19

Beat 10 Common Running Roadblocks

Everyone hits a few bumps on the road. Here's how you can work your way around the most common and perplexing ones.

D r. George Sheehan once famously noted that "Every runner is an experiment of one." What he meant: The experiences of another runner don't necessarily apply to you. This is true to an extent, since an overweight female runner doesn't learn much from reading about the men's world record holder in the 3000-meter steeplechase. But it's also untrue much of the time. Most runners face nearly universal problems as they tackle new challenges: How can I improve my endurance? What workouts will make me faster? What are the best prerace foods?

This chapter tackles 10 of the issues that many runners face at one time or another. You probably won't find that all apply to you, but many will. And the strategies outlined will almost certainly help you improve your running. You might be unique. But when it comes to a simple and historic sport like running, millions have arrived at these cross-roads before, and the lessons they learned will help you surmount the hurdles.

One definition of insanity is doing the same thing over and over and expecting different results. By that standard, there are a lot of runners who could use some serious intervention. They're the ones who sprint from the start, knowing that this time they'll hold that pace to the end. Or the ones who, having done the same run for the past three weeks, figure that today is the day they'll be able to run 30 minutes longer. But even if you're not certifiable, it's likely you've repeatedly hit some obstacles with your running and were left thinking, "There's got to be a better way." Well, there is.

EASY FIXES

Here's how to skip merrily past ten common running problems.

1. Problem: Every time I get really fit or am building my mileage to where I want it, I get injured.
Solution: Allow your body to adapt to a specific fitness level. If you often get injured at a given level of weekly mileage, train at 10 to 20 percent less for at least a month. If you still develop injuries at this lower level, back off again until you find a weekly mileage total that allows you to train consistently for several months.

"The trick is allowing enough time to adapt to a particular volume and intensity level," says Joe Rubio, coach of the Reebok Aggies running team. "Once adaptation has taken place, you can gradually shoot for higher levels of fitness and not get hurt." Unfortunately, this takes what many runners don't seem to have much of: time and patience. Two to three weeks isn't a long time in running; six months to a year is. Allow several months of gradual increase if you're trying to do something ambitious like doubling your weekly mileage.

Bear in mind that mileage and intensity are different stresses that, when combined, increase your workload exponentially. So adapt to them independently. If you want to increase your mileage, "avoid running super-hard workouts," says Rubio. "If it's the time for you to add intensity in the form of hills or speed sessions to develop racing fitness, drop your weekly mileage 10 to 20 percent before adding the tough stuff. That's what elite track athletes do; it allows them to complete the harder workouts that lead to significantly faster race times without increasing their injury risk."

2. Problem: My training has plateaued, and I can't get past 30 minutes or three miles a day.
Solution: Run different mileages during the course of a week. Start by doing one run a week longer than your current limit. The day before, cut your normal run in half to rest up. On the big day, make sure you're running comfortably, not straining; go at least 15 seconds per mile slower than usual. The first time you try this, shoot for an extra mile or 10 minutes. Follow this longer run with another half-the-norm day. Do this once a week for three weeks, each time adding a mile to your longest run, and you'll not only boost your endurance, but your regular-distance runs will seem a lot easier.

If you continue to have trouble extending your distance, run with a friend on your long days. The time will pass much more quickly.

3. Problem: I always slow by at least 30 seconds a mile at the end of a 5-K.
Solution: The three most likely reasons for slowing toward the end of a 5-K are: (1) You lack the nec-

essary aerobic fitness; (2) You haven't done enough long intervals; (3) You started too fast.

Reason 1: If you run less than 20 miles per week or your longest run is less than 5 miles, increase your weekly mileage to at least 25 or 30 miles, and your long run to at least 6. You'll improve your basic aerobic fitness, and this will help you to maintain your pace throughout a 5-K.

Reason 2: If all you do in training is slow mileage—or even if you occasionally do speed-work but seldom include intervals longer than 400 meters—then you won't have the ability to maintain a fast pace for 5 kilometers. You may be able to go out fast for the first mile, and you might even be able to hang in there for the second mile, but the lactate levels in your muscles will rapidly rise during the race, and you'll have to slow dramatically in the third mile. To remedy this, include one or two sessions of long intervals (600 to 1600 meters) per week at your goal 5-K pace for at least five weeks before the race.

Reason 3: If you're well trained, you're simply going out too fast. Run the first mile slower than you have been, so your finish time will improve. If you know your 5-K race pace, run the first mile at that pace. If you don't know it, do this workout: four repetitions of 1600 meters with a one-minute jog between reps. Your average time for the 1600-meter repeats is a good indicator of how fast to run your first mile in the 5-K.

4. Problem: I can't find a goal that works for me—either it's not motivating enough, or I always fail to reach it.
Solution: Find a goal that has two ingredients: impetus to get out the door, and direction about

what to do once you're out there.

Only you can decide what's a motivating goal for you. Does thinking about it get you fired up? Can you visualize yourself beaming because you've attained it? Then you've found a good one. But if it induces no more excitement than the Tuesday morning staff meeting, you need to pick anew. Good goals balance that inspirational quality with being achievable. That is, they take you a bit beyond your comfort zone but no further. Taking 10 minutes off your 10-K time by a week from Thursday is the sort of goal that's only going to break you down and break your heart.

"Make sure you're setting short-term goals that will help lead you to your long-term goals," advises Illinois resident Jenny Spangler, who set the American masters record in the marathon less than two years after giving birth, and knows a thing or two about working toward far-off goals. For example, if your goal is to break 45 minutes for a 10-K three months from now, aim for an 8-K at that pace two months from now. Similarly, if you currently run 25 miles a week and want to get up to 40-mile weeks, set interim goals of comfortably averaging 30, then 35 miles a week.

5. Problem: I run on the treadmill mostly, and it's just boring as hell.
Solution: Ask yourself, "Why am I running on the treadmill?"

Is it because you want to know exactly how far you ran? Or because the calories-burned meter makes you think you are dropping pounds left and right? Simply out of habit? If so, step off the 'mill, and step outside. There's a whole world out there to explore, where the scenery and weather are different every day, and where the time flies when you're having fun.

If you decide that you must run often on a treadmill, use the controls to create workouts that require more mental focus than simply waiting for the time to run out. Some good treadmill options:

Progression runs, in which you increase the pace at set increments (every three minutes, every half-mile, etc.).

Short intervals, such as alternating two minutes at 5-K pace with two minutes slow.

Cruise intervals, such as 10 minutes at half-marathon pace, followed by two minutes easy, followed by another 10 minutes at half-marathon pace.

Simulated hill workouts, in which you keep your pace steady, but you alternate one minute at zero percent incline with one minute at five percent or more incline.

6. Problem: I daydream and lose concentration during long runs and races, and my pace lags substantially.

Solution: Do the kind of training that helps you not only physically, but mentally as well. "In my opinion, interval sessions on the track, more so than any other kind of training, teach you how to be mentally tough," says Keith Dowling, a 2:13 marathoner and a leading American road racer for more than a decade. "It's a pretty unforgiving environment—you get feedback every 200 meters, and you can monitor your pace so you know right away if you've had a mental lapse. After a while, you learn how to readjust your pace almost intuitively."

"When I'm really well prepared," Dowling says, "losing focus in a race just doesn't happen. I'm in the moment."

7. Problem: When I run with others, either I run so fast it feels like a race, or so slowly it feels like I'm not getting a workout.

Solution: Make sure every training session has a purpose. This principle applies not only to the glamorous stuff like track workouts and long runs, but also to running with your buddies. Regularly running within a minute per mile of your 10-K race pace on supposedly easy days can lead to injury. Or it will tire you out for your speed workouts or long runs.

"What I suggest to runners who face the problem of running too fast, too often, with others is simply to schedule specific training runs with specific running friends," says Rubio. "For instance, if you have a friend who stays one step in front of you on every run, chances are that you'll run faster than you should with this person. Reserve runs with 'one-stepper' for days when you've already planned a harder tempo run."

As for too-slow training partners, count your blessings. Running with slowpokes could be just what the doctor ordered. "Easy recovery days are essential," says Rubio. "Many top runners train with someone much slower once or twice a week to slow the pace on scheduled easy days."

8. Problem: I start feeling really tight in the shoulders and upper back during a run.

Solution: Try flexibility and yoga poses that focus your shoulders, arms, and neck. These areas get tensed up from working a desk job or driving a long commute. "Loosening up those areas will make your running feel more fluid," says Pete Pfitzinger, a two-time Olympic marathoner and general manager of the New Zealand Academy of Sport North. If you can afford it, a deep sports massage once a month or more will further loosen your upper body.

Tightness in your shoulders and upper back can also stem from weak muscles or poor running form. "Incorporating core-conditioning exercises into your training routine can help to eliminate both of those problems," Pfitzinger says. "Doing 'striders'—accelerations of about 100 meters—while maintaining relaxed shoulders and arms can also help improve your ability to relax your upper body during running."

9. Problem: I've been doing weekly track workouts for the past couple of months, but I'm not getting faster, and I don't enjoy them.

Solution: "Make sure you are doing workouts that coincide with your goal race length and pace, and also the phase of training that you're in," says Spangler. In other words, while all-out 200-meter repeats will certainly have your lungs and muscles burning, they're not as effective as mile repeats at your goal pace if you're preparing for a 10-K.

If the 5-K is your focus, most of your track workouts should be repeats of 800 or 1200 meters at your goal 5-K pace; aim for 12 laps of hard running in a workout. When you're building toward a half-marathon, alternate between these workouts: One week, do one continuous run of 20 to 30 minutes at your half-marathon goal pace, followed the next week by mile repeats at 10-K race pace.

Also, says Spangler, "people respond differently to track workouts—it takes longer for some people to reap the benefits of interval training." In other words, could be you just need to give it a little more time.

But if your patience has run out and you simply don't enjoy track workouts, says Spangler, "get off the track and do fartlek or tempo runs on the roads, trail, or grass. Run by effort and don't be dependent on your watch." These off-track workouts have the added benefit of making you run fast

Amby Burfoot's Running Round-Up

For the first 10 years of my running career, I had the strangest problem. At least I thought it was strange: I couldn't run fast enough on downhills. Going up, no problem. I pulled away from most of my competitors. But when we crested the hill and headed down the other side, I lost every yard I had gained. And then some. The other runners seemed to sweep past me without effort.

I felt slow and awkward and lumbering on the downhills, when I wanted to feel quick and light. I asked other runners how they handled the downs so adroitly. Few could explain. "I just relax and let go," one friend said. The instructions weren't clear enough for me to figure it out. As a result, I had to experiment on my own.

After many failed attempts, I finally got it right. Now I often fly past the runners around me when we come to a downhill stretch. My secret? I don't know if it will work for you, but here's what I do. When I hit a downhill, I try to imagine that my feet and legs are a bicycle wheel just rolling and rolling and rolling as effortlessly as can be. The moment my forward foot hits the ground, I lift it. I don't stay on the ground and don't push off it; I just lift my foot as quickly as I can. Problem solved.

And once I learned how to do this, I didn't have to practice at all. It's simply a technique that I can turn on as easily as turning on a light switch. You can do the same with the problems you encounter. Just keep trying new approaches until you find the one that works.

on a variety of terrain, just as you need to do in road races.

10. Problem: After a big race, I always get these awful letdowns.

Solution: Choose another goal before you run your big race. "I bypass any major letdown I might feel after a big race by looking ahead to another one," says Dowling "and looking at the challenge of how to prepare for it." Dowling recommends having another meaningful running goal eight to ten weeks away, preferably one centered on a different distance than your just-completed goal (e.g., a fast 10-K if you've done a marathon, or a long trail race after a season of short road races).

And allow yourself to enjoy breaks after your races. "After a marathon," he says, "I might not even run for up to a month. I've worked so hard before the marathon that I look forward to that downtime, to just sitting around watching TV or devoting time to other interests that are easy to neglect when I'm in heavy training. [Dowling plays in a band.] I also use that time to get rid of any nagging pains that might have come up before the marathon so I'm ready to go when it's time to start training again."

[VI]

The Mental Side of Running

Chapter 20

Train Your Brain for Better Performance

How to Think Like a Champion

The more years I run, the more I'm impressed by the mental side of running. In my earlier days I used to think that success in running was purely a matter of finding the right training combination. If you did the right long runs, if you did the right speed workouts, if you worked all the numbers, well, you would be ready to run great.

Of course, I still believe in the importance of training. But now I believe that attitude is even more crucial. Because running will always humble you, as Bill Rodgers put it many times, and you need something to keep you going when the going gets tough.

Now, in many regards, humility is a good thing. It teaches respect, which is where learning begins, and we can all stand to learn something new every day. But too much humility is like too much apple pie—it begins to weigh you down. And runners need to be light, positive-thinking people to overcome the inevitable obstacles they face. This chapter explains how positive thinking can lead to powerful running.

Roger Bannister's historic first sub-four-minute mile, recorded on May 6, 1954, ranks as one of the greatest and most widely known moments in the history of sports. What's less well-known is the intriguing fact that in the next 12 months, four other runners also broke through the previously impossible barrier. Why? Had the human species suddenly evolved into a higher organism, capable of running with greater speed and endurance?

Of course not. The only explanation for the post-Bannister rush of sub-four milers is that four minutes had represented more of a mental barrier than a physical barrier. Knowing that Bannister had run a 3:59, the rest of the world's milers could no longer believe such a time was beyond their reach. They had little choice but to redouble their efforts to run as fast as Bannister and faster.

The makeup of a champion

Champions share many characteristics, none of which are determined by their running speeds. How many of these statements describe your running and your life? A champion . . .

- . . . has the courage to risk failure, knowing that setbacks are lessons to learn from.

- . . . uses a race to gain greater self-knowledge as well as feedback on physical improvement.

- . . . trains thought processes as well as the body to produce a total approach to performance.

- . . . understands his athletic weaknesses and trains to strengthen them.

- . . . actively creates a life of balance, moderation, and simplicity—values that help improve running and life.

- . . . views competitors as partners who provide challenge and the chance to improve.

- . . . understands that running performances are like a roller coaster, with many ups and downs, and that you have to accept both the good and the bad.

- . . . enjoys running for the simple pleasures it provides.

- . . . has vision. A champion dreams of things that haven't been and believes they are possible. A champion says, "I can."

The most successful runners think like champions.

The Bannister story is perhaps the best example in running of this basic concept: Negative thinking limits performance. Turn the thinking around, and suddenly the impossible becomes possible. This doesn't apply just to breakthrough performers, world records, and gold medals. It applies to every one of us, to every race we run, and, indeed, to every situation we face in our lives.

If you can train your mind—and you can—your body will follow. In the rest of this chapter, I'll describe a number of techniques that you can use to improve your performances and increase your enjoyment of running.

BELIEVING YOU CAN

By 1954 more than 50 medical journals had carried articles saying it was humanly impossible to break four minutes in the mile, but Bannister didn't buy their arguments. He refused to limit his own potential. His success proved that we are capable of those things that we are capable of believing. Or, to put it another way, as an athlete, you should always act as if you can. With this positive attitude, you can then find out the truth of your athletic potential by living out the experience.

Far too many of us do the opposite: We decide ahead of time that we can't. We think we're too old, too heavy, not well enough trained, not tough enough, not blessed with the right muscle fibers. The list goes on and on, developing into a litany of negative, limiting language and beliefs. And the outcome is always the same: If you think you can't, you can't.

Henry Ford described both sides as well as anyone when he said, "If you think you can do it, you're right. If you think you can't do it, you're still right." When you believe and think "I can," you activate your motivation, commitment, confidence, concentration, and excitement, all of which relate directly to achievement. If you think "I can't," on the other hand, you sabotage your chances of achieving your goals.

Over the years, I have worked with a wide range of athletes—from Olympians to midpackers—and during those years I've noticed one clear and consistent pattern: The most successful runners think like champions. The "I can" belief forms the foundation of their approach to all things in life. They refuse to accept "I can't" unless they have collected objective data showing that a goal is beyond their grasp. Even then, they don't say, "I can't." They simply reformulate their goals to move them within reach.

The same approach will work for you. It won't necessarily turn you into an Olympic champion, but it will help you to run better and enjoy it more. The "I can" attitude will also allow you to adopt the following mind-sets, all of which are designed to help you unlock the extraordinary potential that each of us possesses as a runner.

BOUNCING BACK FROM FAILURE

To succeed, every runner must learn to deal with mistakes and failures. All champions realize that the path to personal excellence is cluttered with obstacles. Arriving at the top is a process that involves many setbacks. Champions accept this process, understanding that you can't stretch your limits without encountering some rough moments along the way.

I recall the attitude of Herb Lindsay after one of his few losses in 1980, a year when he was the country's top-ranked road racer. When I asked Lindsay how it felt to finally lose one, he said that he would bounce back at the next race and that he considered every loss a lesson in how to become an even better champion. Lindsay didn't get down on himself. He created a personal environment in which failure and losses were acceptable learning experiences that could help him improve.

We have all learned everything we know physically—from walking to running a marathon—by trial and error, so there's no reason to become our own worst enemies when we suffer a setback. From time to time everyone falls short of their goals. It's an illusion to believe that champions succeed because they do everything perfectly. You can be certain that every archer who hits the bull's-eye has also missed the bull's-eye a thousand times while learning the skill.

When you create a mental environment that accepts mistakes, you free yourself to keep trying, to keep extending yourself, to keep taking risks. Sure, you'll have some bad days, but if you accept them as opportunities for growth, you can learn much from the experiences. An accepting attitude helps you perform with greater relaxation, which, as all champions know, is one of the key building blocks of success.

A NEW DEFINITION OF WINNING

To bring out your best, you also need to adopt the champion's true attitude toward winning. There has to be more to running than taking home a medal or age-group award. Philosopher Alan Watts once said, "You don't sing to get to the end of the song." The same applies to running: You don't run to finish or to get it over with.

In his classic work *The Zen of Running*, Fred Rohe states: "There are no standards and no possible victories except the joy you are living while dancing your run ... you are not running for some future reward—the real reward is now!"

That's quite similar to the motto of the modern Olympic Games: "The important thing in the Games is not winning but taking part. The essential thing in life is not conquering but fighting well." If you run with this attitude, the results will take care of themselves. While running, focus on the internal battle. Concentrate on overcoming fear, self-doubt, and other limiting beliefs. Forget about external issues, like your time. Such outward concerns will only deplete your energy, create tension, and slow you down.

APPRECIATING YOUR OPPONENTS

Thinking like a champion also means adopting a new attitude toward your opponents. Traditionally, being a good competitor meant being a good predator. You succeeded most when you attacked and thrashed the opposition. But it doesn't have to be this way.

In the movie *Running Brave*, Billy Mills slows down near the finish of one race, even as a coach stands on the sidelines screaming, "Crush your opponent! Take him for everything! Own him!" But Mills is well ahead of the other runners and understands that he will gain nothing by destroying them. That the real Mills made this choice doesn't mean that he wasn't a fierce runner. In 1964, he won the Olympic 10,000 meters in Tokyo,

considered by many to be one of the biggest upsets in Olympic history.

Obviously, the killer instinct isn't a requirement for optimal performance. It's much healthier and more beneficial to view opponents as partners who, because of their great efforts, afford you the opportunity to raise the level of your own performance. You depend on them to extend your limits. Think about it: How often do you run as fast in training as you do in races? When I race, I often recite an affirmation that reminds me of how my opponents help me reach my potential. The affirmation goes like this: "My opponents are very important to me. Because they are here, I experience greater depth as an athlete."

When we come together to try to reach our potential, such as in a road race, others can only help us. With such a view, you will enter a race more relaxed, focused, and energized. You can't help but perform better as a result of cooperation rather than antagonism.

Curb the will to win

Of course, we all like to do our best, to succeed, to set new personal records. Our performances provide a handy gauge of self-improvement, and the recognition we receive is rewarding. But too many runners suffocate their enjoyment of running by overemphasizing the importance of fast times. About all this does is build up your tension and anxiety, which can't help you run better. In fact, these responses actually interfere with your natural fluidity and speed, thus creating an obstacle to the goal, to say nothing of how such attitudes diminish the fun of running and racing.

SIMPLICITY IN ALL THINGS

The true champion recognizes that excellence often flows most smoothly from simplicity, a fact that can get lost in these high-tech days. I used to train with a world-class female runner who was constantly hooking herself up to pulse meters and pace keepers. She spent hours collecting data that she thought would help her improve. In fact, a good 25 percent of her athletic time was devoted to externals other than working out. Sports became so complex for her that she forgot how to enjoy herself.

Contrast her approach with that of the late Abebe Bikila, the Ethiopian who won the 1960 Olympic Marathon running barefoot. Fancy clothing and digital watches were not part of his world. He simply ran. Many times in running, and in other areas of life, less is more.

Bill Rodgers won his first Boston Marathon in 2:09:55 while wearing a plain white T-shirt on which he had hand-lettered the initials of his track club. When you learn to run simply, you find that you can concentrate on simply running.

Another proponent of such thinking is Mark Nenow, the American record holder for 10,000 meters on the road. Nenow has never been concerned with weight, muscle biopsies, heart rates, or sports science. He's had no grand expectations and therefore has never been devastated by setbacks. He just keeps running.

Bikila, Rodgers, and Nenow stand as perfect examples of a philosophy that Joe Henderson, *Runner's World* magazine's first editor, has expressed on many occasions: "Don't let the planning and analyzing get in the way of the doing and enjoying." It's an approach that would benefit many runners.

The need for change

When you're feeling stale and burned out, it could be because you're overtraining. But it could also be because your mental program needs an overhaul. Do any of the following statements describe you? If so, you should consider ways you can change your thought patterns.

You struggle constantly for external recognition rather than internal satisfaction.

You measure your self-worth as a runner solely on the basis of each performance.

You focus on perfection, an unrealistic goal, rather than pursuing a journey of excellence.

You condemn yourself for failures, setbacks, and mistakes rather than realizing that not only are they inevitable, but they offer good opportunities for learning.

You blame others or uncontrollable circumstances when things go wrong. This leaves you feeling helpless.

You see running as something to conquer.

You have unrealistic goals that result in frustration, disappointment, and distraction.

BALANCE IN YOUR LIFE

Runners who think like champions know when they have done enough. Doing too much, especially in training, is one of the greatest misfortunes that a runner can encounter because it can wipe out all your hard-earned conditioning.

More isn't better. Moderation is better. Olympian Jeff Galloway has used this approach with various marathon training groups around the country. Many of these groups, following a program of training every other day, have achieved marathon-completion rates of 98 percent and higher.

Balance is another side of moderation, and something runners occasionally have trouble keeping in perspective. A few years ago, a national-class client of mine was experiencing the classic signs of burnout and fatigue. He was so obsessed with running that he kept getting injured. I asked him to visit my office to discuss his situation. The following dialogue sums up our conversation.

Me: "How much do you need to train?"

Marty: "I'd train 12 hours a day if I could."

Me: "Marty, you really need to consider having more balance in your life."

Marty: "I would be balanced. I'd do 12 hours of working out and 12 hours of sleep. That would be a perfect balance."

Marty may be an extreme case, but many other runners suffer from overtraining. They believe that they won't excel unless they devote everything to the effort. But there are many examples of the opposite.

Ingrid Kristiansen set her marathon record two years after the birth of her first child. Her interests in family and hobbies other than running provided balance in her life and may have enabled her to compete with less tension and anxiety.

Avoiding extremes will help you run farther, wiser, and longer in life. Adding balance to your running means decreasing injury and burnout. At the same time, you'll find yourself enjoying your running more, feeling more motivated, and looking forward to many more years of productive, fun-filled participation.

THE ZEN–TAO APPROACH

After his superb victory at the 1990 New York City Marathon, Douglas Wakiihuri, born in Kenya and trained in Japan, stated that his marathoning could not be separated from his search for life's truths. Wakiihuri is right. Winning at racing, as in life, is an inner journey without a destination.

Amby Burfoot's Running Round-Up

All of the mental strategies in this chapter can work for runners, as shown through a number of telling anecdotes, but the one I find most compelling from my own experience is the power of simplicity. It rings so true to me, because I have seen it in action so often.

We westerners have a tendency to look outside ourselves for secrets and shortcuts. We place great faith, for example, in the secrets of science. We believe it can teach us how to train and race faster. Maybe it can, and we would certainly be foolish to ignore truths that are revealed to us.

But running is such a basic, nontechnical activity that the greatest truths may be the simplest. You have to train hard. You have to take rest breaks. You have to eat well but not too much. You have to expect some bad days and bad races; all life, after all, follows certain cyclical patterns. Excessive worry and hair-pulling won't do much good. The best way to race well another day is to put today behind you.

You can't change it, so you might as well accept it and move onward. Face tomorrow with a fresh, open, confident attitude. If you believe tomorrow could be the day when everything works out perfectly for you, then that may in fact be the case.

In searching for both athletic and personal growth at the same time, Wakiihuri represents a new breed of champions I call sacred warriors. These runners realize that they will have the most success in their external lives only after they have won the inner battle over self-doubt.

When you adopt a similar attitude, it doesn't mean that you'll run world records or even personal records. You will, however, decrease the pressure and stress you may feel when running. And this can only help you improve your performances and your appreciation of running. By focusing on running as an exciting and fulfilling journey without a destination, you will see that your running can't be anything but successful and rewarding.

You have within you, right now, all that you need to achieve your realistic goals in running. Thinking like a champion will allow you to reach

Post-labor running

Like Ingrid Kristiansen, many other women runners have improved after the birth of their children, despite the obvious fact that children demand incredible amounts of energy and attention. This doesn't have to be a negative factor. Indeed, it's a positive when it means that the runner has added more balance to his or her life. Yes, his. Keith Brantly finally made the U. S. Olympic Team in 1996, after finishing fourth in 1988 and 1992, when he brought his seven-month-old son with him to the Olympic Trials.

that potential. Remember that all your accomplishments are the direct result of your thoughts. When you choose the right kind of thoughts, you can create the running destiny you have always wanted.

Chapter 21

Yes, You Can

Discover How You Can Get the Most out of Yourself

All of us have the feeling that we have more ability than we exhibit, that we could get more out of ourselves if only we knew how to tap our full potential. We see others perform amazing feats, and they don't seem any different or more talented than we are. How do they do it? How can we do the same?

In running, this line of thought can be self-defeating. The truth is that some runners do have more talent than others, and no amount of training or concentration is going to bridge the gap. Because races are based on such hard-edged mathematics—someone finishes in 2 hours, someone in 3 hours, and someone in more than 4 hours—we can't escape the reality of our performances. And it's more important to accept ourselves as we are and to practice the sport for its myriad benefits than to get hung up on changing a 4-hour performance to a 3-hour finish.

Still, we would like to run as fast as we can—to bring out our best—and we know that the mind holds the key to being better. This chapter by Ken McAlpine explores how different athletes have

succeeded in digging deep to reach their maximum running potential.

Sport hurts. When you challenge yourself in a race, whether it's the muscle-busting seconds of a sprint or the muscle-wasting hours of a marathon, you encounter moments when your heart rocks your ribs, your muscles sear, and your mind strains to recall why you're doing this at all. How you handle these painful, pivotal moments during a race often determines success or failure. Some athletes and coaches suggest that the ability to dig deep and persevere is all that stands between you and your potential.

"To do well, you have to push yourself," says two-time Olympic 3000-meter runner PattiSue Plumer, who has made a career of gutsy performances. "You have to keep going. You have to go

Top training tips

Start by recognizing that you can't tap reserves that aren't there. Physiology dictated that you have a finite amount of energy. This energy must be rationed carefully. This may seem like something any dolt would know, but if it were, you wouldn't see a third of every race field burst off the starting line like commuters late for a bus. Experienced athletes parcel out their energy reserves in miserly fashion, knowing full well what will come later.

"As you tire, it takes more effort—physically and emotionally—to pull through the last part of the race," says three-time Western States 100 winner Tom Johnson. "You need to save half of your energy for the last third of the race."

How to measure your energy dispersal? Pay close attention to how you feel. "If it's early in a race and you start feeling the lactic acid build up, and your heart rate's going sky high, those are pretty clear signs that you're using too much energy too soon," says three-time Olympic cyclist John Howard. "It's okay to feel the lactic acid building up late in a race, but early on you should feel loose and comfortable."

Easing back on the throttle early on can sometimes pay stunning dividends. At the 1990 Canadian Ironman, triathlete Erin Baker pared back her effort during the 112-mile bike ride and uncorked a 2:49 marathon run. "If you just take a deep breath, calm yourself down, and bring your heart rate down 10 to 15 beats per minute, you can actually save quite a bit of energy," says Baker. "A little bit saved adds up to much more than you'd think."

beyond what you think you're capable of doing."

Athletes have been pushing the edges of their performance envelopes since the days of the first Olympics in Greece. Through trial and error, the best runners have developed a retinue of physical and mental techniques for coping with, and occasionally stepping through, the difficult moments that beat the rest of us to a smudge.

There are no universal, surefire methods. Pushing through tough times involves performance intangibles—intelligence, desire, sheer pigheadedness—that don't plug neatly into a formula. But the ability to dig deep and persevere can, to some extent, be cultivated, bringing you a step closer to racing and training at your full potential.

PRACTICE HARD

"If you want to learn to run through pain, you have to experience the pain first," states Plumer. "I think the fastest way for most people to improve their performance is by experiencing this pain and learning how to handle it. But most people avoid this."

Plumer recommends at least one intense, race-simulating interval workout a week. Fine, you say, I do intervals. But do your interval workouts really force you to push back your limits? Perhaps your interval sessions have become rote? Local tracks are brimming with runners who can pop off quarters like slot machines. But is that the point?

Traditionally lauded for their physical benefits, intervals offer a crucial psychological boon. Familiarity with discomfort fosters comfort.

"You must experience hurt during training," says 1972 Olympic Marathon gold medalist Frank Shorter. "Then when things get difficult in a race, you just think, 'I've been here before. I know what happens. If I keep up the pressure and the mental intensity, eventually I'll come out of this.'"

BACK OFF FROM PAIN

It happens to us all at some point, but when you do run face-first into pain, know that it is okay to step back a bit. While many athletes see backing off as an overt admission of spineless wormdom, elite runners don't hesitate. When they start to struggle, they ease off the pace, regroup physically, then push on again. No one—at least no one who hopes to finish—grinds on without reprieve.

Shorter points out that races typically take place in surges—hard efforts alternating with bouts of recovery. The winners aren't necessarily the fastest runners, says Shorter; they're the ones who can recover from the surges the fastest.

"The less well-trained you are, the longer it takes for you to recover," Shorter adds. "But if you're trained to any degree, and you slow down enough, you will recover."

So, when your heart feels as though it might burst, and your legs are threatening to turn to cement, the best thing you can do is precisely what you want to do—ease back.

Pushing through difficult moments is largely a matter of maintaining composure. It goes back to relaxation. Experienced runners understand this, which is why they say things like "You fight pain by relaxing and gaining control" and "As the pain intensifies, the response is to become more relaxed." Advice like this may sound silly, especially when your heart is ricocheting about your chest. And, true, relaxing won't make the pain go away, but it will keep you from crumbling.

TAKE A DEEP BREATH

The best way to relax, focus your effort, and maintain your form is through controlled, rhythmic breathing. "Controlling your breathing is crucial," says three-time Olympic cyclist John Howard, echoing a belief voiced by most athletes. "It allows you to focus and concentrate almost entirely on your form. Not a lot of athletes do this. They lose control of their breathing, and they lose contact with their bodies. Their form falls apart. When you lose your form, you're lost."

THE POWER OF YOUR MIND

Ultimately, the ability to cope mentally with tough times may be what separates the best from the rest. Unfortunately, sports psychology and its terminology—such as thought stopping, trigger words, and alternative scripts—tend to turn people off. Before you look away, realize that science has documented a mind-body link. Using sophisticated tools and techniques, researchers have shown that athletes can induce profound changes in their brains during competition, changes that can greatly enhance their performances. Elite archers, for example, can damp down distracting impulses in the left, or analytical, side of the brain, allowing the reflexive, free-form right hemisphere to send arrows flying true. The biology can be complex. Just understand this: It's the foolish athlete who ignores the mind.

"I don't think the average person realizes what sort of impact the mind has on performance," says Leonard Zaichkowsky, a Boston University sport psychologist who has worked with everyone from Little Leaguers to Olympians. "They know it impacts, but at most they might think, 'Well, I read about it once, but it doesn't affect me that much.' Rest assured, it does."

The psychological tactics for pushing on are as varied as the athletes who use them. Many are simply ploys, often outright chicanery, designed to convince the body that it isn't on the verge of meltdown.

BREAK THE RUN INTO CHUNKS

Breaking your run down into mentally manageable chunks is one example. Steve Scott, who has run more than 100 sub-four-minute miles, tackles races lap by lap. On the third lap, when things really start to hurt, his goal might be just to stay with the leaders through that lap. Instead of focusing on the pain, and that it won't be ending anytime soon, he concentrates on the competition and the moment—poof, that lap is gone, and there's only one left.

Ultrarunner Tom Johnson, whose mental hurdles are a bit more daunting, uses the same

The second wind mystery

Ask exercise physiologists about second wind, and you'll get much head-nodding that, yes, this is an intriguing subject indeed. But no one knows precisely why second wind occurs.

"All we can do is speculate," says Robert Murray, Ph.D., director of the Gatorade Sports Science Institute's exercise physiology laboratory in Barrington, Illinois. "Theories can take you from the top of the body—the brain and the central nervous system—all the way down to the bottom, to the biochemistry of the muscle cells. If you talk to 100 physiologists, you'll probably get 100 different answers."

The most common theory goes something like this: When you start exercising, your muscles burn glycogen as fuel. This requires oxygen. Your body has a limited amount of stored oxygen, and it burns it quickly. After that, if your body can't supply enough oxygen to your muscles, the muscles break down glycogen without oxygen, or anaerobically. This produces lactic acid. You're in oxygen debt, and you feel lousy: Your muscles burn, your heart beats quickly. Second wind, that welcome flush of relief, occurs when the body finally begins to supply enough oxygen to your muscles.

"The term 'catch-up' is important when we talk about second wind," says Glenn Town, Ph.D., an Illinois exercise physiologist who once finished 24th at the Hawaii Ironman. "When you go from total inactivity to heading out on a run, you create an oxygen debt. The payback in an unconditioned individual can be uncomfortable."

Because their more efficient systems can supply their muscles with a steady stream of oxygen, fit athletes avoid oxygen debt, says Town, and never experience second wind. Beginners can fend off oxygen debt by easing gradually into a run. Start with a brisk walk, move to a slow jog, and gradually increase your speed from there. This may sound pedestrian, but even fit runners often do the same thing, starting their runs at little more than a shuffle.

When the going gets difficult, Howard focuses on inhaling and exhaling long and steadily. Deep, steady breathing triggers the parasympathetic nervous system, the body's relaxation mode. By contrast, huffing and puffing provoke the energy-burning sympathetic nervous system, the same neurological response elicited when you back over your neighbor's cat.

"You respond either in a controlled, systematic, powerful way, or in a panicked manner, where your body is out of control," says Howard. "Athletes need to learn to use the mind to control the body. That's really what it comes down to. Most of us do just the opposite. We let the body control the mind."

trick. Seventy miles into a run, there's no positive way to think of the last 30 miles. So Johnson focuses on how quickly he can run the next five.

"You need something that you can mentally grasp," says Johnson. "After you've done that five miles, then you reach out and grab another five miles and pull yourself through that."

PAY ATTENTION TO FORM

Another simple and effective ploy: Concentrate on technique. Focus on keeping your stride long and your arms moving straight forward and back. This helps maintain form, and it occupies your mind at a time when pain, fear, and whining pessimism are probing for chinks.

During tough times, sports psychologist Joel Kirsch encourages athletes to focus on their "center"—a spot several inches down and in from the navel that he calls the physical center of gravity. Six-time Ironman winner Dave Scott concentrates on relaxing. Fellow triathlete Scott Molina repeats a mantra: "I can win, I can win, I can win." Whatever the object of focus, the premise is the same. Concentrating wholeheartedly on one thing doesn't leave much room for anything else.

FEEL THE PAIN

Confronted with pain, athletes have employed some odd psychological gambits. Runners are particularly creative. In a seminal study of marathon runners, psychologist William P. Morgan noted some innovative attempts to blot out pain: One woman visualized the faces of two coworkers that she detested, then proceeded to squish them, one face and then the other, every step of the race.

Though it may be therapeutic, Morgan concluded that this sort of practiced disregard—which psychologists term dissociation—doesn't help performance in the long run. He observed that world-class distance runners actually associated with the pain. Paying close attention to their bodies' feedback kept them in touch and allowed them to make the right adjustments during the race.

Not that dissociation doesn't have its place. Morgan interviewed a Boston Marathon runner who thwarted the pain of Heartbreak Hill by imagining that he was a powerful steam engine—his breath coming in puffs of steam, his legs as driving pistons. Dissociation, concluded Morgan, has powerful advantages, but it should be used sparingly. Ignorance may be bliss, but we shouldn't lose contact with the machine.

Concentration on every step of a marathon—or, for that matter, a 5-K—will turn your brain to mush. Your mental approach should be the same as your physical effort—bouts of focus separated by periods of mental meandering. But when things get ugly, best to look in.

"So many people try to get through events by externalizing," says Howard. "They think about tomorrow's dinner or how great it's going to feel to finish. The real athletes are able to perform better by going in, by focusing very closely on what the body is doing. When you don't pay attention to the body, you lose touch. When you lose touch, you lose control."

None of these mind games will help unless you can bring them into play. Unfortunately, most people view psychological skills, if they think of them at all, in the same light as onion dip—something they can whip up in a moment's notice. Not so.

"These are things that you need to practice

before you get into a race," says PattiSue Plumer. "You can't just expect to call them up and have them work. They're skills. Like any other skill, they need to be practiced."

Break down the wall

Much has been made of the wall, and anyone who has ever crashed into it knows why. Your body crumbles, your will turns to mush. At best, your pace falls off to a stagger. At worst, you fall on your face. Ugly? Yes. Inevitable? No.

"I don't believe that there's a wall out there," states six-time Ironman winner Dave Scott. "It's a bunch of baloney. You can control your glycogen stores so that you never hit the wall."

When you exercise, you tap two fuel sources—glycogen and fat. Glycogen is high-octane stuff. It fuels hard effort; as a rule, effort greater than 60 percent of our aerobic capacity demands glycogen. Fat drives us at slower speeds, and it is an almost inexhaustible energy source. Your body's total glycogen stores amount to 2,000 calories; a single pound of fat contains 3,500 calories, and your body is probably more than 10 percent fat.

"Competing successfully in any kind of endurance event boils down to being able to burn fat and spare glycogen," explains Riverside, California, nutritionist Ellen Coleman. "Making your glycogen last as long as it can, that's the secret to endurance." The best way to conserve glycogen and tap fat? Carefully monitor your body's signals and keep an eye on your pace. High-intensity, anaerobic effort gobbles your precious glycogen reserves.

"Treading that fine line between aerobic and anaerobic, that's the way you go fast over the long haul," claims Olympic cyclist John Howard. "You want to keep the anaerobic efforts to a minimum, conserve your glycogen supply, and then, when the end's in sight, really throw the coals on and cross the finish with nothing left."

With practice, you can learn to tap your deepest reserves of strength and energy. You can push yourself beyond what you think you're capable of doing.

"So often you'll hear people say, 'I hit the wall. I ran out of gas. I just couldn't do anything else,'" muses Dave Scott.

"I bet you, psychologically, they could have mustered a little bit more energy," continues Scott. "I think that a lot of athletes are physically capable of pushing through tough times. Maybe they don't succeed because they don't have the ability to provide the mental push."

Perhaps we need to change our outlook—to embrace the pain and hard effort of our sport. It's impossible to paint a pretty picture of running's demands, and Johnson doesn't as he reels off the list of ultrarunning's hurts: "Dehydration, hunger, blisters, aching muscles, pounding joints, swelling body parts. . . ."

Plumer, too, gives testimony to the pain of running when she leans into the final lap of a race, temples tingling, face flushed hot, pain sweeping her frame. Yet she positively bubbles at the thought.

"That's what's so important, so exciting, about sport," she says. "It teaches us to challenge ourselves. It teaches us to push beyond where we thought we could go. It helps us find out what we're made of. This is what we do. This is what it's all about." What we dread, we should relish.

Amby Burfoot's Running Round-Up

I've always been one of those slow-but-steady runners. If I won a lot of races in my day, my success didn't come from any excess of athletic brilliance. It came from discipline and determination, from the fact that I stuck to my programs and goals no matter how slow and sometimes frustrating the progress.

I believed in what I was doing, particularly that the whole was greater than the sum of the parts. Take running the marathon, for example. My goal was always to run a marathon at a five-minute-per-mile pace. Now, when I considered this goal in its entirety, I was overwhelmed by the impossibility of it. Anyway or anytime you look at a marathon, it tends to seem impossible.

Yet every week I ran lots of miles—far more than the 26 in the marathon. And every week I ran a few of those miles faster than a five-minute pace. Not many, but a few. I broke the marathon down into small parts, which seemed much more manageable than the full distance, and I practiced on the parts rather than the entirety. A little mental trick—that's all it was.

And it worked. In the best marathon of my life, I ran the first 18 miles at exactly a five-minute pace. I slowed a little in the last eight miles, but still averaged a 5:08 pace for the full distance, finishing in 2:14. On the one hand, I couldn't believe what I had accomplished. On the other, I realized that I had only succeeded to this degree because I had found a way to believe.

Chapter 22

89 Great Motivational Tricks

Running is easy, but sometimes getting out the door is not. Here's a list of surefire methods.

R unners often focus too much on their legs, lungs, and heart, as if these organs are crucial to their success. Well, of course! You can't run well without strong legs, lungs, and heart. But they are only a part of the process, and a small part at that. Another organ that's usually overlooked is far more important: the brain.

These days everyone knows that exercise and good nutrition are key ingredients in a healthy lifestyle. However, this doesn't for a moment guarantee that everyone establishes and follows the healthy routines. Quite the opposite, in fact, as the obesity crisis points out to us in newspaper headlines nearly every week. People know what they should do. Still, they don't get it done.

Why? Because they haven't established the motivation foundation necessary to a regular workout program. And until you get your brain in better shape, neither will you. Translation: You need to develop a very large bag of motivational tricks to ensure you follow up on your exercise resolutions and goals. This chapter presents dozens upon dozens of quick, get-you-going motivation

zingers. Follow the ones that work best for you, and add to them with a list of your own best motivators.

Work deadlines, sore hamstrings, and a mother-in-law due for dinner. You have lots of reasons to skip your run. These motivating tips, inspiring quotes, and more will help kick you out the door. Pick your fix. Repeat as necessary.

Create a blog where you post your daily mileage, then give out the Web address to your friends and family. Do you really want Aunt Ellen to ask why you skipped your four-miler on Wednesday?

Baby, get a new pair of shoes. Two-time Olympian Shayne Culpepper puts new gear she receives as an elite athlete to good use. "It's fun to break in a new pair of shoes," she says. "Sometimes that's enough to get me excited."

Running commentary: "Running is a big question mark that's there each and every day. It asks you, 'Are you going to be a wimp, or are you going to be strong today?'" —Peter Maher, two-time Olympic marathoner from Canada

Go soft. It's hard to stay motivated with shinsplints, so get off the pavement for a few days and run on a cross-country course or unpaved bike paths.

Look to the past. Emil Zatopek, who won four Olympic golds in his career, was a tough-as-nails athlete known for his intense training methods, such as running in work boots. Competing with a gland infection and against his doctor's orders, the Czech won three distance events—including the marathon—at the 1952 Helsinki Olympics. That stuffy nose doesn't seem quite so bad now, does it?

Forget time. Leave your watch at home once in a while, advises Shane Bogan, who coaches distance runners in the Washington, D.C./Baltimore area. "It's liberating not to be worried about pace," Bogan says.

Think fast. Get a boost by doing this simple

Good-To-Go Playlist: Classic Rock

- "Don't Stop Me Now," Queen
- "Break on Through," The Doors
- "Gimme Shelter," The Rolling Stones
- "Come Together," The Beatles
- "What Do You Do for Money Honey," AC/DC

negative-splits workout: Run for 20 minutes as slowly as you want, then turn around and run home faster. "The long warmup helps you feel great and run faster on the way back," says coach Christy Coughlin of Wilmette, Illinois.

Blaze a new path. "If you do the same runs all the time, it can beat you down," says Olympian Alan Culpepper. GPS systems work great for mapping new routes. Or check out favoriterun.com or usatf.org/routes, which use Google Maps to let you plan and save routes.

Running commentary. "No one can say, 'You must not run faster than this or jump higher than that.' The human spirit is indomitable." —Sir Roger Bannister, the first man to run a sub-four-minute mile

The boston marathon beckons. Think you can get there? (Go to baa.org for qualifying times.)

Race Odd Distances For An Instant PR.
Kennedy Drive 8-K, San Francisco

Run for Alex 2-miler and 5-miler, Bentleyville, Pennsylvania

Six in the Stix II, Newport, New Hampshire

Quad-City Times Bix 7-miler, Davenport, Iowa

Falmouth Road Race 7-miler, Falmouth, Massachusetts

Bigfork Valley Challenge 4.5-miler, Bigfork, Minnesota

Read this. *The Loneliness of the Long-Distance Runner*, a short story by Alan Sillitoe, tells the tale of a rebellious youth in a reformatory who runs in solitude and makes a stand against a system he doesn't believe in. You'll have new appreciation for the power of solo runs.

Play in the street. Skip a dreaded track workout for a fartlek (Swedish for "speed play")

session. After 10 minutes of easy jogging, run hard between two telephone poles, then slow down until you pass three. Then see if you can get to the traffic light before it changes, followed by a jog to the next mailbox. There are no set rules, so make it up as you go along.

The pile of dishes in the sink can wait until the sun goes down. Your tempo run can't.

Run at lunch. Daniel Sheil, a marathon coach in Portland, Oregon, recommends lunch-time runs for two reasons: (1) You get your workout in before the day gets away from you; (2) You get a midday break from work stress.

Running commentary: "The more I run, the more I want to run, and the more I live a life conditioned and influenced and fashioned by my running. And the more I run, the more certain I am that I am heading for my real goal: to become the person I am." —George Sheehan, M.D., beloved former *RW* columnist

That new running watch you want? Buy it—after timing 10 more speed sessions with your old one.

Watch this. In the stirring 1981 Oscar winner for Best Picture, *Chariots of Fire*, two British athletes prepare for and compete in the 1924 summer Olympics. For bonus motivation, download the famous Vangelis theme to your MP3 player for tomorrow's run.

Wear a pedometer on your run. Distance sounds more impressive in steps. Some tricked-out sports watches also record steps.

Buddy up. Not many people can keep up with nine-time University of Colorado all-American Sara Slattery. Luckily, two-time Olympian Shayne Culpepper happens to live down the street. Find your own version of the Olympian next door to run with regularly.

Look to the past. In 1949, 9-year-old Wilma Rudolph learned to walk without leg braces after suffering from polio and spending most of her first years in bed. Rudolph went on to win three gold medals in the 1960 Olympics.

Have a daily goal. Scott Jurek, seven-time champion of The Western States 100-Mile Endurance Run, sets goals not just for big races but also for workouts. "Maybe it is a technique goal, maybe a pace goal, maybe a goal of running faster at the end," he says.

Make a massage appointment for the day after your long run.

Watch this. Baseball had Babe Ruth. Basketball had Michael Jordan. American distance running had Steve Prefontaine. Doesn't matter that he wasn't the best ever—he was the sport's rock star. *Prefontaine* (1997) and *Without Limits* (1998) both capture Pre's cocky swagger. Or check out the 1995 documentary *Fire on the Track: The Steve Prefontaine Story.*

Get yourself a hearty dog who needs lots of exercise. You'll always have a reason for a daily jog.

Run through a spring storm. With rain

Good-To-Go Playlist: Country

- Cocaine Blues," Johnny Cash
- "Ain't Going Down (Til the Sun Comes Up)," Garth Brooks
- "Wide Open Spaces," Dixie Chicks
- "Chasin' That Neon Rainbow," Alan Jackson
- "The Devil Went Down to Georgia," The Charlie Daniels Band

hitting you sideways and the wind whipping your face, you'll feel alive. Just make sure you have a dry pair of shoes for tomorrow.

Read this. The cult classic *Once a Runner*, by talented runner John L. Parker Jr., captures the hard work and dedication required of fictional collegiate miler Quenton Cassidy.

Feel a need for speed. Sometimes you need the thrill of moving your legs as fast asthey can go. To get the wind blowing through your hair, try six to eight 200-meter repeats at your mile race pace.

For emergency use only: Consider taking a short break from running if you think you've got the beginning of an overuse injury or you're truly fatigued. A couple days of rest may be the thing to reinvigorate you. Call it instant running motivation for three days from now.

Exercise improves sexual performance, according to research. Nuff said.

It's never too late to salvage your New Year's resolutions.

Read this. *Pain*, by Dan Middleman. Fictional college senior Richard Dubin attempts to balance hard partying, a complicated relationship, and world-class competition.

Good-To-Go Playlist: Hip-Hop

- "If I Should Die," Jay-Z
- "Get By," Talib Kweli
- "Let's Get It Started," Black Eyed Peas
- "Lose Yourself," Eminem
- "Bombs Over Baghdad," OutKast
- "Get Low," Lil Jon
- "Caught Out There," Kelis

Good-To-Go Playlist: Alternative Rock

- "Beautiful Day," U2
- "Run in Place," The Nadas
- "Seven Nation Army," The White Stripes
- "Take Me Out," Franz Ferdinand
- "Get Free," The Vines
- "Just (You Do It to Yourself)," Radiohead

Go early. Two-time Olympian Shayne Culpepper says that rather than putting off a run, she'll head out even earlier than usual when she's not in the mood to work out. "If I have that extra cup of coffee or I wait an extra half hour, it becomes too torturous," she says.

Look to the past. Billy Mills came out of nowhere in the 1964 Olympics to become the only American to win a gold medal in the 10,000 meters. Mills's PR at the time was nearly a minute slower than that of Australia's Ron Clarke. With 100 meters to go, Mills sprinted ahead, improving his PR and setting a new Olympic record.

If you're really in the mood to change things up, or if you just have nothing to wear, check out the list of clothing-optional races at cybernude.com/nuderuns.

Pay yourself. Set a price for attaining a certain weekly mileage goal. When you hit it, pay up. Keep your mileage money in a jar, and once it accumulates, buy yourself that new running jacket you've been ogling.

Ask a friend to bike alongside you when your running partner isn't available.

Get wet. Log your miles by running in the deep end of a pool while wearing a flotation vest. Break it up by going hard for five minutes, then resting for one minute. Work up to an hour.

Race Results stay on Google forever.

Turn things around. "A poor performance is a strong motivator for me," says elite marathoner Clint Verran. "I can't wait to prove to myself that I'm a better runner than my last showing." Verran also says negative comments from his coaches fire him up. "For me, proving somebody wrong is key."

Been marathoning for years? Maybe it's time to try an ultra. Or the mile.

Become a running mentor. Once you get your neighbor, coworker, or significant other hooked on your favorite sport, they'll be counting on your continued support and guidance—and company.

Feeling tired? Instead of taking the day off, throw some walk breaks into your run. Use the breaks to refuel, stretch out sore muscles, or get inspired by the scenery.

Head for the hills. "When I need a boost, I attack a hill workout," says Greg Meyer, winner of the 1982 Chicago Marathon and 1983 Boston Marathon. "You can't do hills halfhearted." Meyer believes the difficulty of the workout brings out the best in him.

Watch this. In the 2005 Canadian film *Saint Ralph*, a teenager sets out to win the 1954 Boston Marathon, thinking this is the "miracle" required to wake his mother from a coma.

Run for a reason. Do a race for charity. Helping kids with diabetes or women with breast cancer makes it much easier to get out the door.

Dust off your track spikes. Most states have Olympic-style summer games where you can compete in events like the mile or the 400-meter hurdles. If you're really looking for a change of pace, train for a field event like the long jump.

Running commentary: "Workouts are like brushing my teeth; I don't think about it, I just do it. The decision has already been made."—PattiSue Plumer, U.S. Olympian.

Remember that you almost always feel better after a run than before it.

Look to the past. Roger Bannister and John Landy (the only two men to have broken four minutes in the mile at the time) raced at the 1954 British Empire and Commonwealth Games in Vancouver in what was billed as "The Miracle Mile." Landy led for most of the race, but Bannister passed him on the final turn—proving it ain't over till it's over.

Running commentary: "If you want to become the best runner you can be, start now. Don't spend the rest of your life wondering if you can do it." —Priscilla Welch, who won the 1987 New York City Marathon at age 42

Keep a log. Greg Meyer, former Boston Marathon and Chicago Marathon champ, says his logbook keeps him motivated. "I just can't stand to look at my log and see a goose egg for the day," he says.

Make a connection. Fitness-singles.com connects active people looking for love. Get in your run and go on a date at the same time.

Bring home some hardware. Okay, so you're not going to win the Chicago Marathon, but that doesn't mean you can't score a trophy. Find a few small local races where you might be able to compete for the top spots in your age group.

Don't expect every day to be better than the last. Some days will be slower than others, and some days might even hurt a bit. But as long as you're on the road, it's a good day.

If you don't run road races, where will you get all your T-shirts?

Just start. If the thought of running your full workout is too much to bear, just suit up to run around the block. Chances are, once you're outside, you'll start to feel better and put in at least a few miles.

Read this. *Bowerman and the Men of Oregon,* by Kenny Moore. Learn about Bill Bowerman, one of the most famous track and field coaches of the past century and cofounder of Nike. You'll be surprised how the legend initiated his new runners at the University of Oregon.

Run solo and away from the crowds on recovery days. The faster runners on popular routes will make you want to pick up the pace. Alone, you'll be able to listen to your body and reap the recovery you deserve.

Running commentary: "Those who say that I will lose and am finished will have to run over my body to beat me." —Said Aouita, 5000 meter Olympic gold medalist

You're never too old for a gold star, says Sacramento-area running coach Shauna Schultz. Plan your workouts a week in advance, then place a star sticker on the calendar for each day you meet your goal. "Visualizing your progress in this manner is very encouraging," Schultz says.

Become a race director. If you live in a small town with no road races, start your own. Most towns have some sort of yearly celebration in the summer, and you can tie the race to that. Work with local track and cross-country teams to help promote it.

Run an errand—literally. Run to get cash at the ATM, buy that lottery ticket for the mega-million-dollar prize, or return the DVD to the rental store.

Good-To-Go Playlist: Guilty Pleasures

- "Good Vibrations," Marky Mark and the Funky Bunch
- "Toxic," Britney Spears
- "Lovefool," The Cardigans
- "Flagpole Sitta," Harvey Danger
- "Fergalicious," Fergie

Check weather.com. If you know it's going to be 110 degrees by 2 P.M., run early in the morning. Terrible thunderstorms on Saturday? There's your day off. Proactive scheduling now will give you fewer excuses later.

Quit running in circles. Group "point to point" runs are a fun way to mix things up, says Andy Steinfeld, who coaches marathon runners in Maryland. His runners head out for 12 to 20 miles, then refuel at a local restaurant before hopping on the subway to ride back to the starting point.

Watch this. The 1999 docudrama *Endurance* shows how Ethiopian Haile Gebrselassie became one of the best distance runners of all time.

Create conflict. Drew Ludtke, head women's track and cross-country coach at the University of St. Francis in Joliet, Illinois, says his runners are sometimes too social. So he tells them to imagine that the runner next to them just stole their boyfriend, which amps up the competition—and the fun.

Run trails to challenge your body and mind. "Trails are a fantastic way to give your training a change of pace," says Long Beach, California, coach

Todd Rose. Rose advises always running trails with a partner and a cell phone to stay safe.

Be realistic with your training. Sticking to a schedule of three workouts per week feels a lot better than quitting a more demanding plan. Go to runnersworld.com/smartcoach to customize your training program.

Live in the now. Seven-time Western States champ Scott Jurek focuses on the moment to get him through rough spots. "I tune in to my breath, technique, and my current pace, and I stay away from what lies ahead," he says. This is especially helpful when "what lies ahead" is another 99 miles.

Get some perspective. Eritrean-born U.S. runner and 2004 Olympic Marathon silver medalist Meb Keflezighi listens to songs about his former country's struggle for independence from Ethiopia when he needs a boost. "The true heroes are the soldiers," he says, also mentioning American troops in Iraq. "Those are the real tough guys."

Buy a full-length mirror and make sure you look in it every day.

Read this. *Life at These Speeds*, by Jeremy Jackson. When an entire track team is killed on the way home from a meet at the beginning of this novel, star Kevin Schuler, who rode home with his parents, is left to pick up the pieces. Sad but stirring.

Good-To-Go Playlist: Silence

■ Leave the MP3 player at home and see how you like it. Sometimes, the rhythm of your own breathing is the most inspiring thing of all.

Wear gold racing shoes. With those on your feet, you'd better be fast. It worked for Michael Johnson.

Try a tri. Logging a chunk of your weekly miles in the pool and on the bike for a triath-lon can reinvigorate your mind and body—and running.

Sale away. When online running coach (therunningcoach.com) Christine Hinton is feeling unmotivated, she heads out for what she calls a Garage Sale Run. "I take some cash or my checkbook with me and run in search of garage sales," Hinton says. "When I find one, I stop briefly to check out the goods. I tell you, I have found some good stuff that I've picked up later with the car."

Running commentary: "The will to win means nothing without the will to prepare." — Juma Ikangaa, 1989 New York City Marathon champion

A healthy runner is a happy runner. As soon as you feel like you might be coming down with something, pamper yourself: Eat more healthfully (think lots of fruits and veggies), and get extra rest. A little prevention today means you won't be debating next week whether you're too sick to run.

Listening to your feet crunch gravel for an hour can erase a day's worth of stress.

Invest in good gear. For beginners, this may mean a good pair of running shoes to avoid injuries and technical clothes made of fabric that wicks away moisture and prevents chafing. For others, experimenting with the latest GPS unit or shoe pod can be a fun way to track training progress and stay motivated.

Be creative. If the idea of going on your regular four-miler just sinks you further into your recliner, remember that there are other ways to put in some miles—like a pickup game of soccer, flag football, or ultimate Frisbee. A soccer midfielder runs up to six miles in a regulation 90-minute game.

Forget about the big picture every now and then. Put away your training manual and your race calendar. Quit overthinking it. Run for today.

Amby Burfoot's Running Round-Up

As I read these concluding words to this chapter, I've personally logged about 103,000 miles since I began running at age 16. (I'm now 62.) I've also finished the same Thanksgiving Day race for 46 years in a row. When it comes to motivation, I seem to score quite high. How have I managed this? For the most part, it's very simple.

In fact, the KISS system—Keep It Simple, Stupid—has formed a big part of my approach. I don't obsess about the color of my running shoes or the technologies inside. I just pick shoes that feel right when I lace them up and do a test run on the sidewalk. I probably don't own a set of matching shorts and singlets, and I haven't strapped on a heart-rate monitor in about 15 years. Sure, I like digital stuff as much as the next guy, but none of it has ever improved my running, at least not since the invention decades ago of lightweight plastic wrist chronographs.

When I want to go fast, I do, though I don't last as long as I used to. When I want to go slow, which is most of the time, I'm happy to amble along. When I need a walking break, I take one. Time was, I thought that anyone who slowed to a walk ought to be taken out back and shot. Now I see walking as just an activity that occurs at one end of the running scale. Both walking and running involve moving the feet, one in front of the other. It's just that walkers don't move quite as fast as runners. Otherwise, it's the same thing.

I no longer try to run every day of the week. Instead, I try to run more days than I don't run, which usually means four times a week. And I'm not afraid to add other exercise like stationary bicycling (my favorite because I can read and exercise at the same time), swimming, and strength training. I also run and walk with friends as often as possible. That's the ultimate motivational trick, though I understand dogs are good, too. When you have someone else waiting and depending on you, well, that's the surest way to get yourself moving.

Chapter 23

Reach All Your Goals

Whether you aim to improve your training, racing, motivation, injury prevention, or workout consistency, here's the path to follow

Running is a sport overflowing with possible goals. You can aim for faster times on the track, more strength on the cross-country course, or more endurance in the marathon. You can set your sights on a 20-pound weight loss, or an increase in quadriceps strength or hamstring flexibility. You can pick out new goals for every year, every season, and every new age-group you enter.

With so many goals to reach, how do you accomplish them all? The obvious answer: one at a time. Running breeds patience, one of the crucial components of high-level achievement. It also teaches that many small steps add up to a mile, first, and then a 5-K or 10-K or however far you want to go.

Variety is another important ingredient to success in running. You can't spend all your time churning out the miles, and you shouldn't. Instead, you should pick occasional nutrition goals—eat less sugar and saturated fat, for example—and some goals that can only be attacked in the gym. Any exercise that strengthens the tissues and muscles around the knees is a friend to all runners.

From time to time, focus on your knees.

Or pick other goals, such as the ones outlined in the pages that follow, and go for them!

Nobody reaches all their goals, but without having one or two in front of you at all times, you won't achieve any.

GOAL: Run a Six- (or Seven- or Eight-) Minute Mile

No matter how much time you want to knock off your mile, Greg McMillan, founder of the McMillan

Running Company personalized coaching service, says the first step is to increase your stride frequency. You'll develop a lighter, quicker step by running short, submaximal repeats engineered to adapt your neuromuscular system—your body's intricate network of brain, nerve, and muscle. "After even two or three of these workouts, the body seems to adapt, and people are already running faster," says McMillan. After several weeks of boosting your stride frequency, add longer, pace-specific interval work to fine-tune your speed to meet your time goal.

THE PLAN

Twice each week (but not on consecutive days), warm up for 10 to 15 minutes, then begin a series of ten 15-second repeats at 90 percent of your top speed. After each repeat, recover with one or two minutes of easy running. Every week, increase the interval time by five seconds, until you're up to 45 seconds, at which point cut these workouts to once per week and add one of the pace-specific interval workouts below per week for six weeks.

Note: › indicates that you should start at the slow end of the pace range given, then gradually increase the speed of each repeat.

WEEK: 1, 3, 5

Workout: 6 to 8 x 400 meters with 200-meter recovery jog

Six-minute miler: 1:30 › 1:25

Seven-minute miler: 1:44 › 1:39

Eight-minute miler: 2:00 › 1:54

WEEK: 2, 4, 6

Workout: 4 to 6 x 800 meters with 400-meter recovery jog

Six-minute miler: 3:06 › 2:58

Seven-minute miler: 3:38 › 3:29

Eight-minute miler: 4:09 › 3:58

GOAL: Run Negative Splits

Despite the pessimistic name, negative splits—when you complete the second half of a run or race faster than the first—are perhaps the most positive path to running nirvana. "When you run a well-executed negative-split race, it's the best you'll ever feel as a runner," says Jenny Hadfield, coauthor of *Marathoning for Mortals*. But to be successful, you need more than physical ability. "It takes confidence," says Hadfield. "You need to hold back early, with the certainty that you'll have what it takes to turn it on later."

THE PLAN

Find an out-and-back, relatively flat course that will take you approximately 50 minutes to run. On the way out, run at a comfortable, but not easy, pace (about 75 percent of your maximum heart rate). When you hit the turnaround, bump up the intensity to 85 percent. "You're not going all-out, but you're definitely working," says Hadfield. Run this workout once per week in the five weeks leading up to your goal race.

GOAL: Kill the Hills

Running up a hill too fast not only hurts, it can also ruin a run or a race. "You have to think of hills within the context of the whole run," says Hadfield, "Most people freak out and run up the hill as fast as they can. Then they're pretty much done."

The key to running a hilly course well is to hold your effort level steady as the road or trail tilts skyward. If you're wearing a heart-rate monitor, strive to keep the number constant as you leave the flats behind. Otherwise, just think even effort, not even pace, and make peace with slowing down. Hadfield promises you'll be faster over the long haul. "It's not just about how fast you can go up the hill," she says. "It's about how fast you can go up and down the other side. If you're not cooked from the climb, you can make up time on the descent."

THE PLAN

Once a week, alternate between the following two hill workouts.

Even-effort hills: This workout teaches you how to run hills strategically. Find a rolling course the length of a medium-distance run, or use a treadmill to simulate a medium-distance hilly course. After a 10-minute warmup, run at 75 to 80 percent of your maximum heart rate, and maintain this effort level going up each hill. As you crest the hills, open your stride and gently lean into the hill using gravity to pull you down faster without increasing your effort.

Power hills: These hill repeats build strength and stamina. Find a moderately steep hill

that takes you one or two minutes to run up, or simulate such a hill on a treadmill (a three- to five-percent grade). After a 10-minute warmup, run up the hill at a hard pace. Jog very slowly down the back side of the hill. Try five to eight repeats, and add one or two each session, or do the same number but try to run the incline faster as you get fitter.

GOAL: Improve Your Finishing Kick

Many runners think that a strong finishing kick is all about the end of a race. In reality, it's more about how you prepare for and run the beginning and middle of a race. That's because to have a finishing kick, you have to have something left in the tank for the final stretch. "When you go out too hard or you do minimal running at race pace before the event, it's pretty much impossible to finish strong," says Jason Koop, a pro-level coach with Carmichael Training Systems.

"For races up to and including the 10-K, you need to train at your race pace in a series of intervals that eventually add up to the whole race distance," says Koop. "For races longer than 10-K, duplicate pace only, not duration, since you'd need too much recovery at the longer distances."

THE PLAN

Run each of these two workouts once a week, but not on consecutive days.

Target-pace intervals: The goal of this workout is to eventually run your goal-race distance (10-K or shorter) at target race pace in a series of intervals. For example, if your goal is to run a 10-K at a six-minute-per-mile pace, break the distance into six one-mile efforts at six-minute pace separated by three minutes of easy jogging, or 12 half-mile (800-meter) repeats at race pace with 90 seconds of jogging in between. To begin, try running repeats equaling up to half the distance of your goal race. Then add more each week until you reach the whole distance. If you can't maintain the same pace for each repeat, you're building too fast. For longer goals, such as a half-marathon or marathon, practice race pace in one- or two-mile segments as part of longer runs.

Pick-me-up pick-ups: Once a week, during an easy run, throw in four to six 60-second pick-ups, where you increase your pace to a hard (not all-out) effort. Run easy for at least five minutes in between. During the pick-ups, concentrate on increasing your cadence and remaining light on your feet. The goal is to develop leg speed you can call on when the line is in sight.

GOAL: Injury-Proof Your Body

"You have to make prevention a priority," says Mark Fadil, a massage therapist and Team in Training coach. "By the time someone comes in with an injury, there's almost always been a progression that could have been halted earlier."

According to Matt Fitzgerald, online coach (trainingpeaks.com) and author of *Runner's World Guide to Cross-Training*, the key to preventing most running injuries is to increase the strength and stability of three important joint areas: the hips, knees, and ankles. "Most people blame impact for running injuries," says Fitzgerald. "The real problem is how impact can affect joint stability. If you can strengthen and stabilize these areas, impact becomes less of a problem."

THE PLAN

Do this combination of four exercises two or three times per week after an easy run.

For Hip Stability: Single-Leg Romanian Deadlift: Stand on your right foot only with your left leg slightly bent and your arms relaxed at your sides, a light dumbbell in each hand. Tilt your torso forward from the hips and reach toward the floor with both dumbbells. Extend your left leg backward for balance. Now return to the starting position. Concentrate on keeping your abs tight and your posture neutral throughout this movement.

Hip Hiker: Stand with your left foot on the floor and your right foot on a six-inch step or similar elevated surface. Straighten your right leg and pull your left foot up even with your right. Balance for five seconds, then lower your left foot back to the floor, but without putting your weight on it. Do 12 to 20 repetitions, keeping your full weight on your right leg throughout, then work your left hip.

For Knee Stability: VMO (Vastus Medialis) Dip: Stand normally on a stable elevated surface, such as an exercise step that's six to 12 inches high, with your toes even with the edge. Shift your full weight onto your right foot and reach down toward the floor in front of the step with your left foot. Touch your left heel to the floor without putting any weight on it and return to the starting position. Do 10 to 12 repetitions and repeat with the right leg.

For Ankle Stability: Pillow Balancing: Remove your shoes, place a pillow on the floor, and balance on it on one foot for 30 seconds. Switch feet and repeat. At first it might be difficult to last 30 seconds, but you'll improve quickly. Keep it challenging by using a bigger or softer pillow, or by stacking pillows, balancing longer, or closing your eyes as you try to balance.

GOAL: Stay Fit with the Time You Have

Anyone who has all the time they want to run is either a professional athlete or unemployed and childless. For the rest of us, Mark Allen, six-time Ironman champion, has some good news. "By spending a mere 20 minutes in your aerobic zone, at least every three days, you can hold onto your hard-earned fitness," he says.

Sixty minutes a week? Is the man kidding? No, he's not. Ideally, you'd want to shoot for 20 minutes of aerobic exercise every day. But when you can't fit in a daily 20-minute workout, the goal is to not let more than two days of rest go by between workouts. "It's on the third day of inactivity that your fitness really begins to slide," says Allen.

THE PLAN

If you have . . .

60 minutes/week: Three 20-minute runs. For each, run easy for five minutes, then focus on maintaining a high cadence of around 180 footstrikes per minute.

80 minutes/week: Three 20-minute runs as above and add two 10-minute strength-training sessions after two of your runs. "The strength training will help you maintain joint and muscle integrity, which is going to be important when you have more time and can start ramping up the miles again," says Allen.

100 minutes/week: Three 20-minute runs as above and two 20-minute strength-training sessions.

120 minutes/week: Two 20-minute runs, one 40-minute run, and two 20-minute strength-training sessions.

140 minutes/week: Same as 120 minutes per week, but slowly add time to your long run.

160 minutes/week: What are you complaining about?

GOAL: Never Bonk Again

Sometimes you can feel it coming, as if you're running into a pool of steadily deepening water. Other times it hits with all the subtlety of Howard Stern. The bonk. It's the equivalent of your car running out of gas—in the middle of the interstate. The trick is to consume the right amount of calories—at the right time.

THE PLAN

Eat early: "One of the biggest nutritional mistakes I see runners making is back-loading their day," says Nancy Clark, R.D., author of *Food Guide for Marathoners: Tips for Everyday Champions.* Clark notes that even experienced athletes often eat too little at breakfast and lunch, only to find themselves famished in the evening hours. The result? Erratic running performance. Instead, start your day off with at least a 400- to 600-calorie breakfast that's high in carbs but also offers some protein and good fats. Think oatmeal with a dollop of yogurt or some trail mix with nuts and raisins.

Consider time: If you're running for less than an hour, don't sweat it. "Your body has plenty of stored glycogen for up to an hour of exercise," says Liz Applegate, Ph.D., nutrition editor for *Runner's World* magazine. For runs over an hour, fuel up according to your body weight. Two hours before, eat one gram of carbohydrate for every pound. An hour before, top off with another half gram of carbs per pound (for the average runner, that's an energy bar).

Munch on the run: During runs over an hour, eat 100 calories of carbs every 30 minutes from the beginning to maintain your energy levels.

Refuel posthaste: The one-hour period immediately following exercise is when your body is most receptive to refueling, and meals with a four-to-one carbs-to-protein ratio are best for restoring your glycogen supply. "Any sandwich with meat and vegetables should have what you need," says Applegate. Reloading your energy reserves soon after they've been depleted will help ensure that you won't bonk the next time you head out.

GOAL: Run Every Day

You could forgive Mark Allen for skipping a run or two. After all, the man won six Ironman triath-lons, including a record-setting five consecutive victories starting in 1989. Allen, now a 48-year-old business owner and father, still works out at least once every day, alternating between running, lifting weights, and surfing. Here's how Allen keeps his motivation for daily exercise high and his risk of injury low.

THE PLAN

Slow down: "If you want to be a runner for life," says Allen, "90 percent of your training should be in your aerobic zone, which is around 75 percent of your maximum heart rate. That's where you're going to stimulate your systems, rather than wearing them down."

Double up on goals: "To stay motivated year after year, you need to have a clear vision of why you're running. A lot of people decide to run a marathon, do it, and then never lace up their running shoes again. So you need to have life-marker goals, like running a marathon, *and* goals that simply keep you consistent, like running to maintain weight or ensure a high quality of life."

Think body over mind: Allen believes that if you take care of your body—get enough rest, cross-train, eat right—your mental motivation will follow. "So many people dive into running programs with 1,000 pounds of motivation, which usually leads to injury and burnout." When you're feeling great, motivation comes naturally.

Pump it up: "Weight training is a low-stress way to get the strength benefits of speedwork without pounding your body. To stay strong, I recommend two 30-minute weight sessions per week, except in the three weeks before a race."

Amby Burfoot's Running Round-Up

When I was younger, in my early 20s, I wanted to run fast marathons, and I wanted to do them yesterday. Tomorrow just didn't seem soon enough. I had little patience, and I needed to see signs that I was getting stronger and faster on an almost weekly basis. This approach led to some significant breakthroughs, and some disastrous breakdowns.

With age, I got smarter about my goals. Not a lot, mind you. I'm not claiming to be running's Albert Einstein. But the accumulation of years and miles brought a certain wisdom with them. I still wanted to run fast from time to time, but I realized that I couldn't control certain aspects of my training and racing. To an extent, I would have to go with the flow. I took the high tides as far as they would carry me, and tried not to get depressed by the low tides.

Mostly I learned the truth of the old Biblical passage: "For everything there is a season." I began to see that I couldn't be in top shape every single day. Indeed, I would never attain a fitness peak if I didn't accept rest days and longer rest periods as a necessary part of life and running. I also began to understand that I couldn't focus entirely on hard running to get in shape. I needed more cross-training, and even some strength training and stretching. These latter two were never my favorite activities, but I found that I could set modest goals in both arenas, and reap bigger-than-expected rewards. That kept me motivated.

I might not have put all the pieces together perfectly. But I saw that there were more pieces than the narrow focus of my 20s had revealed. And that working toward many small goals was often a smarter approach than chasing one huge, overwhelming goal.

VII

Cross-Training

Chapter 24

Train Better by Running Less

Cross-Train Your Way to Stronger Races

Cross-training can be a tough concept for many runners to grasp. It's not that we don't believe that a variety of workouts is good for us. It's just that we can't figure out where the training time is going to come from. Making time for a 30- to 40-minute run is often difficult enough. How are you going to swim and bike and row and all that stuff?

We probably feel this way about cross-training because of all the attention the Hawaii Ironman Triathlon has received in the past 25 years. The amazing Ironman athletes swim 2½ miles, bike 110 miles, and then finish off with a jaunty little marathon. And to prepare for the Ironman, which takes 9 to 10 hours (or much more for the middle- and back-of-the-pack racers), some triathletes train almost that many hours per day. Who needs it?

Fortunately, no one but an Ironman athlete needs it. The rest of us can benefit from much more realistic doses of cross-training. Still, it's hard to figure out how to begin and how much and what kinds of cross-training to do. These are the questions that are answered in this chapter.

Life used to be simple. Runners ran, and swimmers swam. Bicyclists pedaled, weight lifters grunted, and Ed Sullivan was on TV every Sunday night. Then everything got mixed up. Runners started cycling, swimmers lifted weights, cyclists starting running . . .

The weirdness probably started with the first Hawaii Ironman Triathlon in 1978. Things have gotten even weirder since. Now, it's not unusual to see athletes climbing stairs that go nowhere or cross-country skiing over a gym floor. What next? Some futurist will probably figure out a way to ice-skate without ice.

Strangest of all, while these varied activities may look a bit wacky, they're actually very good for you. By doing them, you'll stretch certain muscles, strengthen others, and burn plenty of calories.

But what exactly is cross-training supposed

to do for runners, you wonder? And, given all the cross-training choices, which are the best ones for you?

This subject has been examined by some of the nation's leading exercise physiologists, debated by numerous elite runners, and discussed in scores of sports-medicine journals. And there's a raging debate on the topic. The controversy involves three major points of view.

1. The do-more, get-fitter theory. Proponents of this position believe that runners should cross-train with exercises and activities that are as close to running as possible. The logic: The stronger you can make your running muscles, the better you'll run.

2. The rest theory. According to this approach, runners should cross-train with sports that are as different from running as possible. The logic: You can burn calories and get a good workout. At the same time, you'll be resting your running muscles and won't be creating the one-sport muscle imbalances that often lead to injury.

3. The specificity theory. Specificity advocates believe that runners shouldn't cross-train—period. It's a waste of time and will only tire you for your next run. When you need a day off from running, take a day off from everything. The logic: Training is sport specific, so the best way to train for running is to run.

No wonder so many runners are confused about cross-training. Who are they supposed to believe, and which theory should they follow? "All of the approaches make sense and could work," says Mike Flynn, Ph.D., an exercise physiologist and one of the nation's leading researchers in cross-training. The trick to optimizing your training program, he explains, is to pick the approach that best fits your current running and fitness goals.

To make your decision easier, we've designed cross-training programs for five different types of runners. Simply find the category that best describes you and follow the suggested advice.

BEGINNING RUNNERS

This is for runners who log five to 15 miles per week.

The basics: If you're running to get into shape, the first thing you need to do is build your cardiovascular system. A strong heart and strong lungs will supply more fuel to your working leg muscles, which will allow you to run without constantly feeling out of breath.

If you're switching to running from another sport, you're probably fit enough to run a few miles without much problem, but don't try to do too much too soon. Running involves more pounding than most other sports, and it takes a while for the muscles, tendons, and ligaments to adapt.

The program: The best cross-training program for beginners is one that mixes running and cross-training in equal amounts. If you're running twice a week, then try cross-training twice a week as well. This will allow you to build your cardiovascular system and muscle strength simultaneously, without undue risk of injury. Another good idea: Since your body may not be prepared to handle more than one hard run a week, split your hard workouts between running and cross-training.

The exercises: As a beginning runner, almost any aerobic activity will help increase your cardiovascular strength. The best exercises are those that also strengthen as many of your running muscles as possible. These exercises will improve the coordination of your running muscles and teach them to process and store fuel more effectively.

INTERMEDIATE RUNNERS

This is for runners who log 15 to 40 miles per week.

The basics: You have developed a strong cardiovascular system through your running. Hence, easy cross-training workouts won't improve your running performance. You need to choose cross-training activities that either provide a very high intensity cardiovascular workout or specifically target your running muscles.

The program: You should be running two to three times as much as you are cross-training. Run for two or three days, and then do a cross-training workout. If you are doing two hard runs a week, select cross-training workouts that allow you to exercise at a moderate pace. You should be using these workouts just to give your running muscles some extra training without extra pounding. If your body can handle only one hard run a week, then one of your cross-training workouts should be an interval or tempo workout (a run that starts off easy, builds to a steady speed in the middle, and then finishes at an easy pace).

The exercises: Cross-training exercises that provide high-intensity, cardiovascular workouts are cross-country skiing, stair climbing, and high-cadence stationary cycling. "Grinding away in a high gear on a bike will slow your turnover,

Get cross-training

The best cross-training exercises for beginning runners are in-line skating, cross-country skiing, and stair climbing. Although circuit weight training won't do much for your aerobic endurance, a twice-a-week program is a good idea. It can help build your body's protection against running-related injuries.

but using a high cadence (over 90 rpms) will keep you quick and allow you to get your heart rate up," says Tim Moore, Ph.D. For muscle-specific workouts, stick with cross-country skiing, in-line skating, and stair climbing.

ADVANCED RUNNERS

This is for runners who log more than 40 miles per week.

The basics: You have probably maximized your cardiovascular conditioning, as well as the strength, efficiency, and coordination of your leg muscles, so cross-training won't directly do you much good. To improve your running performance, you need more quality in your runs. Running coaches and exercise physiologists generally recommend at least two hard runs per week—a shorter interval session on the track and a longer tempo run on the road or trails.

The program: Since both hard running and high mileage can increase your injury risk, your best bet may be complete rest. This will allow your muscles to recover completely for your next run. If you don't want to take days off, you can consider low-intensity cross-training with a sport that doesn't tax your running muscles. This will burn calories, and the variety will keep you mentally

Why weights?

For advanced runners, a twice-a-week circuit weight-training program will also strengthen your leg muscles so that they can withstand the pounding of high-mileage, high-intensity running.

Weight training is also very important for injury-prone athletes, as it helps strengthen muscles, tendons, and ligaments. As a result, the stresses of running are distributed more evenly.

fresh. Some researchers have even found that very light activity may help you recover more quickly than complete rest.

If you choose to cross-train, replace one or two of your easy runs—preferably the ones that come a day after a hard run—with a cross-training activity.

The exercises: Cycling, swimming, pool running, and rowing all will give your running muscles a break and let them recover for your next hard run.

INJURY-PRONE RUNNERS

This is for runners who experience two or more running-related injuries per year.

The basics: Surveys show that two out of every three runners will experience a running injury in the course of a year. "With two to three times your body weight coming down on your legs with every stride, each step you run brings you closer to injury," says Flynn. "And if you have even the slightest biomechanical problem, the risk is even greater."

But this doesn't mean that you can't run. Cross-training can help in two ways. First, it can keep you healthy by allowing you to stay fit without the constant pounding of running. Second, cross-training can help forestall the performance losses that come when an injury keeps you from running. Studies have shown that runners can maintain their running times for up to six weeks by cross-training alone if it is done at the proper intensity.

The program: The best cross-training program for injury-prone runners includes two to four runs per week (depending on how much your body can tolerate) and two cross-training workouts. Both cross-training workouts should target running-specific muscles in order to increase their strength and efficiency without subjecting them to pounding.

The extra training of these muscles through cross-training rarely produces injuries since pounding is the primary injury culprit. But if you're unsure about an exercise, ask your doctor. Also, since many running injuries are induced by high-intensity workouts, don't run more than one of these per week. Looking for more burn? Get it from your cross-training, not from your running.

The exercises: As stated above, injury-prone runners should keep their cross-training work-outs as specific to running as possible. In-line skating, stair climbing, rowing, and cross-country skiing are good choices. Unfortunately, some injuries—stress fractures in particular—don't afford you many cross-training options. In these cases, cross-training in the pool by swimming or deep-water running is the best alternative. These are non-weight-bearing activities that don't stress the legs.

Cross-Training Guide

The chart below provides an outline for your running and cross-training (x-training) workouts. In addition, for almost all runners, several circuit weight-training workouts per week will strengthen the upper body and certain leg muscles. Don't mix circuit weight training with a hard running schedule, however.

BEGINNING RUNNER

Running Days	Running Days, Hard	X-Training Days	X-Training Days, Hard	Best X-Training Activities
2	1	2	1	In-line skating, cross-country skiing, stair climbing

INTERMEDIATE RUNNER

Running Days	Running Days, Hard	X-Training Days	X-Training Days, Hard	Best X-Training Activities
3-5	1-2	2	1	Bicycling, in-line skating, cross-country skiing

ADVANCED RUNNER

Running Days	Running Days, Hard	X-Training Days	X-Training Days, Hard	Best X-Training Activities
5-6	2	0-2	0	Bicycling, swimming, pool running, rowing

INJURY-PRONE RUNNER

Running Days	Running Days, Hard	X-Training Days	X-Training Days, Hard	Best X-Training Activities
2-4	0-1	2-3	1-2	In-line skating, cross-country skiing, stair climbing, swimming, pool running, rowing

GENERAL-FITNESS RUNNER

Running Days	Running Days, Hard	X-Training Days	X-Training Days, Hard	Best X-Training Activities
2	0	2	1	Swimming, rowing, cross-country skiing, bicycling with arm resistance

GENERAL-FITNESS RUNNERS

This is for low- to mid-mileage runners who are more concerned with overall fitness than racing performance.

The basics: Look at any elite runner, and you'll notice that running doesn't do much for the upper body. It also neglects the quadriceps in favor of the calves, hamstrings, and buttocks. Furthermore, after the age of 30, all the muscles in our bodies begin to lose some of their strength and energy-producing abilities. Fortunately, exercise can cut the rate of these losses almost in half.

The program: The best cross-training program for general-fitness runners targets the muscles that running neglects.

"Running is great for the cardiovascular system, but if you're concerned about your overall well-being, you need to cross-train with a range of activities," says exercise physiologist David L. Costill, Ph.D., director of the Human Performance Laboratory at Ball State University in Muncie, Indiana.

For total-body fitness, run twice a week, and do a complementary exercise on one or two other days of the week. In addition, 20 minutes of circuit weight training twice a week will help you condition any muscles that you may have missed.

The exercises: General-fitness runners need exercises that target the upper body and quadriceps. The best choices are rowing, swimming, cross-country skiing, and cycling on a stationary bike that has attachments to work your upper body.

Amby Burfoot's Running Round-Up

As a fanatic, high-mileage runner in the 1960s and 1970s, I was not a quick convert to cross-training. I admired the Ironman triathletes, to be sure, particularly their ability to run a marathon in the 2:40s at the end of a long, exhausting day. But I wasn't about to do any cross-training myself because I couldn't find any evidence that it would make me a better runner.

I still can't. The exercise physiologists, in particular, claim that the only way to become a better runner is by running. Forget all that stair climbing and stationary cycling.

Yet today, I'm an avid cross-trainer, and not because I think that it will make me a faster runner. I cross-train because I think that it increases my total-body fitness and also because I can do a high-quality workout without pounding my legs the way a hard road run does. End result: fewer injuries. A result that any runner, fast or slow, would be happy to achieve.

Fewer injuries may even make you faster because it will allow you to put together a more consistent, uninterrupted training plan. A cross-training program that develops your leg muscles could make you faster by increasing your stride length. And there are now lots of elite runners who claim that cross-training, especially running in a pool, has made them even more successful competitors. All of which sounds great to me. But the thing I like the most is that by mixing cross-training with my running, I'm able to continue running pain-free. As far as I'm concerned, that's even more important than running fast.

Chapter 25

Treadmills to the Rescue
The Many Benefits of Treadmill Training

Treadmills didn't come easily to their present-day status. Nearly twenty years ago, they were considered tinny, cheap, noisy contraptions that cluttered up a basement and didn't serve much purpose. I didn't know any serious runners who owned one.

And if you did, you didn't admit it. The ethic of distance running virtually demanded that you run outdoors, no matter what the conditions. It was supposed to, among other things, put us in touch with our roots. No roofs overhead for the dedicated runner.

Fortunately, that attitude has largely changed. Just as cross-training doesn't make us less of a runner, neither does treadmill running. The advantages of working out on a treadmill, especially from a safety perspective, are too obvious to list. (The day before writing these lines, I heard of a well-known Canadian runner seriously injured when he was hit by a snowplow while running.)

Of course, once you buy a treadmill or decide to use one at a health club, you still have to figure out what workouts are best suited to the treadmill. This chapter should help.

Back in 1980 Benji Durden had a secret. The soon-to-be Olympic marathoner was sneaking over to the exercise physiology lab at Georgia Tech University in Atlanta to do workouts on a treadmill. "I didn't tell other runners I was using a treadmill," recalls Durden. "They would have thought that I was strange. Heck, even the lab guys thought that I was a little nuts."

Today, however, thousands of runners are doing their hills and speedwork on treadmills, instead of on the roads or track. Still, two basic questions keep popping up, mostly from first-time users. Why should I use a treadmill, and how do I use a treadmill? Some coaches, fitness directors, and some of the world's fastest treadmill trainers provided answers.

WHY YOU SHOULD TRAIN ON A TREADMILL

Are you one of those runners who thinks treadmills are only good for rainy days? Well, running on a treadmill offers other training benefits you may not be able to get on the roads. There are many reasons to consider using a treadmill.

Cold. It's January in Michigan, and the scenery looks like outtakes from Ice Station Zebra. So you head to the rec room, pop a National Geographic special about the Fiji Islands into the VCR, then step on your treadmill for a six-mile run.

This is the most obvious reason to use a treadmill. Severe winter weather not only can make it tough to train outside, but also can be dangerous. You probably know someone who prided himself on running every winter day, no matter how miserable the weather was—that is, until he hit an ice patch and ended up on the injured list for two months. "I don't mind the cold too much," says Minnesota's Bob Kempainen, a 1992 Olympic marathoner. "But if it's slippery, I'll get my 10-mile run in on a treadmill. Why risk it?"

Heat. Severe heat is another reason to hightail it to the health club or wherever there's a treadmill inside. Masters runner Carol McLatchie, who lives in Houston, where you can melt your outsoles during the summer, has her treadmill on the back porch next to an air conditioner. She does several summer workouts a week there. "The air conditioner is just a small window unit," she says. "It gets the temperature down to 80 degrees. But that's a lot better than the 95 degrees outside."

Job. Job restraints present other reasons why many train on a treadmill. Sometimes a quick 30-minute run on the company treadmill at lunch is the only way to fit in a workout between meetings.

Durden, who coaches several runners by fax and phone, remembers a particularly busy month when he lived on the treadmill in his office. "I did 23 days in a row on a treadmill," he says. "I was afraid that if I went out on a long run I'd miss a lot of calls. It was either that or take a cellular phone with me. And I didn't know how well the cellular phone would work when it got all hot and sweaty."

Precise pace. World-class masters miler Ken Sparks, Ph.D., an exercise physiologist at Cleveland State University, likes treadmills because they're precise. "They give you a much more evenly paced workout than running on a track," he says. "For instance, if you're doing 400-meter repeats on a track in 90 seconds, you might run the first 200 in 43 seconds and the second in 47. On a treadmill, you can't do that. Each 200 will be exactly 45 seconds."

Hills. Hill workouts are a special feature of treadmill running for McLatchie and 2:34-marathoner Joy Smith, Houston denizens who otherwise would have to drive 90 minutes to find an incline

Trust the treadmill

Budd Coates, health promotions manager at Rodale Inc. in Emmaus, Pennsylvania, and four-time Olympic Marathon Trials qualifier, recalls an evening workout done on a treadmill while watching his baby daughter. "I didn't get a chance to run during the day because of work," says Coates, a 2:13 marathoner. "So I brought my daughter in and sat her down next to the treadmill. And the rhythmic sound of me pounding on the treadmill put her to sleep." (Coates, however, cautions parents: "The belt of a treadmill is like a spoke on a wheel. It's a temptation for kids to put their fingers and hands in there, so be careful.")

made by Mother Nature. Even Durden, a Colorado resident, prefers to run hills on a treadmill.

"You can duplicate your hill sessions from week to week almost perfectly," says Durden. "If you want to do a two percent grade and a one percent recovery, you just punch some buttons. It's very precise and easy to do."

Race-course workouts. Computerized treadmills come with built-in programs that can take you up and down hills or increase the pace and slow the pace during your run. They also let you program your own courses.

Colorado's Matt Carpenter has trained on his treadmill to get ready for the Mount Washington Road Race in New Hampshire. Carpenter programs in the exact grade of the ascent and sets the pace at slightly faster than the course record. One year, Carpenter won the race but missed the record by 33 seconds on a day when rain made the footing slick. "You can't put mud on a treadmill," he says with a shrug.

McLatchie and Smith ran up and down hills before the 1992 Boston Marathon at precisely the grade and length of the Newton Hills, including Heartbreak Hill. Ditto for the U.S. Women's Olympic Marathon Trials. Even though the Trials were held in Houston, McLatchie and Smith didn't want to beat themselves up running the mostly concrete course several times before the actual race. So they programmed their treadmills with the last 6 miles of the race, where freeway ramps provide the only hills on the course.

"We ran that workout on the treadmill once a week for three months before the Trials," says McLatchie. "We would run outside to fatigue our legs, then hit the treadmill for the six-mile program. During the actual race, we felt that our legs knew those hills."

Avoiding the lonely road. Finally, treadmills come in handy for beginning runners and

Using the treadmill to prevent injury

World-class Masters miler Ken Sparks recommends treadmill training to come back from injuries or avoid them altogether. "First of all, there's less pounding of the legs on a treadmill than on the roads," says Sparks. "That's because the treadmill belt gives when you land on it, unlike concrete and asphalt. Second, there's no side-to-side slope on a treadmill as there is on roads. That slope forces you to overpronate (your feet rotate too far inward on impact) and can lead to shinsplints, Achilles tendinitis, and knee problems. And third, on a treadmill, there's no lateral pressure on your knees and ankles as there would be if you were running around a track, and lateral pressure can lead to injuries."

those who don't appreciate the loneliness of the long-distance runner.

"The treadmill, especially one in a fitness center or health club, provides a comfort because instead of venturing out on your own, you're surrounded by a room full of people," says Scott Kinzer, manager of several fitness centers for Procter and Gamble in Cincinnati. Similarly, treadmills are useful for runners who are wary of a solitary jog through the park.

HOW TO USE IT

Like a new pair of running shoes, a treadmill needs to be broken in—or, rather, you need to be broken in to the treadmill. "The first few times on a treadmill, start off slower than you think you should," says Durden. "You need to get accustomed to it so that you don't feel awkward or as though you're going to fall off."

Adds Smith, "You don't just do a 12-mile run

on it right away. You need to get used to the rhythm of the treadmill. Most runners can get used to it fairly quickly, but for some, it's pretty tricky."

Take McLatchie's husband, Jim, for example. "Jim has been periodically banned from the McLatchie treadmill," says Carol with a laugh. "He just can't get the hang of it. He keeps falling off it and getting beat up. One time he fell off and was lying half-stunned, pressed against the wall, while the belt was whipping around and thumping on his leg. Finally, he reached over and unplugged it."

That's an extreme-case scenario. In reality, learning to run on a treadmill is like learning to ride a bike. Once you get the hang of it, it's easy.

Still, there are other things that you need to know about treadmills. "When I'm on the treadmill, I always have this feeling that I'm going faster than on the roads," says McLatchie. "I just don't have the visual cues, like scenery going by, and that throws me off a bit. Another sensation is that when I stop, my equilibrium is off. Something is still moving. It's like I was out at sea, and now I'm on land again. I have sea legs for a few minutes. But you get used to those things."

Here are some other ways to make treadmills enjoyable and worthwhile.

Overcome monotony. The monotony of treadmill training is a big complaint among runners. And dedicated treadmill trainers won't argue with you on that point. Instead, they'll tell you how they've gotten around it. World-class marathoner Ken Martin blasts music on his stereo system while on his treadmill. Durden watches videotapes from previous Olympics. McLatchie's treadmill is next to a window that looks out on her backyard. Smith has a full-length mirror in front of her treadmill so that she can monitor her running form.

Another option is to schedule your treadmill sessions for peak hours at the health club—so you can socialize, or at least have something to look at.

(But be aware that most health clubs have a time limit on treadmills, usually 20 to 30 minutes.) No matter where you are on a treadmill, don't look at your watch. "If I look at my watch, time seems to go real slow on a treadmill," says Carpenter.

There's one surefire way of avoiding monotony on a treadmill. You simply take your cue from Peter O'Toole in *Lawrence of Arabia*, who, after putting out a match between his fingers, explained that "the trick is not minding." And how do you not mind a treadmill workout? Throw in a little pain.

"I never get bored on my treadmill," says Sparks, who treadmill trains alongside garden hoses, rakes, and shovels in his garage. "That's because I know that when I step on my treadmill, I'm going to be doing an intense speed workout."

Similarly, marathoner Don Janicki's treadmill sits isolated in his basement. "I know that when I'm going down there, it's going to be a tough workout," he says. "I actually look forward to it."

BRINGING THE OUTSIDE IN

You can do practically any outside workout inside on a treadmill. Prior to his 2:09:38 second-place finish at the 1989 New York City Marathon, Martin logged all his long runs on a treadmill. "I'd just get into a nice rhythm and stay controlled," he says. "I also thought it was good because I had my drinks right there beside me, so I didn't have to stop to drink, and I could practice drinking on the run."

But Martin's may be a special case. Many runners can't tolerate a two-hour easy run going nowhere. Other workouts, such as tempo runs, hills, speedwork, and specially designed race-course sessions, are more suited to the treadmill. Says British distance coach Brian Scobie, echoing

Sparks and Janicki, "It's much easier to get through a workout on a treadmill simply by structuring it."

Run efficiently. Durden still remembers a structured tempo workout he did on a treadmill in 1980. "It was at a lab in Missoula, Montana, where they were testing shoes for Nike," he says. "In two days, I ran 14 workouts of eight minutes in length at a five-minute pace. I was extremely efficient on the treadmill. And two weeks later, I made the Olympic Team in the marathon."

Smith often covers 10 to 12 miles on her treadmill, but she breaks up the monotony by throwing in two or three two-mile tempo runs (runs that start easy, build up to a steady speed, and then finish at an easy pace).

Coates likes to set the treadmill at a five-minute pace and cruise for 15 to 25 minutes. "It's actually kind of relaxing," he says. "You don't have to check your splits, and you don't have to concentrate on keeping your pace. Because if you don't go at a five-minute pace, you're off the back of the treadmill."

Make speedwork count. Sparks has been running speed sessions on a treadmill since the late 1960s, when he was a graduate student under David L. Costill, Ph.D., director of the Human Performance Laboratory at Ball State University in Muncie, Indiana. "I didn't have much time back then, and some of my workouts would actually be jumping on a treadmill and running a four-minute mile, then jumping off," he says.

Nowadays, on his homemade treadmill, Sparks clicks off 63-second quarter-miles with a one-minute jog in between. But don't try this at home—or at the health club. Most treadmills won't go faster than a 75-seconds-per-quarter-mile pace.

Therefore, you might want to limit your speed sessions on a treadmill to longer repeats, say, 800s or miles.

Choose your hill workouts. "Treadmills can really give you quite a workout," says Janicki, who does hill sessions on his treadmill. Most treadmills allow you to raise and lower the incline for both uphill and downhill running. You can very easily change the slope for short, steep repeats or set it at a particular grade for a long, steady climb. Also, many treadmills come with charts that convert miles per hour to mile pace at certain uphill grades, so you can determine your effort at different treadmill inclines.

Amby Burfoot's Running Round-Up

A dirty, little secret: I've never done a long run on a treadmill. I think that 40 minutes is about my record. I'm sure that I could go much longer, but I just don't have the inclination. For long runs I'll still take the outdoors, even the frigid, icy streets outdoors. I just slow down. I'll go as slow as it takes to make the run feel safe.

Otherwise, I've grown totally addicted to treadmill running. Oftentimes, I find myself running on the treadmill on days when it would be perfectly easy to run outdoors. Why?

Because I like "going for the burn" on a treadmill.

I do interval training—fast/slow running. Or I do 10 to 12 minutes of treadmill running, then an equal time on a stationary bike, then more running (or weight lifting or rowing or stair climbing). I enjoy the variety. I like exercising one part of my body for a while, and then another part. I keep running at the center of the workout but explore other possibilities.

My fast treadmill running serves a purpose, too. It helps me hold on to my leg speed. During the winter I don't do much (or any) fast running outdoors. So a few bursts of speedy running on the treadmill keep me in touch with faster running.

Chapter 26

Training the Whole Body
Set Personal Records with This Unusual Mix

Nothing succeeds like success, and this is a major success story. Not only that, it's a story that I watched unfold up close and personal, as they like to say on TV. This chapter's author, Claire Kowalchik, began the training program that she describes here as a middle- to back-of-the-pack runner.

When she finished the program, she was a lot faster. Indeed, I haven't known too many veteran midlife runners who improved as much as Claire did over a six-month period. Part of her improvement came from pure hard work, the kind that's always capable of helping you lower your PRs.

But most of it comes from the fact that she decided to try a new training program and to stick with it even when the program made her feel slower and more tired before it eventually made her faster and stronger. The program was different, it was difficult, and it took time to adjust to—but it worked. It worked for Claire. And it can work for you.

In just two miles, my workout would be over. A simple cooldown—something I had done hundreds of times before. Piece of cake. Or so I thought.

But after running 100 yards, all the strength and energy just flushed right out of me. My easy cooldown turned into a torturous two miles.

This was my introduction to embedded circuit training, a form of training that draws its name from the circuit-training exercises that are sandwiched between runs. In the weeks and months that followed, I would grow to dread these circuit workouts. At least I dreaded them at first. Later, after I had set PRs of more than four minutes for the 10-K and 19 minutes for the marathon, I had a change of heart.

But before I explain "embedded circuit training," let me back up a bit and tell you more about myself. For one thing, it has taken me years to get to the point where I can call myself a runner. I used to reserve that term for my friends and others who could run 5-Ks in under 20 minutes and 10-Ks in under 42. But not for myself. I didn't feel that I belonged.

When I started running back in the early 1980s, I finished my first 5-K in over 27 minutes. But I kept at it anyway, covering 20 to 25 miles a week. By 1988 I was able to complete the New York City Marathon in 4:05—a glorious but painful experience. I didn't think that I would ever want to run another.

Still, I kept running and eventually got my 10-K time under 50 minutes. Then the Boston Marathon lowered its qualifying time to 3:40 for women in my age group. Boston . . . sigh . . . I had to admit it: Boston was a dream, for me as for so many other marathoners. I decided to aim for the Portland Marathon, six months off, to qualify for Boston.

THE PROGRAM

That was the easy part. The hard part was devising a training program that would get me to a sub-3:40. So I sat down to chat with Budd Coates, the health promotions manager at Rodale Inc. (where I work) and an elite marathoner himself.

We began by going over my previous training and race times. What fitness activities did I do other than running?, Coates asked. None.

Had I been lifting weights at all? No, not in a few years.

How much training had I done in the past two weeks? I told him.

Coates never said, "Sure, you can qualify." Nor did he laugh and tell me to forget it. He simply said, "Okay. I'll write up a training schedule for you and get it to you in a couple weeks." If he could write the program, I figured I could at least try it.

EMBEDDED CIRCUIT TRAINING

This brings me back to where I began this chapter—with the embedded circuit workout. When my training schedule arrived, it included the usual mix of long runs, short runs, hill repeats, speed workouts, and so on. But my eye stopped when it came to an unusual entry. It read, "Run two miles easy, do circuit training, run two easy."

I called Coates to ask for an explanation. He told me that I should run two warmup miles to the fitness center, and then carry on with 30 minutes of circuit weight training. He had developed a special circuit routine designed to build strength in the leg and upper-body muscles that are most used in running.

Between each set of repetitions, I needed to do some aerobic activity for 30 seconds—skipping rope, stair climbing, stationary cycling, anything to keep my heart rate up. After completing the circuit routine, I finished my workout with an easy two-mile cooldown run. Altogether, the embedded circuit workout would take more than an hour to complete. It seemed like a lot.

"But this isn't supposed to be a hard workout," Coates said. "The running is easy, the lifting is easy. Combining the two does make it harder, but doing the workout shouldn't kill you."

The purpose of all the circuit training, he further explained, was to build upper-body strength that running alone couldn't give me. This would prevent my arms and shoulders from tiring during the latter miles of a race. With a better-balanced body, I would run taller, stronger, and faster.

Even more important, Coates continued, was that the circuit training would help prevent injury.

When the upper body tires, a runner tends to lean forward, which puts extra strain on the back muscles, causing the gluteal and hamstring muscles to become tense and tight. This can lead to lower-back and knee problems. With a stronger upper body, I would be able to maintain proper carriage and avoid injury.

The program certainly made sense, and I was eager to try it, though I still had some doubts. Could I do all this? My workout schedule had never before included anything like embedded circuit training.

DIVING IN

Coates pioneered the use of embedded circuit training in the mid-1980s. He had always done circuit weight training in addition to his regular running. He fit it in on his easy days. Since he also ran a few miles on his easy days, this meant that he had to cram in two workouts on what was supposed to be a relatively restful day.

Why not simply combine them? he asked himself at one point. So he did. And one day while running home after finishing his circuit training, he realized that the workout was more than just a time-saver: It was also a new way to prepare muscles for racing. The two-mile cooldown in particular helped to achieve that.

A DIFFERENT APPROACH

Personally, while churning away on various indoor exercise equipment in Coates's laboratory, I felt like a guinea pig. I would be in the fitness center lifting weights, skipping rope, sweating, lifting,

stair climbing, lifting, sweating. . . . Full of determination to get to Boston, I focused on doing all my training right—no skimping, no shortcuts.

Friends would look at me a little strangely as I would zip by—there was no socializing for me. They would come over to the stationary bike where I was pedaling as rapidly as I could and look at me in wonder. "Gee, you're really working hard," they would say. "Are you training for something special?"

"Budd's . . . (pant) . . . trying . . . (pant) . . . to kill me," I'd reply. Then I would run to the bench press: ugh, whew, ugh, whew, ugh, whew. Sweat beaded on my forehead. Grab the jump rope: skip, skip, skip. With the last lift of the dumbbell curl, I would dash out of the gym and head for the fitness trail, feeling all pumped up and powerful from 30 minutes of circuit training.

And then it would happen. I would hit the trail and crash. Fatigue would rein me in and leave me shuffling along to the finish of another embedded circuit workout.

My routine called for two of these workouts a week: Tuesdays and Thursdays. I was always tired afterward, and my enthusiasm was dwindling. And they seemed to wear me down for intervals on Wednesdays. On the track, I would have to shorten 800s to 400s. On other occasions I would cut the number of repeats that I was supposed to do. I would finish a "speed session" and then walk a lap with my head bent in discouragement.

This program isn't working, I thought. This is supposed to be easy. Only my confidence in Coates and my own stubborn tenacity kept me plugging onward.

I ran a few races during the spring but nothing very serious. Then, in midsummer, the time came to test my training in a more focused race. I

Embedded Circuit Training

This training offers the perfect way to use indoor facilities and equipment to build your strength and endurance. To try it, first pick two easy days in your current training program. Then complete the circuit exercises on each easy day.

Remember: Since you're adding a new stress—strength training—to your aerobic running, you can't expect fast results. In fact, you'll probably feel incredibly tired at first. But once your body adapts, you should run stronger and faster than ever before.

Here are guidelines for doing the exercises.

Adjust the weights so that you are able to do 8 to 12 repetitions for the arm exercises, 12 to 15 repetitions for the legs.

When doing leg extensions and leg curls, set the weights at 30 pounds for extensions and 20 for curls, or 20 pounds for extensions and 10 for curls. If you can only lift 10 pounds for leg extensions, then do not do curls at all until you become stronger.

Between all circuit exercises, do approximately 30 seconds of some aerobic activity such as stationary cycling, stair climbing, or skipping rope.

When trying embedded circuit training for the first time, you might want to forgo the aerobic activity between lifts, especially if you have never done any weight training before or if you are a beginning runner. Once you adapt to this training and feel ready for a more challenging workout, add the aerobics.

It's best to do these exercises in the order presented here. Exercises are paired according to the muscle groups that are worked (1 and 2, 3 and 4, 5 and 6, and so on), and the two exercises within a pair must be done in order.

When you feel comfortable with this routine, you can increase the final two-mile cooldown to four miles.

Stop embedded circuit training a week before a short race, a month before a marathon.

The Workout

After running an easy two miles, complete the following circuit exercises:

1. Bench presses
2. Dumbbell flies
3. Lateral pull-downs
4. One-arm dumbbell rows
5. Leg extensions
6. Leg curls
7. Dumbbell presses
8. Lateral raises
9. Shrugs
10. Upright rows
11. Triceps push-downs
12. Dumbbell curls

Finish the workout by running an easy two miles.

decided on a local race, the Longswamp 10-K, with a course that rolled gently through Pennsylvania farmland.

Race day arrived unusually warm. About 200 runners showed up. I had no confidence, no goal, no strategy. I figured that I'd just go out and see what happened. In truth, I feared the worst.

A shout from the race director started us down the road. The early pace felt comfortable. In most of my other races, the first mile felt like hard work that would soon turn to agony as I inevitably slowed down.

At Longswamp, I went through the first mile in 6:50. Gads. That was much faster than my normal 10-K pace, and it felt easier. I glided down the country roads, passing a few runners in every mile. This wasn't work, it was fun. The miles rolled on, and I felt good.

When I reached the final turn, I still had something left, so I sprinted to the finish. I crossed it in 42:20, finishing second in the women's division. More incredibly, I had improved my PR by 4 minutes.

STEPPING UP A GEAR

The next week, I returned to my embedded circuit training with a new sense of confidence. Coates had promised from the beginning that my body would eventually adapt to this new training, and now it did. As I grew stronger, the lifting got easier, and I could run the two miles afterward without any difficulty. The Wednesday speed sessions started going better, too.

It was time, Coates said, to take embedded circuit training to a higher level.

Fortunately for me, this didn't mean a great leap in training—at least not on paper it didn't. I simply increased my postcircuit cooldown run from two miles to four. It didn't sound like much, but it was. Once again, I struggled to finish these workouts and found myself more tired than ever. But once again, I soon adapted and got stronger.

WORTH THE AGONY

Finally, it was time to taper for the marathon. As the training loosened, my emotions tightened. I wanted so much to qualify for Boston. I had worked so hard to prepare. I had even seen the positive results. Still, with the marathon, you always

Be a guinea pig

Embedded circuit training isn't endorsed by coaches and athletes around the country. Its effectiveness hasn't been proven by researchers in studies. But Budd Coates has had success with it, running the second-fastest marathon of his life (2:13:48) at age 30. And other runners at Rodale Inc. have found it equally beneficial. "It's a great workout for the working person," he says. "But you're all basically guinea pigs."

wonder: Can I really run it at my goal pace, especially when that goal is more than 10 minutes faster than my PR?

The week before the marathon, I caught a cold. Depression. I slept. Cut back on running even more. Drank gallons of orange juice, swallowed thousands of milligrams of vitamin C, and plunged ahead with my marathon plans. I went over my race strategy with Coates. To qualify for Boston, I had to run an 8:20 pace or faster. We decided I should aim for something around an 8:10 pace.

TIME TO RUN

Race day finally arrived. The weather was good— cool and overcast. Anxious and excited, I burrowed into the pack of runners. It was time. The gun fired, and we headed through the streets of Portland. I ran the first mile nervously, not having a clue how I would feel or what the split time would be. I passed the one-mile marker in exactly eight minutes. The second mile went up a slight grade, but I never noticed it and hit the mile marker in 15:52. Whoops. Control yourself, Claire.

After the third mile, I relaxed and settled into

my pace, which wasn't easy because I felt so good that I wanted to run faster. I had to hold myself back. The miles floated by. I felt more comfortable running the marathon than I had during any of my long training runs. At one point I thought, "Gee, I'm really running well. I'm a marathoner. I'm a real runner." And I started to cry.

PACING YOURSELF

As well as everything was going, I knew it couldn't last. In both of my previous marathons, the last 10-K had proved incredibly difficult. Yet I contin-ued running strong through 20 miles, then 21, then 22. The runners around me were slowing down. Some began to walk. I passed dozens of them. Sure, I was getting tired. But somehow I kept running smoothly and rhythmically, working my way through miles 23, then 24, then 25. . . .

At last, the final turn and the finish loomed before me. I read the clock—3:33:45. Even after 26 miles, seeing those minutes pricked my desire to run as fast as I could. I reached down for whatever was left and quickened my pace.

I sprinted under the clock just as it turned to 3:34:00, beating my goal by six minutes. I had run a 19-minute PR. And I was headed for Boston.

Amby Burfoot's Running Round-Up

I have to confess, I have never tried Coates's embedded circuit training program, not even after watching Claire cut four minutes from her 10-K time and almost 20 minutes from her marathon time. But I've done somewhat similar programs, enjoyed them, and found that they worked.

One summer in particular, I became seized with the idea of making my training more fun, more varied, and more "organic." My training was organic, as opposed to mechanical, because I didn't go into a gym and work out with weights and fitness equipment as Claire did. But I did do many of the same exercises, and I got very good results.

Basically, I spent two or three afternoons a week running on the pleasant, rolling green campus of a college near where I lived at the time. I didn't do continuous running, however. I did discontinuous running—that is, I would jog for a while, then do an exercise; jog, do an exercise; jog, do an exercise.

The exercises included short hill sprints, pull-ups on a tree branch, stretching, bounding, sit-ups, and other calisthenics. I probably never ran for more than three minutes at a time, but my work-outs lasted 40 to 60 minutes. They were invigorating, they were difficult, they took place in a pleasant environment, and they provided a refreshing break from continuous runs.

Best of all, I raced well that summer and fall. Circuit training teaches us that there are many forms of interval training—not just classic, grinding interval training but also discontinuous interval training that includes different kinds of exercises to make the whole body stronger and fitter.

Chapter 27

Get Great Abs Now

All it takes is a combo commitment to: (A) regular exercises and (B) a lower-fat diet

A washboard stomach isn't just about vanity. It's about being a stronger, faster runner. Here's a simple diet and exercise program for shedding fat and revealing your inner six-pack. It won't necessarily land you on the cover of *Runner's World* or any other health, fitness, or muscle magazine, but it can and will make you look better while it also improves your running.

As with so many other areas of improved physical conditioning, the key is commitment. Finding your inner abs doesn't require excruciating workouts. It simply takes weeks and possibly months to get toned up to the point where a little extra muscle and a little less fat combine in that oh-so-picture-perfect manner that will make you want to go swimsuit shopping. Go ahead, you deserve it. And you'll look just as good in your racing shorts and singlet the next time you line up for a local road race.

Yes, *Baywatch*-worthy abs look great. But they do more than give you the courage to run without a singlet. By increasing the stability of your hips, pelvis, and knees, they relieve strain on your muscles and reduce the chances of injury. And by minimizing wasteful movement at the joints, they

enable you to run faster, stronger, longer. As a runner, you probably think you're well on your way to owning these kinds of abs, and you may be right. Running is the best fat-burning activity around, and lowering your body fat makes muscles appear more defined. But poorly conditioned abs won't pop from even the leanest physiques, which is why core-strength exercises that build your midsection are key.

That's part one of our plan. Part two is paying closer attention to what you eat. Even if you run 50 miles a week and do 500 crunches a day, your belly won't budge if you reward yourself with heaping bowls of pasta and cream-cheese-laden bagels. Trimming calories is the only other way to shed the fat covering your six-pack. Adopt the following abs workout and diet, and you'll be ready to run or race better than ever—singlet optional.

PART 1: YOUR ABS WORKOUT

There are dozens of ab exercises you can use to strengthen your midsection; the most effective ones are those that have the most functional carryover to running. These five exercises are the best of the best. Each will benefit your running in a different way. Do one set of each move, two or three times a week, and build up to two or three sets, three times a week.

1. Oblique Bridge

Benefit: Strengthens the muscles involved in maintaining lateral stability at the hips, pelvis, and spine.

Technique: Lie on your side with your ankles together and your torso propped up by your elbow. Lift your hips up until your body forms a diagonal plank from ankles to neck. Hold this position for 20 seconds, concentrating on not allowing your hips to sag toward the floor. Reverse sides. Progress by extending how long you hold the position. To increase the challenge, do lateral leg lifts from the bridge position.

2. Stick Crunch

Benefit: Strengthens the abdominal wall and improves the stability of the pelvis and lower spine during running.

Technique: Lie on your back, bend your knees, and draw them as close to your chest as possible. Grasp any type of stick (such as a broom handle) with both hands, positioned shoulder-width apart. Begin with your arms extended straight toward your toes. Now squeeze your abdominal muscles and reach forward with the stick until it passes beyond your toes. (This is a very small movement—just a few inches.) Pause for one second and relax. Do 15 to 30 repetitions.

3. Lying Draw-In with Hip Flexion

Benefit: Ab muscles stabilize the pelvis during alternating leg movements.

Technique: Lie faceup with your head supported by a pillow or foam roller. Begin with your hips and knees bent 90 degrees and your thighs perpendicular to the floor. Engage your deep abs by drawing your navel toward your spine. While holding this contraction, slowly lower your right foot to the floor, return slowly to the starting position, and then lower the left foot. If you find this easy, you are failing to hold the contraction. Lower each foot 8 to 10 times. Progress by adding repetitions.

4. Supine Running

Benefit: Strengthens the lower abs and hip flexors with a running-specific leg action.

Technique: Lie faceup with your arms at your sides. Begin with your legs extended and your feet raised two inches above the floor, heels together. Press the small of your back into the floor. Draw your left knee toward your chest while keeping your right leg extended and off the ground and your lower spine in contact with the floor. Return to the starting position and then draw your left knee in. Repeat 8 to 12 times with each leg.

5. Hip Twist

Benefit: Strengthens the muscles that prevent excessive trunk rotation during running.

Technique: Lie faceup with your palms flat on the floor. Extend your legs toward the ceiling, with your feet together, toes pointed. Tip your legs

12 to 18 inches to the right by twisting at the hip, so that your left buttock comes off the floor. Fight the pull of gravity by maintaining stability with your abs and obliques. Pause for a moment, then return slowly to the starting position, again using your core muscles to control the movement. Repeat on the left side. Do eight to 10 repetitions on each side.

PART 2: YOUR ABS DIET

To get great abs you need to lose body fat while maintaining your lean muscle mass. That means consuming just enough calories to nourish your muscles without expanding your waistline. To do that, imagine you've already achieved a lean body, and your goal now is to keep it. If you currently weigh 160 pounds but you'd like to drop 10 pounds, you should eat enough calories each day (about 2,400 for an active person) to sustain 150 pounds of body weight. Because it takes just two calories to sustain a pound of body fat for one day, you just need to trim two calories a day for every pound of excess body fat you're now carrying (or 20 calories daily to go from 160 to 150).

Easy, yes. Fast, no. By following this formula you'll eventually lose 10 pounds of body fat, but it could take more than two years. To speed up the rate of return, you'll need to cut more calories. Not too many, or you'll begin to deplete your muscle carbohydrate stores and compromise your post-workout recovery. But with the strategies outlined here, you can trim anywhere from 100 to 700 calories per day without hurting your running or constantly listening to your stomach growl—and see results in three months. And yes, chocolate is involved.

Smart swaps

By merely replacing some of the foods you currently eat with lower-calorie alternatives, or even by simply adjusting the proportions of foods you're already eating, you can trim several hundred calories from your daily intake and start getting leaner. Here are some examples of how to eat for a trimmer waistline. Even if you don't eat the exact foods listed here, you can still apply these calorie-cutting principles to your own diet.

BREAKFAST

Instead of: 1 cup Wheaties cereal with 2% milk; Grande Starbucks Caffe Latte with nonfat milk
Eat this: ½ cup Wheaties with fresh strawberries and 2% milk; Tall Starbucks coffee with half-and-half and sugar
Rationale: Due to their high fiber and water content, fresh fruits fill more space in your stomach with fewer calories. By adding fruit and reducing the portions of other foods, you can trim calories and still feel satisfied. (Cut 20 more calories by replacing 2% milk with skim.) Coffee drinks made with syrup and milk are calorie bombs, especially in larger sizes. For a lean caffeine fix, drop to a medium coffee sweetened with half-and-half and sugar.
Calories saved: 186

SNACK

Instead of: High-calorie energy bar
Eat this: Kettle Valley Real Fruit Bar
Rationale: Energy bars are convenient and tasty snacks, but they can pack a lot of calories and are dismissed by some nutritionists as "candy bars in disguise." Choose a bar with 150 calories or fewer, eat half, and save the rest for tomorrow—or look

for a leaner choice. Kettle Valley Real Fruit Bars contain ½ cup of fruit and no added sugar or preservatives.

Calories saved: 90

LUNCH

Instead of: Turkey sub; 1 serving of baked potato chips

Eat this: Turkey wrap; baby carrots dipped in light ranch dressing

Rationale: One of the few positive legacies of the low-carb craze is the popularization of wraps as an alternative to sandwiches. Tortillas have fewer calories, and it's easier to stuff them with veggies. Most "light" alternatives to snack chips are still relatively high in calories and low in overall nutrition. Instead, try baby carrots dipped in light ranch dressing. Carrots contain fiber, which will keep you feeling full longer.

Calories saved: 134

SNACK

Instead of: Trail mix (2 parts nuts to 1 part dried fruit)

Eat this: Trail mix (1 part nuts to 2 parts dried fruit)

Rationale: While trail mixes that contain nuts and dried fruit are quite nutritious, those with more nuts than fruit are heavy on calories. A one-ounce serving of mixed nuts contains 175 calories and ¼ cup of dried fruit contains 100 calories, so to make this snack significantly lighter, choose a mix with more fruit than nuts.

Calories saved: 116

DINNER

Instead of: Chicken (4 ounces) and vegetable (¾ cup) stir-fry with white rice (1 cup)

Eat this: Chicken (3 ounces) and vegetable (1 cup) stir-fry with brown rice (¾ cup)

Rationale: You can lower the number of calories in almost any meal by increasing its vegetable content and shrinking its meat and starch content. Lighten it up further by swapping a refined grain for a whole grain. You can make this substitution to other meals by adding more veggies and subtracting cheese from pasta dishes, burritos, and pizza. Also, choose whole-wheat pastas and breads.

Calories saved: 87

DESSERT

Instead of: Fruit sorbet

Eat this: Dove dark chocolate (one piece, .28 ounces)

Rationale: Some desserts have fewer calories than others, and sorbet is lighter than most. But dark chocolate is the world's best dessert by far. Dark chocolate releases mood-boosting serotonin in the brain, so just a single 50-calorie piece can satisfy you better than a whole bowl of sorbet. And the antioxidants in dark chocolate are good for the heart.

Calories saved: 100

Measure of Success

There's an expression that many coaches and dietitians use: "What gets measured gets managed." In other words, if you're trying to control a factor in your life, you'll get better results if you measure it frequently. This principle certainly applies to your midsection. Measuring your body fat allows you to pursue the goal of getting leaner objectively. The easiest way to measure your body fat is to use a body-fat scale. These devices, such as those made by Tanita and Taylor, use bioelectrical impedance (an electrical impulse sent through your body) to estimate body fat with excellent accuracy. They cost roughly $40.

The American Council on Exercise offers these body-fat percentage guidelines:

	MEN	WOMEN
essential fat	2-4%	10-12%
athletic range	6-13%	14-20%
fitness range	14-17%	21-24%
acceptable range	18-25%	25-31%

Once you determine your current percentage, set incremental goals to improve it, checking your progress every two weeks. If you are currently above the acceptable range, set a modest initial goal of moving into this range. If you're in the middle of the acceptable range, work to move into the fitness range. Don't automatically aim straight for the bottom of the athletic range. Not everyone can safely get there, and no one gets there overnight. And don't go below essential fat levels (the amount of fat that's necessary for optimal health).

There is no specific body-fat percentage associated with six-pack abs, but by actively reducing your body-fat percentage through good nutrition and core conditioning you will develop a set of abs you can be proud of.

Amby Burfoot's Running Round-Up

Runners have a mostly well-earned reputation for being leaner and more sinewy than your average Joe or Jane. This comes from all the high-calorie burning that every training mile requires, and it carries many health benefits with it. It doesn't, however, guarantee that you'll ever attain the six-pack abs of your dreams.

Take me, for example: Despite decades of trying, I've never achieved the striated muscle look. My weight's fine—at a very healthy level—but the muscles have never managed to find their way to the surface and give my body the contours that, let's face it, most of use would love to have. In my case and many others, I think, there's a modest genetic barrier. My mother was muscular but my father was shaped like an apple—round in the mid-

dle. I've fought hard to avoid the roundness, but I've never been able to replace it with flat, rippling muscle.

And that's okay. I still recognize the inherent value of core training, and I do more of it with each passing year. Looking good is nice. But functioning at a high level is even more important. Core exercises might help me run stronger and faster. Even more important, they offer protection against the debilitating back injuries that strike so many Americans, in part because of our bad posture and too many hours sitting at a desk. (Like I'm doing right now.)

So I plan to stick with the abs exercises. Even if no one ever asks to take a photo of my taut muscles.

Chapter 28

Abs-olutely the Best Core Exercises for Runners

The U.S. Olympic Marathon medalists follow this routine. You should, too

Training to run is a simple activity, and homo sapiens has had plenty of time to get good at it—like 2 million years. For that reason, breakthrough workouts don't come along very often. Paavo Nurmi did even-paced workouts in the 1920s, the Germans invented interval training in the 1940s, Arthur Lydiard popularized long runs in the 1960s, and Jack Daniels added scientific Nurmi-like workouts ("tempo runs") in the 1990s. That brought us just about to the end of the road.

But then in the late 1990s and through the first decade of the new millennium, runners discovered core training—a form of strength training that focuses on the front, side, and rear of the hip and stomach/back regions. No one has yet proven that core training makes you faster, but the logic behind the workouts is almost irrefutable. Running consists of the legs moving back and forth, while the upper body rotates to balance and stabilize the motion of the legs.

And what connects the lower and upper bodies? Your core, of course. So if you strengthen your core, there's a very good chance your lower and upper body regions will work together more efficiently. That's not a guarantee of better running, but it is a very good recipe.

Every Monday through Saturday at 5 p.m. you can find them, some of the best runners in America—including Meb Keflezighi, Deena Kastor, and Ryan Hall—grunting and groaning together on the carpeted floor of Snowcreek Athletic Club in Mammoth Lakes, California. Under the blare of a techno beat and the watchful eye of coach Terrence Mahon (whom Meb has dubbed "Dr. Pain"), the members of Team Running USA work for 45 minutes toward a common goal: building stronger abs and backs that can only be described in one way—elite.

Intense core training has become essential for elite runners for good reason: It improves efficiency and endurance as it lowers injury risk. Dan Browne, a 2004 Olympic marathoner and a regular carpet-dweller at the 5 p.m. sessions, is quick to cite the benefits he's experienced since beginning a regular regimen: "When I'm running, some of the muscles that used to fatigue don't get tired as quickly, letting me run stronger and longer."

The secret is stability. That's because core strength is the primary force that controls motion in the hips and spine when you run. Think back to when you were learning to ride a bike. You'd wobble and maybe fall until your dad or mom placed a hand on your back. When you run, your core acts as that steadying hand. The stronger the muscles, the more stable your center—and the more efficient your running will be.

A strong core also helps address overuse issues. "If we don't have a strong center, other muscles have to stabilize us," says Toni Dauwalter, a physical therapist whose clients include 2004 Olympic 1500-meter specialist Carrie Tollefson. Over time, the extra work can lead to injury. Mahon cites a litany of problems relating to the lack of that steadying hand: patella tendinitis, piriformis syndrome, sciatica pain.

This is precisely why nearly every top runner busts through some core moves. But there is no industry standard. Routines run the gamut from old-school to cutting-edge. Brian Sell, who finished third in the U.S. Olympic Marathon Trials, grunts through 150 sit-ups a day. Tollefson does exercises typical of gym classes: planks and curls. And Shayne Culpepper, a 2004 Olympian at 5000 meters, performs Pilates.

And then there's the routine followed by Team Running USA. In 2006, strength and condi-tioning coach Dennis Kline of the University of Wisconsin–La Crosse overhauled the squad's ab workout, creating a regimen that targets not just the abdominals but also the back, hips, and glutes (see "Core Curriculum," page xx). The program combines static exercises that improve overall strength and muscular endurance with dynamic moves that teach the core and legs to work together. "We're mimicking the running motion," says Kline. "So we use some exercises that engage the core while using the legs."

Josh Cox, who joined the group last July, had never done something so intense on a regular basis. "I was really sore my first week," he admits. Meb, who also initially struggled with some of the exercises, now has impressive strength—and an eye-popping six-pack to prove it. "It's hard work," says Keflezighi, "but in order to be the fastest, you have to be the fittest."

SUPPORT CREW

Your core—the roughly 30 muscles that connect your legs to your hips, spine, and rib cage—have a tough job. Namely, to work synergistically to stabilize your torso. This is particularly demanding when you run, since 60 percent of your body shifts in about .02 seconds, says Dennis Kline, who designed Team Running USA's core program. Here are the primary stabilizers and how they function when you run.

Obliques. These muscles rotate your torso and work with the transversus abdominis to support your center during movement.

Rectus Abdominis. This muscle is the fitness aesthetic: The contours of the contracted rectus abdominis form the almighty "six-pack." While it helps stabilize your core, its main function is to flex or curl the trunk.

Elite Advice

Mix it up. "Add a few moves during planks to keep yourself entertained and challenged. I alternate lifting a foot for the middle 20 seconds or so. Sometimes I do planks on a stability ball. It's fun to try to balance on those."

—Carrie Tollefson, 2004 Olympic 1500-meter specialist

Transversus Abdominis. This deepest of the abdominal muscles wraps laterally around your center, acting like an internal weight belt.

Psoas Major/Iliacus. Better known as the hip flexors, these muscles lift the thigh toward the abdomen and limit excess motion of the hip joint.

Erector Spinae. This collection of three muscles (not shown) straightens the back and, along with the multifidus, a short muscle, supports the spine.

CORE CURRICULUM

Chances are you can't keep up with the mega talent on Team Running USA—but you can copy their core routine. Kline adapted the routines for everyday runners, as shown on the following page. The two workouts, Base Fitness and Dynamic Strength, work in concert. The Base exercises develop muscular strength, endurance, and balance; the Dynamic moves build power. Translation: You'll be able to run stronger and longer.

Like the elites, you'll alternate between these two routines. Follow the Base workout for four weeks, then the Dynamic routine for three. For phase two, return to the Base workout for a week, this time performing repetitions of each move instead of holding the positions. Then shift again to the Dynamic

routine, continuing that three-week, one-week cycle. Do your core work three times a week. During peak training, drop to one or two days. Cut out the workouts entirely two weeks prior to a big race.

BASE FITNESS

Plank/Side Plank

Lie in a push-up position with your forearms on the ground, keeping your body in a straight line, your elbows directly below your shoulders, and your abdominals pulled in (top, right). Hold. Shift to your side, keeping the elbow directly under your shoulder and both feet on the floor, top foot in front. Lift your hips until your body is in a straight line. For all variations, start with 30 seconds, build to two-and-a-half minutes.

Phase Two: Hold plank as you have been, but lower and lift into a side plank for four sets of six reps, holding each rep for a count of four. The plank was originally used to test lower-back strength, says Kline, and if you can hold it for two-plus minutes, your likelihood of having lower-back problems is low.

Payoff: Develops abdominal and lower-back muscles that support and stabilize the middle of your body.

Bird Dog

Start on your hands and knees, back flat. Raise an opposite leg and arm to hip and torso height. Hold for 10 seconds, build to 30.

Phase Two: Perform four sets of six reps with each side, holding each rep for a count of two.

Payoff: Strengthens the muscles along the spine, the upper back, and the glutes.

Back Extension

Start face down on a Roman chair with your legs hooked, and lift your torso up until it's parallel to the ground; your back should be straight, not arched. Hold. Start with 45 seconds, build to three minutes. (The focus is on muscular endurance, not pure strength, so don't add additional weight.)

Phase Two: Do four sets of six reps.

Payoff: Improves strength and muscular endurance of the erector spinae and other back extensors.

Swiss Hip Extension

Start sitting upright on a stability ball, then walk your legs forward and bend backwards from the hips so the ball travels up your spine until it reaches your shoulder blades. With your arms extended out to the sides, lift your hips up until your torso is parallel to the floor. Then lift one knee about 45 degrees, lower it, then lower your hips toward the floor, and repeat on the other side for one set. "Don't be frustrated if you can't do this well at first," says Kline. Do three sets of five to seven reps, with two minutes rest between sets.

Phase Two: Same as above.

Payoff: Mimics the running motion, but on an unstable surface (the ball), engaging the hip flexors (psoas, iliacus) and extensors (glutes) to work together with the abs and back to stabilize the body.

DYNAMIC STRENGTH

Dumbbell Walkouts

Holding a pair of moderately heavy dumbbells (about 10 pounds more than you'd use for biceps

curls), take small steps forward for 10 seconds and backward for 10 seconds. Breathe naturally. Do three sets, with one minute rest between them.

Payoff: The weights help activate the core to stabilize it as you walk, the same action you want to occur when you run.

Erect Lateral Bends

Place a pole or bar across your shoulders and hold with both hands. Keep your weight on your heels, your knees slightly bent, and tip your body to the side, taking the bar down toward your ankle without bending forward at the waist. Repeat on the other side. Try to keep a tempo of three seconds down (lowering the bar to the side), one second back up to a standing position. Do three sets of five reps on each side, with two minutes rest.

Payoff: Builds muscular strength and endurance in the obliques and the quadratus lumborum (a deep back muscle).

Turkish Get-Up

Lie on your back, and raise a light dumbbell (about the weight you'd use for shoulder presses) with

Amby Burfoot's Running Round-Up

In my family, the wife is the big core-training advocate. She goes to classes twice a week, and always comes home moaning and groaning. A couple of days later, however, she's proud as can be. She shows off her firm middle and tempts me to give it a pinch.

I've always wanted to have muscles and rock-hard abs, but they've always escaped me. I'm trying nonetheless. I've got a couple of favorite core exercises that I do for about 5 to 10 minutes a day at home, and I also try to remember to get down on the carpeting in my office for a few extra minutes at mid-morning and mid-afternoon.

We've got one of those Swedish exercise balls in the corner of our living room, and every once in a while I walk over to sit, bounce, and try a few things. Not much, to tell you the truth. I'm kinda afraid of the thing—afraid I'll fall off and hurt myself. I like to do more core work from a firm platform—my own hands and knees and feet—rather than a roly-poly surface. But I definitely am doing the exercises. They simply make too much sense to ignore them.

your right arm held above you. Then stand up, keeping your arm straight the entire time. Lower back down, finishing the move the way you started. "No matter how you stand up and get down, this recruits many of the core muscles," Kline says. Do three sets of five reps (with each arm), with two minutes rest between sets.

Payoff: Gets the core and legs working together, because holding a weight above your head activates your entire core while your leg muscles are busy getting you up and down.

BODY CURLS

Hang from a pull-up bar, palms facing away from you. Without using momentum, use your core to curl your body up until your knees are between your arms (you'll be almost upside down). Hold a second, then lower slowly. If these are tough, drive one knee up to initiate the move, says Kline. Start with one to two reps, build to four, then add a second set, with 90-second rests in between.

Payoff: Works total body flexion—the abdominals, hip flexors, latissimus dorsi (the back), and biceps.

DOUBLE LEG HOPS

This is essentially a standing broad jump. From a standing position, jump as far as you can; use your arms to pull yourself up. When you land, jump again for a total of three without stopping. Do three sets, with two minutes rest in between.

Payoff: Forces the hips to work in concert with the core muscles to stabilize the trunk from push-off to landing.

Elite Advice

Stick with it. "You're not going to feel good the first few weeks doing this core workout, but once you get past that, you'll experience the benefits. You'll feel stronger and you'll find yourself holding correct form longer when you run."

—Josh Cox, a 2:13 marathoner

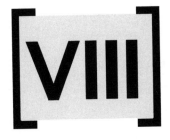

Weight Loss
for Runners

Chapter 29

Your Personalized Diet Program

Everyone's different, and everyone has to find their own unique road to a healthy weight

Not all runners want to lose weight, but many runners do, and there are two good reasons why: Losing weight, within reason, will make you faster; and losing weight will make you healthier.

As a general rule, every pound you lose will help you subtract about two seconds per mile from your running or racing pace. That is, if you lose 10 pounds, you should be able to run 20 seconds per mile faster. That's a significant difference. Of course, when you weigh less, you can also run the same pace more easily, which will help you run farther with less effort and lose more pounds.

That's a big motivation for the thousands who take up running because they have heard that it's one of the most effective ways to lose weight, and especially to keep the pounds off. Virtually no other activity burns as many calories per minute as running. Given our busy lives, that's a huge benefit. What's more, research performed by the physicians associated with the

National Weight Control Registry has shown that serious exercisers are more successful than anyone else at maintaining a healthy weight once they achieve it. In other words, they don't yo-yo back to their former fatty selves.

Losing weight isn't just about looking good. For the four runners on this and the following pages, dropping pounds is a way to ward off health problems, end years of yo-yo dieting, boost confidence, and, well, run faster. With the help of a team of nutritionists and coaches, we've put together all the information you need to lose anywhere from five to more than 25 pounds. These four runners are stepping up to the starting line, ready to change their lives and lose weight for good. Are you?

KATE SANDERS

Wants to lose: 25+ pounds

Reason: Stop a lifelong cycle of weight gain and loss

She's had some success with the Atkins and South Beach diets, but for Kate Sanders, losing weight and keeping it off has been a constant struggle. The event planner knows the basics of nutrition and training from poring over books and magazines, but something still isn't clicking. "I try not to eat too many processed foods, I don't eat fast food, and I eat as many fruits and veggies as I can, but I can't get below 163," she says. Sanders, who started running in 2000, is currently logging about 15 miles a week before she begins preparation for her next half-marathon. "I realize I'll never be an Olympic athlete," she says. "But I do have the power to be fit for the rest of my life."

Starting weight: 170

Target weight: 140

Racing goal: To run the Napa-to-Sonoma Wine Country Half-Marathon in less than two hours, beating her best time by 22 minutes

Kate's Coaches

Tony Williams, owner of Always Running in Seattle (alwaysrunning.com) and Nancy Clark, R.D., author of *Nancy Clark's Food Guide for New Runners* (nancyclarkrd.com).

The Nutrition Plan

"There are times when I'm working that I get so hungry, I'm shaking," says Sanders, who often forgets to eat while she's managing an event, then snacks on high-calorie catered food afterward. That's Sanders's major problem, says nutritionist Nancy Clark: Sanders typically creates a massive calorie deficit during the day, then gets so hungry she overeats later on. Clark wants to overhaul Sanders's habits by making sure she eats at least four times a day and doesn't go more than four hours without eating. Here's how.

DETERMINE HOW MANY CALORIES YOU NEED

Clark uses the formula below to calculate the number of calories clients should consume daily to gradually lose weight while still being able to maintain energy to exercise. Keep in mind that 3,500 calories equals one pound of body fat.

1. Multiply your goal weight by 10.

2. Add 20 percent of that number if you sit at a desk all day; 50 percent if you're moderately active; or 70 percent if you're moving all day.

3. Add the number of calories burned during your workouts (see "What's Your Sweat Worth?" on page 211).

4. Reduce the total by 15 percent.

KEEP A STEADY PACE

Aim for four small meals a day that are about the same number of calories. To help evenly distribute your calories, think of each meal as a bucket. Make sure you have at least three types of food in each bucket: fruits and vegetables, grains, and protein like low-fat dairy and lean meats. Of the calories in your diet, 55 to 65 percent should be from carbs (whole-grain breads, fruits); 10 to 15 percent from protein (chicken, tofu, beans); and 20 to 30 percent from unsaturated fats (olive oil, walnuts).

TRACK INTAKE

Go to calorieking.com to learn how many calories a food has and to loosely count them. "Round to the nearest 50," says Clark. Post a calorie list on your fridge for the 20 foods you eat most often.

The Bucket System

Sanders needs about 2,200 calories a day to lose weight. Here's what that looks like.

Breakfast (600 calories)

Bowl of cereal: 1 cup granola or 3 cups Cheerios (300 cal)

1 cup 1% milk (100 cal)

Banana (100 cal)

8 ounces OJ (100 cal)

Lunch (600 calories)

2 slices whole-grain bread (200 cal)

3 ounces turkey (150 cal)

1 ounce low-fat cheese (100 cal)

Lettuce, tomato, mustard as desired

1 cup low-fat yogurt (100 cal)

10 baby carrots (50 cal)

Second lunch (3 or 4 p.m.) 400 calories

4 graham cracker squares (150 cal)

2 tablespoons peanut butter (200 cal)

Decaf latte with ½ cup 1% milk (50 cal)

Dinner (600 calories)

6-ounce chicken breast (300 cal)

1 sweet potato (100 cal)

2 cups broccoli (100 cal)

2 Fig Newtons (100 cal)

The Training Plan

"You look at Kate, and you see a runner," says coach Tony Williams. "She has a fluid, easy stride." Williams wants Sanders to run, cross-train, and work on her core to maximize her calorie burn and give her enough strength and endurance to eventually run up to six days a week. To start, she will run three or four days a week, cross-train three times, and do a thrice-weekly core routine. She has one rest day a week. As summer approaches, Sanders will run more, cross-train less, and focus on these four strategies.

GET A PHYSICAL

"Biomechanical issues in people who need to lose more than 25 pounds are exacerbated by their weight," says Williams, who sees lots of heavy runners with IT-band problems and plantar fasciitis.

SPEED UP AND SLOW DOWN

Once a week, do a tempo run, which will help boost calorie burn. Slow down for weekly long runs (which should be at least 30 minutes of easy effort) so your body uses fat, not carbs, for energy.

QUICK TIP

BEWARE OF LIQUID CALORIES

Sodas, juices, store-bought smoothies, and coffee drinks have nearly enough calories to constitute a meal.

KEEP STATS

Log your daily workouts and weight. The sense of accomplishment is hard to beat when you look back and see that you can cover the same two miles two minutes faster and you weigh 12 pounds less.

DOUBLE UP

One weekend day, do a moderate run of 40 to 60 minutes in the morning. In the afternoon, ride a recumbent bike for 30 minutes. You'll burn extra calories and get blood flowing to your muscles, which will help speed your recovery.

JIM DOLAN

Wants to lose: 20 pounds

Reason: Stave off diabetes and cardiovascular disease

What a difference

A week of workouts for Sanders, then and now

	THEN CALORIES BURNED	NOW CALORIES BURNED	CALORIE DIFFERENCE
MONDAY	Off	45 min recumbent bike, moderate (mod) + 15 min core 347+106=453	453
TUESDAY	2-mile run, easy (11 min/mile) 246	3-mile run, easy (11 min/mile) 369	123
WEDNESDAY	Off	3-mile run, mile 2 at tempo (9 min/mile) + 15 min core 385+106=491	491
THURSDAY	3-mile run, easy 369	45 min recumbent bike, hard 405	36
FRIDAY	Off	Off	0
SATURDAY	Off	6-mile run, easy + 15 min core 738+106=844	844
SUNDAY	5-mile run, easy 615	a.m: 4-mile run, easy; p.m.: 30 min recumbent bike, mod 492+231=723	108
TOTAL CALORIES BURNED	1,230	3,285	

CALORIE DIFFERENCE: EXTRA CALORIES BURNED: 2,055

With two sets of twins (ages 8 and 3), a three-hour round-trip commute to New York City, and a job as an accountant that demands 10-hour days, Jim Dolan has his plate full. But he knows keeping his weight down is imperative; his family history includes heart disease, diabetes, and cancer, and he's on statins for high cholesterol. So three days a week, Dolan takes a 5:13 a.m. train to run on a treadmill before work. It's no surprise, though, that his nonstop lifestyle doesn't lend itself to good eating habits. "The people at McDonald's by my office know me by name," laughs Dolan, a six-time marathoner with a PR of 4:06. Yet he realizes he needs to kick those habits for his kids. "As much as I want to run Boston, I have the bigger picture of living a healthy, long life in mind," he says.

Starting weight: 186

Target weight: 165

Racing goal: Run sub-3:35 at the Philadelphia Marathon in November to qualify for the Boston Marathon

Jim's Coaches

Jason Koop, pro coach at Carmichael Training Systems in Colorado Springs (trainright.com) and Ilana Katz, M.S., R.D., owner of Optimal Nutrition for Life in Atlanta (onforlife.com)

The Nutrition Plan

"I love sweets," admits Dolan. "And when I sit down to have a few potato chips, the next thing I know, the whole bag is gone." While junk food is an issue with Jim, nutritionist Ilana Katz is more concerned with getting Dolan to eat less, more often. That, plus fewer stops at the drive-thrus and some prepa-

ration for the day's meals, should put Dolan well on his way to dropping 20 pounds.

STOCK YOUR OFFICE FRIDGE

Load up with healthy snacks, so you'll forgo the Hershey's Kisses on your coworker's desk. Try packets of cottage cheese, yogurt, low-sodium V8, almonds, baby carrots, and sugar-free puddings.

LIMIT DIET SODAS

Dolan drinks as many as three cans daily. Katz suggests cutting back substantially. "Studies have shown that those who use artificial sweeteners tend to lose less weight than those who don't," she says.

THE POWER OF ELMO

Katz wants Dolan to adopt a nutrition strategy based on eating less more often (ELMO for short). So he'll have six or seven small meals a day with no more than three hours between meals. "If you wait too long, your metabolism drops and fat-storage mode sets in, so your tendency to overeat is strong," she says. Katz recommends eating one serving of carbs and protein together, six times a day. And she caps bread at one serving a day. "That will make room for higher quality carbs, such as legumes, brown rice, and potatoes," she says. Keep fats to three servings—one of which should be a daily tablespoon of ground flaxseed, which Katz suggests adding to a smoothie (see below), because it provides fiber and omega-3 fatty acids. Only one processed food (meaning it comes in a box or packet, like chips) per day, and it should be 250 calories or less.

5 a.m. Half a PowerBar or equivalent energy bar (around 125 calories with about 7 grams of protein)

8 a.m. Protein shake (see recipe below) made the night before. Freeze it and let it defrost during your workout.

10 a.m. Yogurt and a piece of fruit

12:30 p.m. Chicken sandwich on whole-wheat bread with tomatoes, cucumbers, and lettuce. "Veggies are unlimited," says Katz. Top it with cheese or dressing for one of the daily fats.

3 p.m. 10 to 15 Wheat Thins and two ounces of string cheese

5 p.m. 20 raw almonds (which provide healthy, unsaturated fats) and baby carrots

8 p.m. Grilled salmon, brown rice, and stir-fry vegetables

WHEY COOL SMOOTHIE

    4 tablespoons whey protein powder
    1 banana
    ½ cup frozen strawberries
    1 tablespoon ground flaxseed
    6 ice cubes
    8 ounces water
    Optional: packet of Splenda or a few drops of almond or vanilla extract

Blend and serve.

The Training Plan

"Jim is an experienced, talented athlete, who isn't limited by potential but by life circumstances," says coach Jason Koop. "He can't train more, because that will take away from his family and job." So Koop devised a program focusing on specific facets of Dolan's running, reaping maximum benefits from the four days he has to exercise.

CROSS-TRAIN FOR FUN

Dolan likes to lift weights, so Koop keeps it in his schedule. "It doesn't interfere with his running and gives him motivation to get to the gym," says Koop. Limit your cross-training to an easy intensity.

SIMPLIFY THE CALENDAR

Dolan wanted to go for a sub-four spring marathon, then aim for a Boston qualifier in the fall. Koop advised him to do both at the same time in Philly so he won't have to ramp up, race, recover, and repeat the process again.

SAY NO TO MULTITASKING

Dolan's old schedule was typical of many runners: intervals on Tuesday, tempo on Thursday, long run on Sunday. His body became efficient at churning out these workouts, so he wasn't burning many calories. "With a lack of time, it's important to focus on one aspect of running for an 8- to 12-week block and nail that before moving on," says Koop, who prefers to train the systems you need least for an event first, then hone in on more important aspects of preparation. If you're training for a marathon, focus first on speed, then tempo, then distance. If you have a 5-K on the horizon, flip the order. The schedule below is for a marathoner familiar with speedwork, who has six months to train and lose weight.

[Weeks 1–8] Speed: Why Intervals and other speedwork jump-start your weight loss by burning through calories at a high rate.

How Reps of two- to four-minute intervals at 5-K race pace (about 95 percent effort), totaling 15 to 20 minutes. Start with either 6 x 3 minutes or 5 x 4 minutes. Your recovery jog should be as long as your intervals, and be run at least two minutes per mile slower. Gradually work up to 40 minutes of speedwork. Separate interval days with two days of easy running.

[Weeks 9–16] Tempo: Why Tempo runs improve lactate threshold, letting you run faster for longer.

How Start with 2 x 10 minutes at tempo (slightly faster than half-marathon pace, or 85 percent effort), with five minutes recovery in between. Each week, add five to 10 minutes to the intervals or run the same amount of time continuously; try this succession: 2 x 10; 1 x 20; 3 x 10; 1 x 30; 2 x 20; 1 x 40. Recover for half the time of the interval. Do tempo runs two or three times a week, with a rest day in between.

[Weeks 17–24] Distance: Why Building endurance is the most important preparation for the marathon. By this point, your base pace will be significantly faster than it used to be, which burns more calories per minute.

How Priority is still on quality over quantity. Your weekly long run should be a maximum of 18 to 20 miles, running one minute per mile slower than your goal marathon pace. Create a schedule that builds incrementally toward that distance and peaks with your longest run three weeks before the event.

What's your sweat worth?

Whatever your pace and weight, here's your calorie burn per hour.

	130 POUNDS	160 POUNDS	190 POUNDS
12 MIN/MILE	472	582	691
11 MIN/MILE	532	655	734
10 MIN/MILE	591	727	864
9 MIN/MILE	650	800	950
8 MIN/MILE	709	873	1,036
7 MIN/MILE	827	1,018	1,209
6 MIN/MILE	945	1,163	1,382

The Head Game

How to keep going when weight loss gets tough

Find a partner. If you don't have a network of active friends, seek out a running group or training partner at rrca.org.

Commit to the long run. Research shows you're more likely to maintain weight loss if you lose slowly. Dropping pounds the right way will take at least six months—and a lifetime of healthy habits.

Stay flexible Too much stress in your life may push you to abandon your running and weight loss goals. It's okay to eat a little more one week. Rest assured, you can pick up where you left off.

Run the numbers. A sustained 10 percent weight loss will reduce lifetime medical costs of an overweight person by as much as $5,300.

LAURA DAVIS

Wants to lose: 15 pounds

Reason: Boost confidence and become a dedicated runner

A beginning runner who uses a run-walk method, Laura Davis was pleased about finishing her first half-marathon last spring. "I trained with a group and made some great friends," says the physician's assistant. "Plus, I experienced the runner's high and got in great shape." Problem is, the pounds she took off in training crept back on when nothing else was on the horizon. Her less-than-stellar diet doesn't help either. (She drinks coffee at 8 a.m., then doesn't eat until around 2 p.m.) While she's motivated to take on another

half, Davis, like many beginners, lacks confidence in her abilities. Still, she's tasted what life is like with running as an essential part of the day and wants more. "I'm ready for that lifestyle change," she says.

Starting weight: 175
Target weight: 160
Racing goal: To run Flying Pig Half-Marathon in Cincinnati in less than 2:30, beating her PR by more than 30 minutes

Laura's Coaches

Christine Hinton, RRCA-certified coach in Crofton, Maryland (therunningcoach.com) and Lisa Dorfman, M.S., R.D., University of Miami sports nutritionist and adjunct professor in the department of exercise sciences (runningnutritionist.com)

The Nutrition Plan

"Laura is one of the easiest and hardest clients I've seen," says nutritionist Lisa Dorfman. "She's easy because her diet has so many places to improve, and she's hard because she has to rethink all her eating habits." Dorfman plans to lay a nutritional foundation for Davis, teaching her what foods to eat when. "Once she nails that, not only will the weight come off, but her running will improve easily, too."

BEFORE AND AFTER

A study from the University of Massachusetts looked at people who maintained at least a 30-pound weight loss over one year and found those who kept the same caloric intake all week during the following year were 1.5 times more likely to maintain their weight than those whose calories fluctuated. Davis's food diary revealed she ranged from 1,000 to 1,600 calories. While it might seem counterintuitive, eating only 1,000 calories a day won't help the scale budge. "If you undereat, it becomes difficult to lose weight because your body holds onto any bit of food it can to simply survive," says Dorfman. Davis's calorie total should be about 1,700 daily. To stay consistent all day, she needs to eat 300 to 400 calories at her meals and 150 to 250 at her snacks. Below is an example of how Davis's new diet differs from her old.

Breakfast

Before (about 1,240 cal): 2 cups of coffee with cream and sugar

After (about 1,700 cal): 1 cup fat-free yogurt, 1 cup strawberries, 1 piece of toast with 1 tablespoon jam

Snack #1

Before (about 1,240 cal): None

After (about 1,700 cal): Apple with fat-free cheese slices

Lunch

Before (about 1,240 cal): Chicken & Vegetable Lean Cuisine, water

After (about 1,700 cal): 6" turkey sub with lettuce, tomato, and other veggies; 1 apple

Snack #2

Before (about 1,240 cal): 5 Hershey's Kisses

After (about 1,700 cal): Half a low-sugar energy bar

Dinner

Before (about 1,240 cal): Broccoli casserole, black-eyed peas, 2 rolls, Crystal Light

After (about 1,700 cal): 5 ounces grilled fish, salad greens, 1 cup peas or beans, 1 cup broccoli

Snack #3

Before (about 1,240 cal): Handful of Craisins

After (about 1,700 cal): Nothing

The calorie difference for each meal is 460 cal

EAT BREAKFAST

A study from the University of Colorado, which tracked about 3,000 people who maintained at least a 30-pound weight loss for more than one year, found that 78 percent of them ate breakfast every day. Only four percent never had breakfast. Although the two ends of the spectrum had the same daily calorie intake, those who ate their Wheaties engaged in more physical activity.

CUT OUT NIGHTTIME SUGAR

Even though Davis's 10 p.m. snacks of Craisins are relatively benign, eating sugary foods right before bed is not a good call: Her body won't quickly burn any of the calories from the snack. "You should eat a minimum of two hours before you go to bed," says Dorfman, who adds that sugar-free Jell-O and an eight-ounce fruit smoothie are good evening snacks, if you need one.

Run the numbers. For every two-pound gain in weight, the risk of developing arthritis increases nine to 13%.

The Training Plan

During her first half-marathon, Davis used a three-minute:one-minute run-walk ratio, so she's physically ready for her more ambitious goal, but still anxious about pushing herself. "Laura is underestimating what she can do," says coach Christine Hinton. "She's very capable of eventually running for 30 minutes straight. If she does that, the pounds will drop right off." Hinton will ramp up Davis's weekly mileage over 13 weeks to 25 miles, including some challenging but doable runs.

KEEP MOVING

Run four days a week, and cross-train two for 30 minutes. Even on a day off "you still need some level of activity," says Hinton. "Walk your dog, park your car far from where you work."

SET WEEKLY CHALLENGES

Davis's weekly schedule increases slowly from a 3:1 run-walk ratio to 14:1, then running for 30 minutes straight (walking as needed). Likewise, add weights or reps when strength training. "Your body adapts quickly," says Hinton. "Switch it up to maximize the burn."

FEELING THE NEED FOR SPEED

Four types of speedwork, listed from easiest to hardest:

Strides. 10 to 15 seconds of picking up the pace on flat ground. "Stay in control; it's not an all-out sprint," says Hinton. "Concentrate on your form and moving your legs faster."

Fartleks. Pickups for any length of time (for example, 30 seconds or to the next telephone pole). "They build speed and strength," says Hinton.

Straightaways. On a track, sprint the straightaways and walk or jog the turns. Begin with four laps total of speedwork.

Ladders. On a track, sprint 100 meters, jog or walk 100; sprint 200, jog or walk 200; work up to 400, then come back down to 100.

ED TAM

Wants to lose: 5-10 pounds
Reason: Reach his peak racing potential

Don't hate Ed Tam because he's fast. At the 2007 Philadelphia Marathon—his first 26.2—he clocked a 3:09:40, capturing a Boston qualifier. Even more enviable: The financial analyst followed a plan that included no speedwork and averaged three to four days of training a week. Looking forward to Boston, Tam wants to be like pro-cyclist-turned-marathoner Lance Armstrong. "Lance shaved almost 13 minutes off his second marathon by training harder and losing weight," says Tam. "I think if I employ a similar strategy, I can sneak in under three hours." Potentially holding Tam back are 60-hour work weeks, a love of anything that involves the words pizza or beer, and less than seven hours of sleep nightly. "I realize my goal is ambitious," says Tam, "but I think it's possible."

Starting weight: 168

Target weight: 160

Racing goal: To run a sub-three-hour Boston Marathon

Ed's Coaches

Matt Russ, head coach and owner of The Sport Factory in Atlanta (thesportfactory.com) and Amy

Bragg, R.D., L.D., director of performance nutrition at Texas A & M University Athletics in College Station, Texas (teamnutritioncoach.com)

The Nutrition Plan

As if his speedy inaugural marathon wasn't enough to make you jealous, Tam's eating habits aren't that bad, either. "He's good about eating nutrient-dense foods, like brown rice, avocados, whole-wheat bread," says dietitian Amy Bragg. All

The Half-Marathon Plan

Getting through the first four weeks

	WEEK 1 3:1 RUN-WALK	WEEK 2 4:1 RUN-WALK	WEEK 3 5:1 RUN-WALK	WEEK 4 5:1 RUN-WALK
SUNDAY	2 miles, easy	2 miles, easy	2 miles, easy	3 miles, easy
MONDAY	XT*	XT	XT	XT
TUESDAY	2.5 miles, easy w/ 4 strides	3 miles, easy w/ 6 strides	3 miles, easy w/ 6 strides	3 miles, w/ 4 30–60 sec. fartleks
WEDNESDAY	XT or off	XT or off	XT or off	XT or off
THURSDAY	2.5 miles, easy w/ 4 strides	3 miles, easy w/ 6 strides	3 miles, easy w/ 6 strides	3 miles, easy
FRIDAY	Off	Off	Off	Off
SATURDAY	5 miles	6 miles	7 miles	5 miles

* Cross-training (XT): at least 30 minutes of easy to moderate effort. Can be strength training, yoga, Pilates, or something aerobic (swimming, elliptical, rowing, cycling).

he really needs to concentrate on is cutting out junk calories. Just a few tweaks to his otherwise healthy diet will get his weight down five to ten pounds by the time he gets to the starting line at Beantown.

FUEL UP PROPERLY

Usually when Tam goes out before a morning run he doesn't eat, because when he does, he spends more time in a porta-potty than he'd like. Bragg suggests something mild and GI-friendly, such as a Carnation Instant Breakfast. "Preworkout is when you can actually benefit from refined carbs like a bagel or plain toast," says Bragg. "Not eating, especially before a tough workout, almost guarantees a bonk."

CAVE TO CRAVINGS

On long-run days, Tam is pulled toward pizza, greasy Chinese food, or other take-out indulgences. Fine, says Bragg, but partake only once a week. "Think of it as a reward for your work."

ORDER WISELY

In restaurants, Tam often goes for high-fat meats, so Bragg steers him instead toward chicken and fish and anything that includes the word "loin," which indicates it's lower in fat than other cuts. Get two vegetable sides with your entree.

HIT THE PILLOW

"Ed is operating on constant sleep deprivation," says Bragg. "When you're overtired, you make bad food decisions." What's more, she adds, when you're bleary-eyed and craving a Milky Way,

often what you really need is a nap. Aim for at least seven hours (eight is better) of sleep nightly.

LAY OFF THE BOTTLE

Tam's answer to Bragg's question about what is holding him back from losing weight? "Too much beer." As in 12 lagers weekly, which he usually drinks on the three nights a week he goes out. While that's not a terribly unusual amount for a single guy in the Big Apple, there's a reason most guys have beer bellies. He's decided to limit his nights out to just once weekly before Boston. "Alcohol provides unnecessary calories and disrupts sleep," seconds Bragg, "and neither is particularly helpful during an intense training period."

AVOID DOUBLE-DIPPING

On long runs Tam needs to keep his tank full with either a sports drink with electrolytes and carbs (like Gatorade) or a nearly no-calorie electrolyte drink (like Nuun) and carbs from Gu; there's no need to wash down a Gu with Gatorade. "For runs less than an hour, you don't need anything but water," says Bragg. Tam uses one Gu an hour into long runs, then one every 45 minutes."Perfect," says Bragg.

The Training Plan

Coming into his Boston preparation, Tam averaged 15 to 20 miles weekly, which put him in a precarious position: He needed to properly train for Boston by upping his weekly mileage to at least 50, while also cutting calories to lose weight. "If runners focus too much on weight loss during the ramp-up for a race, the quality of their workouts will suffer tremendously," says coach Matt Russ. The good news is that Tam will drop pounds with just a few training changes.

INCREASE THE MILES

Tam needs to add a fourth day of running (a five- to eight-miler with some 100-meter strides to increase his turnover) to up his calorie burn and boost his endurance.

MONITOR YOUR HEART RATE

When it gets harder to whittle off inches, using technology is invaluable. "Doing a max effort to find your ranges, then sticking to them, will help you get faster," says Russ, who likes

Four Weeks of Sleekness

How Tam will kick-start his weight loss and training

	WEEK 1	WEEK 2	WEEK 3	WEEK 4
MONDAY	Off	Off	Off	Off
TUESDAY	*TH: 5 x 7 min. @ 7% w/ 5 min. recovery	*TH: 4 x 10 min. @ 8% w/ 5 min. recovery	*TH: 4 x 12 min. @ 8% w/ 7 min. recovery	*TH: 4 x 10 min. @ 8% w/ 10 min. running @ 1% between hills
WEDNESDAY	5 miles	Off	5 miles	4 miles
THURSDAY	10 miles	10 miles	8 miles	11 miles
FRIDAY	Off	Off	Off	Off
SATURDAY	4 miles	5 miles	4 miles	7 miles w/ 8 x 100 meters
SUNDAY	12 miles	13 miles	8 miles	15 miles

*TH=Treadmill hills; start and end each with a 10-minute warmup and cooldown.

the Garmin Forerunner 305 because both runners and coaches can see elevation, pace, and heart rate.

HEAD FOR THE (FAKE) HILLS

Russ suggests moderate hills on the treadmill, like five x seven minutes of climbing at seven percent incline (with five minutes recovery) or four x twelve minutes of climbing at eight percent (with seven minutes recovery). Your effort should be moderate, between 4 and 6 on an exertion scale of 1 to 10.

KEEP ON TRACK

Tam's plan integrates weekly speedwork that ranges between 5 x 600 meters to 3 x 1600 meters. Varying the distances and days you do this speedwork will help keep your body challenged.

GO LONG MORE

While first-time marathoners usually don't hit double-digit runs until the weekend, Tam's plan has two weekly runs that are a minimum of 10 miles. The math is simple: The more you run, the more you lose.

Amby Burfoot's Running Round-Up

A few years ago, in my 50s, I decided to see if I could lose some weight. This surprised a few of my current friends who considered me pretty slim just the way I was. But I remembered my old self—the one who had weighed 20 pounds less when he was in college, at a time that he ran the best races of his life.

I didn't expect to get all the way back to my college weight, but I did manage to pare off 10 pounds, and it made a big difference in how I felt and ran. I felt lighter, more nimble, and more energetic. And I began running faster than I had run in 15 years. Was I excited about this? You bet!

Every slightly thinner dieter has a couple of nutrition tricks that worked for him or her. Here are mine. I ate a high-fiber oatmeal breakfast every morning and tried to include sources of fiber—salad and beans, for the most part—in all my meals. I ate smaller portions of pasta and rice, and larger portions of vegetables in my frequent stir-fries. And I focused mightily, if not always successfully, on cutting down the calories I consumed in the evening, after dinner. I don't think any of these strategies did the trick alone. Rather, weight loss comes from constant vigilance and many small changes.

Chapter 30

The Ultimate Runner's Weight-Loss Plan

How to melt the pounds away with the right combination of exercise and nutrition

There's no such thing as a guaranteed weight-loss plan. If there were, the world would be full of healthy, lean people. It's not—in fact, all the trend lines are heading in the wrong direction—so we can be sure that no one has yet found a surefire, double-your-money-back approach to paring off the pounds. But running comes close.

The reason running works so well is simple mathematics. Running burns roughly 100 calories for every mile you cover, and more than that if you weigh more than 140 pounds to begin with, as many runners do when they take up the sport for the health, the weight loss, the challenge, or whatever your motivations are. At the same time, running doesn't increase your appetite; many people find that it decreases their food cravings.

The result? You burn more calories, and consume fewer. As everyone knows, that's the formula for losing weight, as easy to say as it is devilishly difficult to achieve. One key to success is to make sure you adopt a nutrition plan that's as good for your workouts as it is for your weight loss. That's the focus of this chapter.

DIETER'S STRATEGY: Eat low-fat foods. RUNNER'S STRATEGY: Eat the right fats.

Though the fat-free craze peaked in the 1990s, many dieters still avoid oils, butter, nuts, and other fatty foods. Their logic: If you don't want your body to store fat, then don't eat fat. Many dieters also know that one gram of fat packs nine calories, while protein and carbohydrate both contain just four calories per gram. Dieters can stretch the same number of calories a lot farther if they eat mostly carbs and protein in place of fat.

But having fat in your diet isn't a bad thing, and that notion is catching on again. "I think it's a pretty antiquated thought now that we need to eliminate fat to lose weight," says Jonny Bowden, Ph.D., author of *The 150 Most Effective Ways to Boost Energy Naturally*. In fact, studies have shown that eating moderate amounts of fat can actually help you lose weight. The key is to make sure you're eating the right kinds. Saturated and trans fats are unhealthy because they raise your levels of LDL (so-called bad cholesterol). Trans fats may also lower your HDL (or good cholesterol) levels and increase your risk for heart disease—not to mention weight gain. But unsaturated fats (which include mono- and polyunsaturated) have important benefits. Here's why runners should include these fats in their diet.

1. Keep you satisfied: Unsaturated fats promote satiety, reduce hunger, and minimally impact blood sugar. That's important because if your blood sugar dips too low, you may experience cravings, brain fog, overeating, and low energy, making it "fiendishly difficult to lose weight," says Bowden.

2. Protect heart health: Unlike trans fats, monounsaturated fats found in vegetable oils (such as olive and canola) and avocados have the added power to help lower LDL cholesterol and reduce your risk of heart disease.

3. Reduce injury: Unsaturated fats can help stave off injuries, such as stress fractures. A 2008 study in the *Journal of the International Society of Sports Nutrition* found that female runners on low-fat diets are at increased risk of injury—and a sidelined runner can't burn as many calories.

4. Decrease joint pain: Bowden adds that omega-3 fatty acids—which are a type of polyunsaturated fat found in fish (particularly in salmon), walnuts, and ground flaxseed—possess anti-inflammatory properties that can help soothe knee, back, and joint aches and pains that plague many runners. Translation: You'll hurt less and run more.

Real runner testimonial: "I added salmon, avocados, walnuts, and flax to my diet," says Abi Meadows of San Antonio. "The results were unreal: Over the next six months, the weight came off, and I noticed a huge jump in energy."

Drop 5 Pounds in 4 Weeks

Starting to lose that extra weight can be easier than you think. One pound of body fat equals 3,500 calories, so to drop 5 pounds you need a calorie deficit of 17,500. Here's how to reach that five-pound loss in just four weeks.

DIETER'S STRATEGY: Develop a running routine and stick to it. RUNNER'S STRATEGY: Mix up your routine with new types of workouts.

Anyone trying to lose weight knows that he or she needs to work out on a nearly daily basis—and that's not easy. So to stay on track, dieters develop a workout routine (that often includes lots of steady, slowish runs) and then stick to it no matter what. "People are comfortable doing what they know," says Pete McCall, an exercise physiologist with the American Council on Exercise.

While running an easy three-miler a few days a week is better for weight loss than doing nothing, there is a smarter approach. Break out of your routine by boosting your intensity and doing different types of workouts (like a weekly long run or a day of cross-training) to challenge your body and burn more calories. "It's a lot like city driving versus highway driving," says McCall. "When running a long, slow distance, your body becomes really efficient at using oxygen. The more times you do the same distance, the easier it gets and the fewer calories you burn. Sprinting is like starting and stopping a car,

which uses more gas." Plus, trying something new can add fun and excitement into an otherwise dull workout.

Real runner testimonial: "I started biking to and from work five days a week—and the extra pounds came off in just six months," says Buck Hales of Oak Park, Illinois. "I continue to bike to supplement my runs, and use other cardio machines three to four days a week. I'm still a runner through and through; mixing things up helps keep it that way."

Break Out of a Rut

A 150-pound runner doing a four-miler at a nine-minute pace burns about 480 calories. But you can torch more calories, speed weight loss, and spark up your workouts by swapping that four-miler

CHANGE IT UP	ROUTINE CALORIE DEFICIT	CHANGE-UP CALORIE DEFICIT
Swap out two days of regular running for two days of speedwork	440	1,760
Add three miles to your weekly total	300	1,200
Cut 400 calories from your daily intake	22,800	11,200
Every week add one session of cross-training on a day when you don't run	500	2,000
Every week add one session of strength training on a day when you don't run	400	1,600
TOTAL CALORIE DEFICIT	24,440	17,760 (five pounds)

Estimates are based on a 150-pound person who runs four days a week, logging 15 to 20 miles total, running at a nine-minute-per-mile pace.

with one of these high-intensity runs, one to three times a week.

RUT BUSTER: INTERVALS

What: Alternating sprints of a certain distance (such as 400 meters) with recovery laps; often done at a measured track

Why: Sprinting at high speeds makes your body work harder and burns up to 30 percent more calories to keep up with the demand.

How: 4 x 400 meters hard (max speed), separated by an easy 400-meter recovery lap

8 x 200 meters hard, separated by an easy 200 meters

4 x 100 meters hard, walking back to the start between sprints to recover

Calories burned: 700

RUT BUSTER: FARTLEK TRAINING

What: A less formal version of intervals; the term means "speed play" in Swedish.

Why: Like interval workouts, fartlek sessions make your body burn more calories to match the demand of running faster.

How: While out for a 45-minute run, pick a tree or mailbox about 50 meters away. Run hard (max speed) until you reach it, and then slow down until you're recovered. Continue alternating periods of hard running with recovery.

Calories burned: 540

RUT BUSTER: HILLS

What: Running uphill for a period of time

Why: Hills require more force to overcome the angle of the incline, leading to a challenging cardio workout; it's also a great way to strengthen the larger muscles of the legs.

How: Find a steep hill 40 to 80 meters long. Follow this sequence, each time running up the hill and jogging back to recover. Start with 10 reps, progressing to 20:

five runs at 50 percent max speed

two to three runs at 80 percent max speed

one sprint at max speed

Calories burned: 600

DIETER'S STRATEGY: Cut out carbohydrates to lose weight. RUNNER'S STRATEGY: Have quality carbs in every meal.

In the past decade, the Atkins diet and other low-carb spin-offs have become as popular as 100-calorie snack packs. It's understandable why dieters would find these plans attractive: Just eat high-protein, high-fat foods—and shun carbs—to drop pounds. "The theory behind reducing carbs is that it helps control blood-sugar and insulin surges," says Jonny Bowden, Ph.D. "When you eat a high-carb food, insulin carries the sugar to muscles. But if your muscles don't use the energy, it gets stored in fat cells," leading to weight gain.

It's a different story for runners, however. We

need carbs because they're our main source of glucose, a sugar that our brains and muscles use as fuel. Most glucose is stored in muscles and the liver as glycogen and used as energy when we run. But the body can only store a limited amount of glycogen, so if you haven't eaten enough carbs, you'll literally run out of fuel.

Keeping carbs in your diet will have a domino effect, says Barbara Lewin, R.D., owner of Sports-Nutritionist.com: Your energy levels will stay high, your workouts will improve, and you'll have more zip throughout the day. All this leads the way to a greater calorie burn and weight loss. Just keep in mind that "the kind of carbohydrates you eat makes all the difference in the world," says Bowden. Here's a quick guide to choosing the right ones for the right times.

1. Slow-burning carbs: These are high in fiber and are slowly digested. They keep your blood sugar steady, provide long-lasting energy, and should be a staple of your diet. Get them in oatmeal and other whole grains, beans, lentils, fruit, and vegetables.

2. Fast-burning carbs: These are digested quickly, are low in fiber, and have a greater effect on your blood sugar. They provide a quick hit of energy that's useful to runners right before working out, but they should be eaten in moderation. Get them in pasta, white rice, white flour, potatoes, and cornflakes.

Be careful not to get the majority of your calories from carbs all the time. "I call it the flu diet," says Lisa Dorfman, R.D., University of Miami sports nutritionist and adjunct professor in the department of exercise sciences. "Everything is bland and white." Research supports a colorful diet: A recent study published in the

American Journal of Clinical Nutriti[ ] eating colorful berries twice a day f[ ] helps lower blood pressure. "Eat a[ ] ors daily," says Dorfman, "so that you can b[ ] assured you're getting enough fiber and protein to help steady blood sugar and feel more satisfied after eating."

Real runner testimonial: "I gradually introduced whole grains into my diet, foods like whole-wheat English muffins and pita bread, and my energy skyrocketed," says Jessica Trumble of Albuquerque, New Mexico. "Now I make sure to eat carbs, especially in the morning because it helps fuel my day. My runs are easier, I don't tire during my workouts as much, and I've lost weight."

DIETER'S STRATEGY: Cut 500 calories a day to lose one pound a week. RUNNER'S STRATEGY: Reduce calorie intake based on personal needs.

You've probably heard of the 500 Rule: Slash 500 calories a day to lose one pound a week of body fat (one pound of body fat equals 3,500 calories). "It's a nice, clean rule," says Lewin, and for a lot of dieters, cutting 500 calories a day will help them lose weight—at least for a while. The problem for runners, though, is that slashing that many calories can be too much—especially if you're training hard. "Cutting too many calories can be your worst enemy," she says. "It can lead to plummeting energy levels. You might not be able to work out as well or maintain muscle mass; you're setting yourself up for failure." So rather than cutting 500 calories, runners should work to identify the number of calories they personally need to eat to lose weight, says Lewin. Here's how to find that number.

1. Count calories: Track your intake by keeping a detailed food journal for one week, says Lewin. Write down everything you eat, and note your energy and hunger levels on a scale of 1 to 10 (nutritiondata.com and calorieking.com provide calorie counts for most foods, making it easy to do the math).

2. Trim—don't slash: "Start by cutting about 300 calories a day," says Leslie Bonci, R.D., director of sports nutrition at the University of Pittsburgh Medical Center. "It's a more doable number and is more likely to reflect a drop in body fat." As long as you're running, you'll still hit a 500-calorie deficit per day and lose about one pound a week.

3. Tweak it: If you cut 300 calories and maintain your energy levels, but the number on the scale hasn't budged, it's time to reduce your intake gradually, says Bonci. You can also adjust for training. Racking up miles for a marathon? Add calories back in. Having an easy week? Reduce your intake further.

Small Changes, Big Rewards

You don't need to make drastic adjustments to your calorie intake to start dropping pounds. Small substitutes here and there can add up and lead to major weight loss. Jennifer Ventrelle, R.D., owner of a private weight-loss practice in Chicago called Weight No More, suggests these simple food swaps for a day of meals to help cut calories while keeping your energy levels high.

Swap Out: Bagel with cream cheese: *360 calories*

Swap In: Whole-grain bagel with peanut butter and a cup of yogurt: *325 calories*

Swap Out: Starbucks Grande Latte: *190 calories*

Swap In: Starbucks Grande Skinny Vanilla Latte: *130 calories*

Swap Out: Clif Bar: *250 calories*

Swap In: High-fiber, high-protein granola bar, such as Kashi GoLean Crunchy Bar: *180 calories*

Swap Out: Subway six-inch roast-beef sandwich on white with mayo, cheese, and veggies: *400 calories*

Swap In: Subway six-inch roast-beef sandwich on wheat with mustard, no cheese, extra veggies, and apple slices on the side: *340 calories*

Swap Out: Four-ounce pork chop and salad with apples, walnuts, and goat cheese: *485 calories*

Swap In: Four ounces of pork tenderloin and a mixed green salad with apples and walnuts (hold the cheese), and a half cup of brown rice: *380 calories*

Swap Out: One cup of vanilla ice cream: *290 calories*

Swap In: Half cup of vanilla ice cream with one cup of raspberries: *205 calories*

Original daily intake: 1,975 calories
New daily intake: 1,560 calories
Total daily savings: 415 calories

DIETER'S STRATEGY:
Eat diet food.
RUNNER'S STRATEGY:
Eat real food.

Many dieters walk the aisles of the grocery store feeling more anxiety than pleasure. They want to buy foods that will help them lose weight, provide nutrients, and make it easier to practice portion control—but aren't sure what to choose. So they gravitate toward foods that make those promises, zeroing in on products that are part of a weight-loss program or feature words like light, low-fat, reduced-calorie, diet-friendly, or low-carb. "People think they need a certain diet program or diet products to be successful," says Elaine Magee, R.D., author of the book *Food Synergy*, and these foods promise success.

But all too often, the opposite is true, says Magee. Runners can accomplish the same weight-loss goals while eating whole, real foods that taste better, provide more nutritional value, and are more satisfying. "When you go for healthy whole foods," says Joy Bauer, R.D., author of *Joy's Life Diet: Four Steps to Thin Forever*, "such as lean proteins, boatloads of vegetables, fresh fruits, whole grains, nuts and seeds, and low-fat dairy, you tend to get satiated on the right amounts." That means it will be easier to keep portions under control and gauge how many calories you're taking in. "Many dieters also end up feeling deprived because they think they have very few choices," says Magee. But when you realize that you have a nearly limitless range of healthy, whole foods, that feeling fades away—along with the desire to overindulge.

Just make sure to choose "less dense" food such as vegetable soup and turkey sandwiches over "energy dense" foods such as hamburgers. Less dense foods have a higher water content than fats

and carbs, explain researchers in a 2007 *American Journal of Clinical Nutrition* study, which found that people who lower their energy density lower their weight. A more recent study from the same journal found similar results: Those who eat a lot of energy-dense foods weigh more, have a higher intake of trans and saturated fat, and eat fewer fruits and vegetables.

Sticking to a real-food diet does take a bit more time than pulling out a low-fat frozen dinner entree. But with proper planning, runners can minimize the work. "Stocking your freezer and pantry with healthy staples, like seasonal fruits and whole grains, ensures you have plenty of ingredients on hand," says Magee. "And when you find simple, healthy recipes that work for you, hang onto them," so you'll have ideas for quick meals when you need them. After you've been filling your plate this way for a while, "you'll start to feel empowered," Bauer promises, and that will have a positive effect on your running, your weight loss, and your attitude toward food.

DIETER'S STRATEGY:
Avoid strength training to keep from adding on pounds.
RUNNER'S STRATEGY:
Balance running and strength training.

Dieters often shy away from strength training, such as lifting weights, out of a fear it will make them bulk up. Others are intimidated by going to a gym. But for many dieters, the reason is simpler: They know one hour of intense cardio burns more calories than one hour of strength training. If you're pressed for time, it would seem that intense cardiovascular exercise would provide more bang for your buck, leading to a greater weight loss than pumping iron.

Yet the truth is that taking the time to add strength training to your routine a few days a week has a number of counterintuitive benefits that can help boost your weight loss. Studies have shown that strength training can improve body composition by helping you maintain or increase your lean body mass and can decrease your percentage of body fat, helping you look leaner and burn additional calories. Here's how it works.

1. Muscle burns more calories: "Fat burns almost nothing at rest," says exercise physiologist Pete McCall, "whereas muscle uses oxygen. If you increase lean muscle mass, you'll increase the body's ability to use oxygen and burn more calories." Your body typically uses about four and a half to seven calories per pound of muscle every day. If a 160-pound runner with 20 percent body fat increases his muscle mass and lowers his body fat to 15 percent, he'll burn an extra 36 to 56 calories a day at rest—simply by adding muscle.

2. You'll be more efficient: Strength training can help you run faster, longer, and more efficiently. A study published last year in the *Journal of Strength and Conditioning Research* showed that runners who add three days of resistance training exercises to their weekly program increase their leg strength and enhance their endurance. Obviously, runners with better endurance can run longer—and burn more calories. You'll also be able to recover faster from those long runs because strength training makes your body more efficient at converting metabolic waste into energy. "It's like being able to convert car exhaust into gas," says McCall.

3. You'll be less injury-prone: "If you increase your strength, you'll also increase your joint stability, reducing your risk of repetitive stress injuries," says McCall, citing a study in the *Journal of Strength and Conditioning Research*, which showed that incorporating moves such as squats, single-leg hops, and ab work into a workout can not only prevent lower-body injuries, but also improve performance as well. Leg exercises are particularly important when it comes to reducing injury: These exercises strengthen muscles around the knees and hips, two areas that often cause problems for runners.

Real runner testimonial: "I added a three-days-on-one-day-off strength-training routine to my regimen, focusing on two muscle groups at a time," says Tom Parnell of Boston. "I believe that lifting weights helped me drop about half of the 40 pounds I eventually lost—plus I got stronger, faster, and haven't gotten injured."

DIETER'S STRATEGY: Drop pounds fast by focusing on short-term goals
RUNNER'S STRATEGY: Lose pounds slowly and have a post-loss plan

For many dieters, their sole motivation is to lose weight as fast as possible. Maybe it's for an upcoming college reunion or to look good in a bathing suit. Either way, the "lose weight fast" strategy often leads dieters down a dangerous path. They slash calories or work out like a fiend to shed pounds as quickly as possible. Then, once they hit their goal weight, they think they're done. They slowly go back to their old habits, and soon enough the pounds start to creep back on.

By avoiding some of these drastic measures, runners can gradually shed pounds and reach their goal weight. But what happens next? "So often we say, 'Hooray, I hit my goal weight. I'm done,'" says Denver-based weight-loss coach Linda Spangle, R.N., author of *100 Days of Weight Loss*. "That's the absolute biggest mistake and prevents you from maintaining long term." Just as you shouldn't stop training once you reach a running goal, keeping the weight off is a daily fight, demanding vigilance and effort. Here's how to address many of the issues that arise while trying to maintain your new body so that 10 or 20 years from now you're still lean, happy, healthy—and running.

1. Keep at it: Most members of the National Weight Control Registry, a group of about 5,000 people who have maintained significant weight losses, continue high exercise levels and some form of a reduced-calorie diet—two principles that got you to your new weight. "You can slowly increase your total calories if you remain very consistent with exercise—but do it gradually," says Spangle, so that you don't risk going overboard.

2. Step on the scale: A 2008 literature review published in the *International Journal of Behavioral Nutrition and Physical Activity* examined the results of several studies on self-weighing and weight gain. The conclusion: People who weigh themselves daily or weekly lose more weight—and keep it off—than dieters who rarely step on a scale.

3. Get support: Finding some social support—from a mentor, friend, or a running group—adds a sense of accountability and helps keep off the pounds. The right kind of Web-based support helps, too. A 2007 study in *Obesity* showed that an online, therapist-led behavioral weight-loss Web site led to greater weight loss than a self-help commercial site.

4. Get enough sleep: Research has linked sleep loss to obesity and suggests that people who don't get enough may weigh more. And a recent study in the *American Journal of Clinical Nutrition* found that people who get less sleep eat more snacks, especially high-carb ones. Without enough sleep, your energy levels, immune system, and mood drop; the only thing up (besides you) will be your appetite. But that doesn't mean you should cut out your morning runs to stay in bed. Routine is key for weight loss. Consider going to bed an hour earlier or try switching your workouts to later in the day.

5. Mind emotional eating: Eating food for comfort or out of boredom is the number one reason people regain weight, Spangle says. Plus, according to a 2008 *Nature* study, emotional eating often triggers binges. Austin-area fitness blogger and former trainer Carla Birnberg tells her clients to ask themselves, "Does a bowl of steamed chicken and broccoli sound good?" If the answer is no, you're not hungry for food as fuel.

6. Keep your motivation high: Create a list of the reasons you wanted to lose weight—and keep adding to the list ("I want to be a good role model for my kids"; "I want to feel young"). It helps you remember the lasting pleasures and benefits of slimming down. "It feels so good to be comfortable in your new body," says Joy Bauer, R.D., "even if every day is a bit of a struggle, it's a struggle worth fighting because of the payoff."

Amby Burfoot's Running Round-Up

Because we are all unique individuals, we ultimately have to find our own best path to running and healthy-weight maintenance. This chapter has provided many pointers, but you still have to supplement with approaches that work best for you. When I was younger, for example, I ran many dozens more miles per week than I do now, and I got a lot of my daily calories from fruit juices. On a warmish day, I would often drink a half-gallon or more of orange juice.

That was good for me then, but wouldn't be today, since OJ is filled with natural sugar calories, like all fruit juices. I have a weakness for sweet juices, and it took me a long time to wean myself from tall, cold glasses of OJ. But eventually I did, because I had to find a lower-calorie drink. These days, lightly carbonated water is my favorite, though many of my friends prefer "flat" water in bottles or from the tap.

I've also had to drastically curtail my ice cream consumption. I now consider it a special summer treat, not a daily delight. In its place, I generally eat cut-up apples with cinnamon and other spices sprinkled on top. Sometimes I'll add a little vanilla- or fruit-sweetened yogurt. These lower-calorie options seem to work well with my more modest weekly running mileage of about 20 to 25 miles. It's all a matter of balance, and it doesn't matter how you get there. As long as you do.

Chapter 31

Eat Smarter, Lose Weight, Run Stronger

Take our quiz to make sure you understand the principles of good nutrition and weight loss for runners

The world of nutrition is full of potholes, complicated concepts, and rampant misinformation. Even runners who spend a fair amount of time educating themselves about optimal sports nutrition will occasionally grow confused. After all, there's just so much to keep up with these days, from the research journals to the thousands of blogs by seemingly well-intentioned and well-informed experts. On occasion, it's a good idea to stop, breathe deep, and review what you think you know.

That's the purpose of this chapter, with its question-and-answer format. It's light reading (thank goodness!) but chock-full of useful advice that you can take to the supermarket or the kitchen table. Some of the questions might seem easy to you, but others are certain to challenge. I particularly like the questions on "serving size." I think a better understanding of this key idea can help you eat healthier and lose weight at the same time (if that's your goal). Good luck with the quiz. I hope you

score in the "impressive" category, or even better.

Whether you want to lose weight, feel more energetic, or fuel your love of running and perform better, you need to know your food. Take this quiz to test your nutrition knowledge and eating habits—then learn a few ways to dine smarter. But don't stop there. After you've taken the quiz and learned the answers, use this new information to shop smarter and improve your diet. Your workouts and your races will appreciate the difference.

As you take the quiz, note your responses on a sheet of paper. On page 232, you'll find the answers and explanations you're looking for.

1. How many servings are in a cup of pasta?
   A. Half a serving
   B. One serving
   C. Two servings
   D. Three servings

2. How large is a single portion of meat?
   A. A deck of cards
   B. A slice of Wonder bread
   C. A hockey puck
   D. A big, fat porterhouse steak

3. What does a single serving of most cereals look like?
   A. A softball
   B. A clenched fist
   C. A golf ball
   D. A bicycle helmet

4. What is the ideal size for a dinner plate?
   A. 9-inch diameter
   B. 10-inch diameter
   C. 12-inch diameter
   D. It really doesn't matter, as long as you fill it only halfway.

5. Do you know how many calories you consume in a day?
   A. Hmm, I have no clue.
   B. More or less, but I hardly think about it most days.
   C. Sure. I have a fairly accurate knowledge of my daily caloric intake.

6. Which has the most calories?
   A. 1 cup of Kellogg's Bran Flakes
   B. ½ cup of Kellogg's Frosted Flakes
   C. ¼ cup of Kellogg's Mueslix
   D. ¼ cup Bear Naked Granola

7. Pound for pound, which of these meats has the least fat?
   A. 95% lean ground beef
   B. Ground turkey
   C. Skinless chicken thigh

8. How many calories are in a venti (24-ounce) Starbucks' Strawberry Cream Frappuccino?
   A. 560
   B. 770
   C. 850

9. Which has more vitamin A?
   A. One cup of Wheaties
   B. One cup of cooked peas
   C. One sweet potato
   D. One cup of kale

10. What is the best source of vitamin K?
    A. Spinach
    B. Broccoli
    C. Carrots
    D. Vitamin what?

11. Do you take a multivitamin?
    A. Yes, every day
    B. Yes, several times a week
    C. Never

12. How many servings of fruits and vegetables should you consume every 24 hours?
    A. 3 to 4 servings
    B. 5 to 9 servings
    C. 9 to 11 servings
    D. More than 12

13. What is the maximum number of energy bars you should consume in one week?
    A. Three per week
    B. One per day

C. As long as they are high-fiber and low-sugar, you can eat as many as you like.

14. How many servings of dairy should you consume daily?

A. Two servings a day, preferably in the morning

B. Two to three servings, spaced throughout the day

C. Active people need three to four servings a day.

15. How much alcohol did you drink last night?

A. None. I rarely, if ever, drink at all.

B. A glass or two of wine

C. More than three drinks; same as always

16. It's okay to eat fast food every day if:

A. The rest of your diet is balanced, low in fat, and high in fiber from vegetables, fruits, and grains.

B. It is never okay to eat fast food daily; twice a month at most.

C. Your diet is low-calorie for the rest of the day.

17. How often do you eat sweets?

A. At least twice a day

B. Every night

C. Several times a week

D. Only on special occasions

18. What is the ideal ratio of carbohydrates to protein for an energy bar?

A. 2 to 1

B. 3 to 1

C. 5 to 1

D. It depends on whether you're eating before or after exercise.

19. What percentage of a runner's calories should come from protein?

A. 25%

B. 10%

C. 30%

D. 5%

20. How often do you run on a completely empty stomach?

A. Never

B. Almost never

C. Almost always

D. Always

21. What is the best way to refuel after a five-mile run?

A. With a low-sugar granola bar

B. With a generous plate of pasta

C. With a milk shake

22. What is your favorite snack to consume during a long run?

A. A granola bar

B. A handful of pretzels and some water

C. Gatorade or another sports drink

23. Approximately how many calories should an active man/woman eat per day?

A. 2,200 calories/1,900 calories

B. 2,600 calories/2,200 calories

C. 2,900 calories/2,400 calories

D. 3,000 calories/2,500 calories

24. If you're trying to lose weight while running, should you cut calories from your diet?

A. Yes. Any way you can cut calories while running is the fastest way to lose weight.

B. No. Just increase your mileage or pace.

C. Yes, as long as you don't skimp on calories consumed during or right after a workout.

25. How much fluid should active people consume each day?

    A. Men need 125 ounces, women need 90 ounces

    B. Eight cups a day

    C. As much as you need to quench your thirst

    D. Six cups a day, excluding coffee and other diuretics

ANSWERS

Give yourself four points for each correct answer, unless noted otherwise below. Then check the "Scoring" section to see how you did and where you need to make changes in your nutritional approach.

1. C. Most people guess lower, and as a result eat more refined pasta than they need to. Here's a better approach: Fill your pasta plate with half the pasta you normally eat now, and the other half of your plate with steamed veggies. You'll get all the carbs you need, along with a lot more vitamins and phytonutrients, such as the antioxidants that are plentiful in many vegetables.

2. A. It's easy to make smart food choices and still sabotage your diet by ignoring serving sizes. To make matters tougher, portions keep growing. "Many people assume muffins are healthier than doughnuts, for example," says Leslie Bonci, R.D., director of sports nutrition at the University of Pittsburgh Medical Center. "It's a good assumption, but muffins used to be two inches in diameter. Today they can be more than four inches, which means they've tripled in calories."

3. B. Nutrition consultant Susan McQuillan, M.S., R.D., advocates using body parts for measurement (presuming you don't have hands like Yao Ming). "Your fist is about a cup, which is a serving of cereal or vegetables," says McQuillan, author of *Low-Calorie Dieting for Dummies*. "An ounce of nuts, or two ounces of chips or popcorn, fits in the cup of your open fist. Your palm is roughly the size of a three-ounce serving of meat. Your thumb from the tip to the second joint is about the size of one ounce of cheese."

4. A. Fifty years ago, American plates were smaller (much like they are in Europe today), and as they have grown larger, so has the collective American waistline. Bigger plates lead to more eating, because they make portions look smaller. "Choosing smaller plates, glasses, and bowls will help train your body to get used to smaller sizes," says Bonci.

5. C. (two points for picking B) For those of us who resist studying nutrition labels, a good rule of thumb for cutting calories is to eat wet foods over dry ones, says Bonci. "Drier foods have a higher calorie density. They don't take up a lot of room in the stomach, so we need to eat a lot of them before feeling full." Cushion the blow of cookies, chips, and other dry foods by combining them with wet ingredients. Eat salsa with your chips. Have a glass of skim milk with your cookie.

6. D. Cereal is delicious, healthy, and more calorie-dense than many people realize. "The calorie costs of Mueslix and nut-and-grain-packed granolas like Bare Naked are huge," says Bonci. "The serving sizes are two or three tablespoons. Of course, no one is eating that little."

7. A. Many assume otherwise, but ground poultry generally has more fat than red meat, because it often contains dark meat and skin. Choose ground breast meat, or look for the words "low-fat." And lean cuts of beef—which include round, chuck, sirloin, and tenderloin—are a healthy, high-protein alternative. Select packages marked 90 percent lean or higher.

8. B. Brace yourself: Some Frappuccinos have more than 20 times the calories of a cup of joe (only 35 to 40 calories with a quarter cup of milk). Of course, fancy coffee drinks are hardly the only perpetrator. Fast-food sodas, large glasses of juice, and oil-can-sized energy drinks are packed with calories. Even an innocent-sounding bottle of Vitamin Water contains 300 calories.

9. C. One baked sweet potato contains about twice the Daily Value of vitamin A. Other good sources of this nutrient (which promotes bone growth and helps regulate your immune system): cooked carrots and spinach.

10. A. (two points for picking B) Spinach and other leafy greens are the best sources of vitamin K, which protects your heart and builds bones. And unfortunately, it's one of many nutrients that runners tend to be deficient in. Why? In many cases, runners simply shy away from foods they don't like (say leafy greens) or limit their intake of red meat, oils, and fatty foods—a healthy habit to be sure, but one that can lead to shortfalls in key nutrients, says Bonci. "Vitamin D can be difficult to get because it's found in foods like liver and egg yolks, which aren't at the top of most runners' lists." Two other problem nutrients for runners who limit oils and fats: vitamin E and zinc.

Creating a Food Diary

Yes, it's possible that you have dietary habits you likely don't even know you have. "Food diaries are very eye-opening when people are trying to get a handle on their eating," says Leslie Bonci, R.D. That's true whether you're trying to lose weight or better understand your eating habits. Rather than spend $250 on a nutritionist, here's how to create your own diary.

Log the details: Bonci has clients create six columns in their food logs: the food, the amount, the time it was consumed, how many minutes it took to consume, where it was eaten, and reason for eating it. "Being detail-oriented is really important for people trying to change habits," she says. Everything—even small bites—counts.

Go long (enough): A five-day food diary is long enough, but be sure to include a weekend in the diary. "Many uncover that their alcohol intake really spikes on the weekend, for instance," says Bonci.

Look for clues: Common mistakes diaries turn up include: unconscious snacking; consuming too many packaged foods; eating too much at night; and ingesting too much salt.

11. A. "I look at multivitamins as an insurance policy—and it's great to take one daily," says Bonci. "But I tell athletes that they still need to do their part by eating real foods." At the other extreme are supplement junkies, who overfortify with nutrient-enhanced energy bars and shakes. Problem is, getting an excess of certain vitamins and minerals can be unhealthy. For example, too much chromium can interfere with the absorption of zinc. And excess iron can cause liver damage.

12. B. While meeting the FDA recommendation of five-to-nine servings of fruits and vegetables a day may seem daunting, there are many easy ways to boost your intake of these important foods. "People forget about spaghetti sauce, vegetable soup, pickles, V8, raisins in cereal, even the peppers and onions on a pizza," says Bonci. "These all count."

13. A. Athletes who pound energy bars on a daily basis do so with the best of intentions; after all, most are rich in fiber and vitamins, and contain an ideal mix of carbs to protein. But when these processed bars start to replace real food, it's time to worry, says McQuillan. Bonci urges her athletes to consume bars, which are often dense with calories, in stages. "Split them in half," she says, "so you have something for pre-run and post-run fuel."

14. B. It is important to consume at least two to three servings of dairy a day, but our bodies can absorb only about 500 milligrams of calcium at a time. That's roughly what's in one cup of yogurt, so space your dairy throughout the day.

15. A or B. According to a study in the *Journal of the American College of Sports Medicine*, serious recreational runners drink more alcohol than sedentary folks. And a glass or two a night is widely recognized as a healthy part of a balanced diet. More than three, however, and you're likely compromising your health and athletic performance. Plus, alcohol can interfere with runners' already higher hydration needs. Try diluting your cocktail with seltzer, and alternate a glass of water between each alcoholic beverage.

16. A. Hey, we all lead fast-paced lives, and there's a time and a place for fast food in those lives. Like once a day, perhaps. As long as the fast foods you pick are generally healthful, and not huge portions of fat, salt, and sugar masquerading as foods. The key is balance and moderation. You can afford to eat fast foods as long as you don't overdo them or rely too heavily on them. For example, at lunchtime you could choose a high-protein, low-fat sandwich, along with a salad that's not drowning in a fatty dressing.

17. D. (three points for picking C; two for choosing B) "If you routinely eat a nutritious, well-balanced diet, then you can fit in sweets or fast food every day, in small amounts," says McQuillan. "The trouble is, most people go overboard. A cup of ice cream is very different from the whole pint." Too many simple sugars "provide the raw material for the manufacture of triglycerides—fats that circulate in your bloodstream that experts now believe are as important as cholesterol when it comes to risk of heart disease, not to mention weight gain," she says.

18. B. An energy bar with a 3-to-1 ratio of carbs and protein perfectly answers your pre-workout and post-run fuel needs. Too many carbs can slow down digestion, causing discomfort mid-workout. (The carbs, by the way, should come in the form of dried fruit, cane juice, or honey, rather than simple sugars.) And a bar with a 3-to-1 ratio supplies plenty of protein to meet your body's post-run demands. The many protein bars on the market are intended more for meal replacements, and while they can serve as an alternative to mindless snacking, they should be used sparingly.

19. C. In spite of the recent protein craze, Bonci still sees many runners skimping. "They all know how important carbohydrates are, but they don't realize that they lack protein and fat in their diets." Most nutritionists advise at least a half gram per pound of body weight. Simple ways to up intake: eating bean dip with your corn chips, adding cheese to your vegetarian chili, or spreading peanut butter on your celery or banana.

20. A. (three points for picking B; one for choosing C) Even though nutritionists harp on the importance of eating before training, many runners still head out the door on empty—and then overeat later. How come? "Lack of planning," says Bonci. "Runners forget or wait until the last minute. I tell my athletes to think about their run one hour before." Aim for a small amount of easily digested carbohydrates so the fuel will be available during your run. Afternoon and evening runners should eat a snack one or two hours prior to exercise; this is as simple as a banana, a handful of cereal, or a bagel.

21. A. Postrun replenishment doesn't require a lot of food, either. "Runners think they need to refuel with large amounts of carbohydrates, like a huge plate of pasta, but all you need is something like a reduced-sugar chewy bar, a half cup of cereal, or a single granola bar," says Bonci.

22. C. During a long run (the only kind that demands midworkout nourishment), stick to wet-

Sudden Impact
4 easy ways to eat better—today

1. Start serving dinner on smaller plates.
2. Eat a snack an hour or two before every run.
3. Take a multivitamin.
4. Eat low-fat dairy twice a day.

ter foods, says Bonci. "A sports drink is my first choice, since it provides fuel, fluid, and electrolytes. But for those who like more calories, opt for gels or honey sticks; these aren't dry and they leave the stomach quickly."

23. B. Very active women need to consume about 17 calories per pound; similarly, active men require about 20 calories per pound.

24. C. "I don't encourage runners to actively try to lose weight while increasing mileage, as it usually results in fatigue, delayed recovery, and sometimes increased risk of injury," says Bonci. "You can slightly trim down the amount eaten at the meals that are not around the time of exercise, however." And don't skip the post-run fueling window: It will help ward off a late-night hunger attack.

25. A. If you're drinking to quench your thirst, you're probably not drinking enough. All types of fluids count (the obvious exception is alcohol); whatever it takes to get your intake near 100 ounces daily.

SCORING

0 TO 20 POINTS

Look on the bright side: You're still alive. It wouldn't be an awful idea to read the advice above and make some changes today.

21 TO 40 POINTS

The bad news: You don't have the best eating habits. The good news: It's easy to improve your score (and your health) with a little extra effort.

41 TO 60 POINTS

Decent—you surely know how to read a nutrition label and eat smart. But that doesn't mean you can't boost your food IQ.

61 TO 80 POINTS

Impressive. You must have strong knowledge— and good habits. With a couple of changes, you can be a nutrition superstar.

81 TO 100 POINTS

You're either a closet nutritionist or a freaking genius. Either way, we toast your future—it's probably going to be a long one.

Amby Burfoot's Running Round-Up

Here's an idea to help you make practical use of the information in this chapter. Review the questions and answers, and select five things that struck you as particularly important to your own nutrition goals. Turn these into five action plans, write the actions on an index card, and put the card on your refrigerator. There's no better place to grab your attention every day.

Then turn the plan into reality. Often, it's best to initiate just one new action at a time. For example, you might want to focus on Answer 20—the need for a quick, energizing snack before your workouts. Buy some energy bars or Fig Newtons or your favorite fruit, and make sure to eat a little before your runs. You'll be amazed by how much stronger this makes you feel.

After you've succeeded on one front, move to the next. Rome wasn't built in a day, and you don't need to make wholesale changes to your diet in a day. In fact, don't even try. You're likely to feel overwhelmed very quickly. Instead, make gradual nutrition changes and watch how they slowly add up to substantial improvements. The same as your training does.

[IX]

The Half-Marathon

Chapter 32

Build Both Your Speed and Your Endurance

The half-marathon demands the perfect combination of muscular and aerobic conditioning

Some runners are defined by a single race. Roger Bannister was the first to break four minutes in the mile, and Abebe Bikila won his first Olympic gold medal running barefoot over the cobblestoned streets of the Appian Way in Rome. Ryan Hall might not belong at quite the same level as Bannister and Bikila, but his big breakthrough race ranks way up there.

In it, he smashed a longstanding American record, announced to the world that he had arrived as a road runner, and added more fuel to the already blazing popularity of the half-marathon distance. Since Hall's astounding performance, half-marathon races have continued their explosive growth.

The distance is halfway to the full marathon, but all-the-way terrific as a race goal for any runner. And Hall's training, engineered by his brilliant young coach, Terrence Mahon, has served as a model for many runners.

Ryan Hall was so pumped after his record-breaking performance at the Aramco Houston Half-Marathon in early 2007, he didn't even bend over to catch his breath. He just started hugging people: his coach, his wife, Sara, and his parents. As they were celebrating, the second-place finisher was still nowhere in sight.

Hall crossed the line in 59:43, taking a minute and 12 seconds off an American half-marathon mark that had stood for 22 years (Mark Curp's 1:00:55 in 1985). In doing so, he joined a select group of world-class athletes who have broken the one-hour barrier for 13.1 miles. "I remember thinking, I'd love to go under an hour at some point," says Hall. "So to do it in my first try was huge for me."

It seemed an unlikely scenario: In his first attempt at the distance, a baby-faced 24-year-old, who had specialized in the mile and 5000 meters at Stanford University, blows away a record that was almost as old as he is—with no one within a quarter-mile of him.

How'd he do it?

THE LONG HALL

For his first half-marathon, Hall trained like a marathoner. In fact, he ran Houston as preparation for the Flora London Marathon on April 22, where he finished seventh in 2:08:24—the fastest-ever U.S. debut marathon.

That's one of two approaches taken by his coach, Terrence Mahon, who describes the half-marathon as an "in-betweener." It pushes runners who focus on 5-Ks and 10-Ks to test their endurance and helps marathoners learn to call upon their speed reserve. Its "in-between" status may also explain its popularity: More than half a million people finished a half-marathon in 2006, and it's the fastest-growing road-racing distance, according to Running USA.

"I've fine-tuned two models," Mahon says. "I take 10-K training and extend it out, or use a marathon program and take down the long runs a bit." The 5-K/10-K runner building up to a half stays sharp with faster-paced intervals, but longer recovery times, than marathoners. The marathoner tackles slower intervals with shorter recovery and longer long runs as preparation for both the full and half-marathon. The best plan for you depends on your strengths and goals (see "What's Your [Half] Type?" on page xx).

Both approaches emphasize the same key workouts: tempo and race simulation runs. Getting used to the comfortably hard pace of tempo workouts, says Mahon, helps you run a fast half. For Hall, extending his tempo run to 12 miles (from 8) made the difference in his preparation for Houston. "Tempos teach you how to gauge your energy," says Hall. "And they really got my legs used to the pounding."

Hall, who lives in Mammoth Lakes, California, with his wife, also a professional runner, trains at altitude, where his tempo pace is roughly 4:55 per mile, 10 seconds slower than it would be at sea level. Altitude compounds the importance of pacing because if you go out too fast, you'll quickly find yourself in oxygen debt. "It's hard to regroup from that," says Hall. "I can't tell you how many times I've gone out way too hard on tempo runs. But if you do enough of them, you find the gear you know you can just stick to."

Hall did long tempo runs every other week as part of a two-week training cycle. On the alternate weeks, he did shorter, faster tempos and—more important—long runs called race-simulation workouts. On these 16- to 20-mile runs, Hall ran the first half at a comfortable pace and the second half at marathon pace, which teaches patience.

Hall maintained his speed with weekly interval sessions, such as two miles at half-marathon pace, one mile at 10-K pace, and a half-mile at 5-K pace, repeating that sequence twice. But he didn't obsess about his splits like he did when he was racing on the track. "I'm not trying to PR in the workout every single time," he says. "My mentality with intervals is to go out there, put in the work, and whatever it is, it is."

A RECORD FALLS

Before Houston, Hall got caught in a snowstorm, missed his flight, and arrived in town, frazzled, late in the day before the race. He and Mahon drove the course, spotting landmarks Hall could use to break up the race in his head.

Mahon's bigger concern, however, was holding Hall back through the first mile. "Ryan is pretty aggressive, and he has to control himself at the start," says Mahon. "You can burn a lot of energy in that first mile." The plan was for Hall to go out at about a 4:35 pace—and absolutely no faster than 4:30. He opened in 4:38, which turned out to be one of his two slowest miles that day. "When I saw that he did what he needed to, I knew he was going to be fine," says Mahon.

Hall covered the next two miles in nine minutes, and led the field by 41 seconds at the 5-K mark. His form never broke—until he started waving his arms at the end to urge more cheers from the crowd. "A ton of emotion came out in the last 100 meters," says Hall. "I've had this belief that God has given me a gift to run, and I can run at a world-class level. I've seen glimpses of it, but never felt like I was starting to arrive. To see that dream begin to come true is unreal, like a little kid finally walking into a major-league baseball stadium."

On the following pages, Ryan Hall offers his advice on training for and racing your best half-marathon.

DURING TRAINING

Don't be afraid of mistakes. That's what training is—practice for the real thing. "You've got to expect you're going to screw up sometimes," says Hall, who frequently goes out too hard on tempo runs. "When I do, I think this is good practice for when I go out too fast in a race and have to regroup."

Simulate race conditions. If you want to run fast on the roads, skip the track and do your interval workouts on the roads.

Know the purpose of each workout. Make the hard runs hard and the recovery runs easy, says Hall. Many runners make the mistake of running too hard on their easy days, which is counterproductive. You'll only tire yourself for the quality days that really matter.

AT THE RACE

Inspect the course. Familiarize yourself with landmarks, so you have some mental breaks in addition to the mile markers. Look for places to run the tangents if you're going for a PR.

Let the terrain dictate your pace. If you want to average seven-minute miles, it's okay to run 7:10s up the hills and 6:50s down, rather than expending extra energy forcing yourself to stick to 7s the entire way.

Run the mile you're in. "Focus on the moment," says Hall. "I avoid thinking about how far I have to go early in the race, because that can be overwhelming. Late in the race I try to forget about how far I have gone, because that would give me an excuse to give in to fatigue."

FOR MERE MORTALS

Of course, few runners can train and race like Hall. But you can still set a personal record with this 10-week plan, which follows the same principles as

Ryan Hall's routine—minus the five-minute miles and 120-mile weeks.

In this training plan, you can choose between two different programs: an extended 10-K (or "short") program, or a modified marathon (or "long") program. To determine which is best for you, see "What's Your (Half) Type?" on page xx. The short program includes slightly fewer total miles, but faster repeats and tempo runs, which will keep your speed sharp for shorter-distance events. Longer long runs and slower tempo and interval paces characterize the long program, building a solid endurance base for runners with a marathon in their near future. Both approaches will prepare you to finish the half and finish fast. (The short program is best for first-timers because the long run does not exceed 14 miles.)

Build up to an eight-mile long run before starting either program. Consult the Pace Guide for details of each workout, and warm up and cool down for a mile before and after each interval and tempo session. Monday is always a rest day.

PACE GUIDE

WORKOUT: TEMPO

Short program: Run moderate-paced tempos at half-marathon goal pace*; hard tempos at half-marathon goal pace minus 10 to 15 seconds per mile.

Long program: Do moderate tempos at half-marathon goal pace* or slightly slower; hard tempos at half-marathon goal pace or slightly faster.

WORKOUT: RACE-SIMULATION RUNS (RACE-SIM)

Short program: Run the first half comfortably, then drop down to your half-marathon goal pace plus 20 to 30 seconds per mile.

Long programs: Same as short program

WORKOUT: INTERVALS

Short program: Run your repeats at 10-K race pace; drop to 5-K race pace the last three weeks.

Long program: Run your repeats at half-marathon goal pace; drop to 10-K race pace the final three weeks.

WORKOUT: LONG AND EASY RUNS

Short program: Comfortable pace, or 50 to 90 seconds slower than your half-marathon goal pace

Long program: Same as short program

***Goal Pace:** Don't know your half-marathon goal pace? Try this: Run for an all-out mile and add 20 percent. For example, if you run a mile in seven minutes, your half-marathon goal pace would be 8:24 (7 x 1.2 = 8.4, which is 8:24 pace).

What's your (half) type?

Use this quiz to decide which program is best for you.

According to Terrence Mahon, who coached Ryan Hall to his breakthrough 13.1-mile debut, you can approach the half-marathon in one of two ways—extend a 10-K program, or modify a marathon program. Whether you should use a short or long program depends on your strengths, preferences, and goals.

1. Which race scenario best describes you?
- A) You struggle in the middle, but outkick other runners with a fast final quarter-mile sprint.
- B) You pass a lot of people during the middle miles.

Most runners know intuitively if they're geared toward speed or built for endurance, says Mahon. Your body responds to workouts in your strength area, meaning doing those runs enhances your training.

2. Which workout are you more psyched for?
- A) Fast 400-meter intervals
- B) A two-hour easy run or a long tempo workout

Doing what you like increases your motivation.

3. Which workout leaves you feeling more beat up the next day?
- A) Long tempo runs
- B) Short sprints

"If I give short, hard intervals for Ryan, he fatigues and it takes a couple days to recover," says Mahon. Needing more recovery time can affect the quality of your other key workouts.

4. What races are on your calendar this summer and fall?
- A) 5-Ks and 10-Ks
- B) A full marathon

Like Hall, who knew he'd run the London Marathon just three months after his half, your goals should factor into your decision on whether to use the short or long training program.

Answer Guide: If the majority of your answers were "a," the short program is best for you; if "b," go with the long program.

13.1 TRAINING PLAN

WEEK 1

Tuesday: Short Program: 5 x 800 meters at 10-K pace; recover after each repeat for half of the interval time. Long Program: 6 x 800 meters at half-marathon goal pace; recover after each repeat for a quarter of the interval time

Wednesday: Off, cross-train (XT), or easy run of 30 to 45 minutes

Thursday: Easy run: 30 to 45 minutes

Friday: Tempo Run (moderate): 4 miles, plus a mile warmup and cooldown

Saturday: Off, XT, or easy run of 30 to 45 minutes

Sunday: Short: Long run, 8 miles. Long: long run, 10 miles

Totals: Short: 23 to 35 miles. Long: 25 to 37 miles

WEEK 2

Tuesday: Short: 5 x 1000 meters, 2 minutes rest between each Long: 5 x 1000 meters, 1 minute rest between each

Wednesday: Off, XT, or easy run of 30 to 45 minutes

Thursday: Tempo (hard): 20 minutes, plus a mile warmup and cooldown

Friday: Off, XT, or easy run of 30 to 45 minutes

Saturday: Race-Sim: 9 miles, 6 easy/3 at goal race pace plus 20 to 30 seconds

Sunday: Easy run: 30 to 45 minutes

Totals: Short: 22 to 35 miles. Long: 22 to 35 miles

WEEK 3

Tuesday: Short: 7 x 800 meters; recover for half of the interval time. Long: 8 x 800 meters; recover for a quarter of the interval time

Wednesday: Off, XT, or easy run of 30 to 45 minutes

Thursday: Easy run: 30 to 45 minutes

Friday: Tempo Run (moderate): 5 miles, plus a mile warmup and cooldown

Saturday: Off, XT, or easy run of 30 to 45 minutes

Sunday: Short: long run, 10 miles. Long: long run, 12 miles

Totals: Short: 27 to 39 miles. Long: 29 to 41 miles

WEEK 4

Tuesday: Short: 2 miles at 10-K pace, 2 x 1 mile at 5-K pace, 2 x 800 meters at slightly

faster than 5-K pace, with 5 minutes recovery after the 2-mile and 3 minutes recovery after the miles and 800. Long: 2 miles at half-marathon pace, 2 x 1 mile at 10-K pace, 2 x 800 meters at 5-K pace, with 3 minutes recovery after the 2-mile and 2 minutes recovery after the miles and 800

Wednesday: Off, XT, or easy run of 30 to 45 minutes

Thursday: Tempo (hard): 25 minutes, plus a mile warmup and cooldown

Friday: Off, XT, or easy run of 30 to 45 minutes

Saturday: Race-Sim: 10 miles, 6 easy/4 at goal race pace plus 20 to 30 seconds

Sunday: Easy run: 30 to 45 minutes

Totals: Short: 25 to 39 miles. Long: 25 to 39 miles

WEEK 5

Tuesday: Short: 6 x 1000 meters; recovery is half of the interval time Long: 7 x 1000 meters; recovery is a quarter of the interval time

Wednesday: Off, XT, or easy run of 30 to 45 minutes

Thursday: Easy run: 30 to 45 minutes

Friday: Tempo Run (moderate): 6 miles, plus a mile warmup and cooldown

Saturday: Off, XT, or easy run of 30 to 45 minutes

Sunday: Short: long run, 12 miles. Long: long run, 14 miles

Totals: Short: 30 to 42 miles. Long: 33 to 45 miles

WEEK 6

Tuesday: Same as week 4

Wednesday: Off, XT, or easy run of 30 to 45 minutes

Thursday: Tempo Run (hard): 30 minutes, plus a mile warmup and cooldown

Friday: Off, XT, or easy run of 30 to 45 minutes

Saturday: Race-Sim: 11 miles, 6 easy/5 at goal race pace plus 20 to 30 seconds

Sunday: Easy run: 30 to 45 minutes

Total: Short: 27 to 41 miles. Long: 27 to 41 miles

WEEK 7

Tuesday: Short: 5 x 1200 meters; recover for half of the interval time. Long: 6 x 1200 meters; recover for a quarter of the interval time

Wednesday: Off, XT, or easy run of 30 to 45 minutes

Thursday: Easy run: 30 to 45 minutes

Friday: Tempo Run (moderate): 6 miles, plus a mile warmup and cooldown

Saturday: Off, XT, or easy run of 30 to 45 minutes

Sunday: Short: long run, 14 miles. Long: long run, 16 miles

Totals: Short: 32 to 44 miles. Long: 34 to 46 miles

WEEK 8

Tuesday: Short: 5 x 1000 at 5-K pace; 3-minute recovery. Long: 6 x 1000 at 10-K pace; recover for a quarter of the interval time

Wednesday: Off, XT, or easy run of 30 to 45 minutes

Thursday: Tempo Run (hard): 35 minutes, plus a mile warmup and cooldown

Friday: Off, XT, or easy run of 30 to 45 minutes

Saturday: Race-Sim: 12 miles, 6 easy/6 at goal race pace plus 20 to 30 seconds

Sunday: Easy run: 30 to 45 minutes

Totals: Short: 27 to 41 miles. Long: 27 to 41 miles

WEEK 9

Tuesday: Short: 5 x 800 at 5-K pace; 3-minute recovery. Long: 6 x 800 at 10-K pace; recover for a quarter of the interval time

Wednesday: Off, XT, or easy run of 30 to 45 minutes

Thursday: Easy run: 30 to 45 minutes

Friday: Tempo Run (moderate): 6 miles, plus a mile warmup and cooldown

Saturday: Off, XT, or easy run of 30 to 45 minutes

Sunday: Long run, 10 miles

Totals: Short: 27 to 39 miles. Long: 27 to 39 miles

WEEK 10

Tuesday: Short: Tempo Run. 1-mile warmup, 20 minutes at half-marathon goal pace plus 10 to 15 seconds. Finish with 4 strides and a mile cooldown. Long: Same as short program

Wednesday: Off, XT, or easy run of 30 to 45 minutes

Thursday: Intervals: 6 x 400 between your 5-K and 10-K pace; recovery equals interval time

Friday: Easy run: 30 minutes

Saturday: Off

Sunday: RACE!!!

Totals: Short: 24 to 31 miles Long: 24 to 31 miles

Amby Burfoot's Running Round-Up

Ryan Hall proved to be the glamour boy of American distance running in the late 2000s, setting records not just in the half-marathon but also in the marathon. And no wonder. That first half-marathon in Houston in January 2007 proved the perfect stepping-stone.

Many other runners who didn't appear on the covers of popular running magazines also followed Hall's approach. It soon turned out that the half-marathon wasn't just a great way to get in shape for the marathon. It's a terrific focal point for any racing distance from the 5-K to the marathon.

You can use half-marathon training to build endurance. You can use it to build speed. Or you can use it as the ideal maintenance program for those times (whether for family or business or other reasons) when you simply can't concentrate on being your best.

If you revert to your half program at those times, you'll be more than halfway to your final goal when you decide to ramp up. In fact, you'll be about 80 percent there. Half-marathon training is that effective.

Chapter 33

Take the Half-Marathon Challenge

Can you get in shape for a 13.1-miler? We say yes! And here's how.

It's hard to believe, but just a few years ago the half-marathon racing distance was virtually unknown to many runners. They ran 5-Ks and 10-Ks and the marathon, of course, but no one bothered to enter 13.1-milers. Then someone flipped a switch.

Now the half-marathon is the fastest-growing race distance, and more popular than its twice-as-long big brother. Why? There is a host of reasons, the following being the most important: The half is a serious distance that requires serious commitment and talent, but doesn't beat you up the way the marathon does; you don't have to do those super-long runs of 18-22 miles that can leave you fatigued all weekend; and the half is a great building block to the marathon, which remains a major goal of many runners.

No wonder everyone wants to enter the half-marathon, which now attracts more racers annually than the 26.2-mile race. It has proven especially popular among women runners who are seeking a challenge, but don't think they're ready for the marathon. Soon, though. Very soon.

THREE RUNNERS. TEN WEEKS. 13.1 MILES.

As a runner, you're constantly searching for the next big breakthrough. Wherever you fall in the pack, you long to run faster, go farther, or get fitter—just like Deb Dyle, Valdi Sapira, and Kate Hoof. They represent three types of runners: a beginner, an ex-runner, and an age group champ. We followed them for 10 weeks as they reached for their next running milestone in the half-marathon. To help them along, we enlisted a team of experts—Toby Tanser, a renowned running coach in New York City; Leslie Bonci, a nutritionist for several professional sports teams; and physical therapist and veteran ultramarathoner David Balsley—to evaluate them, design their training, and teach them what it takes to conquer 13.1 miles. Their experiences will help you meet your next running challenge.

The Beginner

Name: Deborah Dyle

Occupation: Full-time mom

Goal: Become a runner for life

Age: 34

Place in the Pack: Beginner

Deb Dyle had two very good reasons to take up running: her 10-year-old son, Evan, who has autism, and her 9-month-old son, Jake. "I just want to be healthy," says Dyle. "I want to be around as long as I can for both my boys—and I know running is going to help."

Caring for her kids, though, left little time for Dyle to take care of herself; she weighed 172 pounds, 37 pounds overweight. And with a family history of hypertension and diabetes, Dyle knew she had to get fit. She began by taking two-mile walks with her sons. She gradually added intervals of running, extending them by one minute per week. Within two months, she could run five minutes for every minute of walking. Four months later, she had lost 20 pounds and finished two 5-Ks. "I'm a whole different person because of running," she says. "I have more energy, I'm less stressed, and I actually look good in jeans again!"

But Dyle knew that the half-marathon, and making running a lifetime habit, would require a stepped-up commitment. She also had to squeeze training into an already packed schedule. Despite everything she was juggling, Dyle

was determined. "I want to do things right and build a nice solid base to keep running for the rest of my life."

EXPERT ANALYSIS

Diet: Deb had already cut back her eating in order to lose some weight, but because she'd done that, she wasn't getting enough of the healthy fuel that she needed to maintain a steady level of energy. She also wasn't eating any vegetables. I recommended that she eat regular meals, especially breakfast. I also suggested she add more high-quality carbs, like brown rice and whole-grain bread, which are easy to prepare. —*Leslie Bonci*

Training: Debbie is a real fighter, and that gave me great assurance that she was going to lay a good foundation. With beginners, you don't want to blow it by building up too fast, too early. Also, she talked a lot about including her sons in exercise, so it was important to make time for that in her schedule in a way that didn't affect her preparation for the race. —*Toby Tanser*

Strength: Deb didn't do any stretching or strength training, so she needed to add that to her training program. I also recommended that she wear softer shoes, so she didn't worsen some sciatica and back problems that she's struggled with in the past. —*David Balsley*

THE PLAN: BUILD SLOWLY

On her first long run, Dyle went 30 minutes longer than Tanser had prescribed. A-plus effort? Hardly. Classic mistake? Yes. Tanser has seen scores of new runners push too much too soon, get injured, and quit before they reach the starting line. "The body needs to get miles under the belt to build a foundation," he told her. "You must have patience."

After that, Dyle advanced in baby steps. Tanser had her do hills, intervals, and long runs, but modified them so she wouldn't get intimidated—or hurt. He had Dyle work on speed on the treadmill so she could see what certain paces felt like. He added walk breaks to her long runs and gradually increased the time between walks. He scheduled plenty of time for rest so she could recover and continue her walks with her sons.

This slow build boosted Deb's stamina and gave her another essential tool: confidence. Three weeks before the race, she stunned herself by running 12 miles, a distance that once had seemed impossible.

DYLE'S 10-WEEK SCHEDULE

WEEK 1

Monday: 2 miles easy

Tuesday: 3 x 10 min. medium, with 2-min. breaks

Wednesday: 30-min. walk

Thursday: 5-min. walk; 20 min. hard; 5-min. walk

Friday: Rest

Saturday: 8.5 miles easy, with 2-min. breaks every 12 min.

Sunday: 1- to 2-hour hike

WEEK 2

Monday: 2 miles easy

Tuesday: 3 x 12 min. medium, with 2-min. breaks

Wednesday: 30-min. walk

Thursday: 25 min. medium

Friday: Rest

Saturday: 8.5 miles easy, with 2-min. breaks every 20 min.

Sunday: XT

WEEK 3

Monday: 3 miles easy

Tuesday: 4 x 10 min. medium, with 2-min. breaks

Wednesday: 30-min. walk

Thursday: 30 min. medium

Friday: 2 miles easy or rest

Saturday: 9 miles easy, with breaks every 20 min.

Sunday: XT or rest

WEEK 4

Monday: 3 miles easy

Tuesday: 3 x 12 min. medium, with 2-min. breaks

Wednesday: 30-min. walk

Thursday: 25 min. hard-medium

Friday: 3 miles easy

Saturday: 8 miles easy, with no breaks

Sunday: Rest

WEEK 5

Monday: 2 miles easy

Tuesday: 4 x 12 min. medium, with 90-sec. breaks

Wednesday: 30-min. walk

Thursday: 30 min. medium, hills

Friday: Rest

Saturday: 10 miles, with 3 1-min. breaks

Sunday: XT or rest

WEEK 6

Monday: 2 to 4 miles easy

Tuesday: 4 x 10 min. medium, with 80-sec. breaks

Wednesday: 30-min. walk

Thursday: 35 min. medium, hills

Friday: Rest

Saturday: 11 miles, with 4 1-min. breaks

Sunday: Rest

WEEK 7

Monday: 4 miles easy

Tuesday: 4 x 12 min. medium, with 100-sec. breaks

Wednesday: 30-min. walk

Thursday: 35 min. medium, hills

Friday: Rest

Saturday: 12 miles; try not to take breaks

Sunday: Rest

WEEK 8

Monday: 3 miles easy

Tuesday: 4 x 15 min. medium, with 2-min. breaks

Wednesday: 30-min. walk

Thursday: 40 min. medium

Friday: Rest

Saturday: 8.9 miles, with no breaks

Sunday: Short hike

WEEK 9

Monday: 2 miles easy

Tuesday: 5 miles easy, 1 mile hard

Wednesday: 30-min walk

Thursday: 20 min. medium

Friday: Rest

Saturday: 6 miles easy

Sunday: Short hike

WEEK 10

Monday: 3 miles easy

Tuesday: 4 miles medium

Wednesday: 30-min. walk

Thursday: 2 miles medium

Friday: Rest

Saturday: Race

Sunday: Rest

<table>
KEY
</table>

KEY

Easy: 12 to 12:30 min./mile
Medium: 10:20 to 11:05 min./mile
Hard: 9:40 to 10 min./mile
XT: Cross-training
Breaks: Walk breaks

RACE DAY

During the half-marathon, Dyle focused on enjoying the event. She talked with other runners and took in the scenery. She didn't worry about her time—just finishing. Tanser had advised her to run slowly for the first 11 miles. Then, if she felt good, she could pick up the pace for the final two miles. The strategy worked. She averaged 11:30 pace for the first 11 miles, then pushed the final two miles to finish in 2:25:19. "I feel great," Dyle said afterward. "Let's run another!"

BEYOND THE FINISH LINE

Since race day, Dyle has continued running at least three days a week, keeping up her speed and hill work. She went on to finish a 5-K in 29:40, averaging 9:30 per mile and improving her 5-K PR by 6 minutes. She dropped to 132 pounds and made plans for a sprint triathlon and another half-marathon. When Dyle reflects on her first half-marathon, she most values the love for running that she developed. Along with the training basics she learned, she says that enjoyment will "help me continue running for the rest of my life."

The Weight-Loss Guy

Name: Valdi Sapira
Occupation: Physician
Goal: Reclaim a running life
Age: 45
Place in the Pack: Ex-runner

Valdi Sapira first became a runner in the mid-1990s, but only after he had ballooned up to 287 pounds during his residency training prior to becoming an emergency-room physician. He went on a medically supervised diet, started exercising, lost 100 pounds, and took up running at the urging of a friend. "I did three miles and fell in love with it," says Sapira. Over the next decade, he did seven marathons (his PR: 4:38).

But a couple of years ago, 5-foot-7 Sapira fell off the exercise wagon. "It was almost like a post-marathon depression that wouldn't go away," he says. Plus, there were the 12-hour shifts he was putting in at the hospital. The grind didn't help his eating habits, either, which caused him to gain back nearly all the weight he had lost. Sapira wanted to make a comeback—and lose the weight—but didn't know where to begin. When he tried to start running again last year, he hurt his knee.

Sapira faced a quandary common among runners who struggle with their weight: how to enjoy the pound-shaving benefits of the sport without getting injured in the process. He hoped training for a half-marathon could help him make a safe start and get his eating habits in check. "I've always done well when I'm challenged," he says, and he aimed to finish in three hours.

EXPERT ANALYSIS

Diet: With Valdi, I didn't use the word diet; I called it "appropriate fueling." I didn't want him restricting his food too much, which he's done in the past, without success. During his hospital shifts, he'd go for long stretches without food, become ravenous, and overeat. I suggested that he eat every three to four hours, focusing on nutritious foods that would help keep him fuller for longer, such as vegetables, fruits, and soup. —*Leslie Bonci*

 Training: In most cases, I send my runners outside. I sent Valdi indoors, as I knew he would be looking for any reasons, like the weather, to avoid running. Because of his excess weight, I didn't want to overload his joints. To keep him burning calories, I had him do the StairMaster. He enjoys it, so I hoped it would seem like more of a reward than a chore. —*Toby Tanser*

 Strength: Valdi was pretty strong and flexible, but due to his extra weight, he shouldn't be running on hard surfaces. Also, he needed to change his shoes more frequently than other runners might. Because of his weight, he will probably wear out a pair in about 175 miles. —*David Balsley*

THE PLAN: A CAUTIOUS COMEBACK

Despite having run full marathons in the past, Sapira had his doubts about the half. "I was worried that I couldn't do it," he admits. "I wasn't 277 pounds when I did those marathons." Tanser eased Sapira back by having him run mostly on the treadmill, which would be easier on his joints than the roads—and cushion his ego. "While I like running outside," he says, "there's the whole 'shake and jiggle' issue."

The downside? Sapira would have to log epic sessions on treadmills and StairMasters. One day he spent two hours, 41 minutes on the treadmill; another he went 80 minutes on the StairMaster.

Eating changes were a big part of Sapira's half-marathon preparation. Bonci advised him to eat smaller meals more frequently and include carbs, protein, fats, fruits, and vegetables. She also had him plan his eating so he'd have energy when he needed it most: for runs or long shifts. It worked. "I used to just get up and run, and I'd feel jet-lagged," Sapira says. He found that grabbing a bite a half hour before running "really helps."

As his diet changed and workouts intensified, he starting losing weight. Other people noticed, and his confidence soared. "Once that starts happening," Sapira says, "you're really high."

GETTING BACK ON TRACK

Sapira's training was designed to max out his calorie burn without putting too much pounding on his joints. A sample week:

Monday: Rest, but walk every chance you get

Tuesday: 6 x 9 min. medium, with 90-sec. breaks; 2% grade

Wednesday: Rest, but walk every chance you get

Thursday: 6 x 9 min., with 60-sec. rest at medium speed

Friday: Rest, but walk every chance you get

Saturday: 2 hours, 41 min. easy

Sunday: 60 min. hard on StairMaster

KEY

Easy: 11:45 to 12:15 min./mile

Medium: 11:05 to 11:30 min./mile

Hard: StairMaster, 8-10 on a perceived-exertion scale of 1-10

RACE DAY

To help Sapira reach his three-hour goal, Tanser advised him to shoot for a negative split (second half faster than the first). The strategy, and the ultralong workouts he did on the treadmill and StairMaster, paid off with a time Sapira never expected: 2:30:12. He tackled the hills with ease, which he credited to being much slimmer. Perhaps the highlight, though, was how much he enjoyed stepping back into racing again. "I'd like to do Boston," he said later with a smile, "although I'll probably let the Kenyans win."

BEYOND THE FINISH LINE

Sapira didn't leave the half-marathon as his peak performance. He finished a 5-K in 30:28 and a 10-K in 60:28, successes he credits to the weight he lost (51 pounds) and stamina he had built. Training for the half-marathon helped him start his comeback. Now Sapira runs with his 5-year-old son, Josh. "That's the kind of thing," he says, "that really keeps you going."

The PR Seeker

Name: Kate Hoof

Occupation: Teacher

Goal: A 1:30 PR

Age: 38

Place in the Pack: Speedster

Kate Hoof hadn't always been a runner gunning for PRs. In high school, Hoof and her sister, Ritamarie, decided they needed to lose weight and figured running would be the best way to do it. Their first time out, they could barely make it one lap around the track. But Hoof kept at it, and when she started placing and winning her age group in local 5-Ks in her early 30s, she began focusing on her finishing times and her distance. She has completed five half-marathons, with a personal best of 1:37.

"Once you have a time in mind, it becomes a mental thing that you have to break," says Hoof. "It becomes bigger than it really is."

Hoof wanted to lower her 13.1-mile PR by seven minutes. While she wasn't daunted by the goal she'd set for herself, she needed to make her already rigorous training more effective and gain some confidence along the way. "That's a big goal if you have four or five months to train, and a huge goal if you're trying to do it in 10 weeks," Tanser said at the outset of her training program. "Kate would have to spend some time in the fast zone, learning to deal with lactic acid and what speed feels like, as well as spend some time recovering so her body could repair itself."

EXPERT ANALYSIS

Diet: Kate eats well; she just had to focus on making sure that she's fueling up enough—especially before and after she runs. Kate is a salty sweater, so she needed to work on increasing sodium in her diet to keep her electrolytes in balance. She also needed to work on protein intake and adding a little more fat to her diet. —*Leslie Bonci*

Training: Usually you advance in small increments. Kate wanted to take off a big chunk of time. I had to teach her how her body should feel at a much faster pace. I had to make sure her speedwork was tough enough so that when she ran at race pace, it felt within her reach. Also, I wanted her to work on her running form to develop faster footwork and turnover. —*Toby Tanser*

Strength: Kate is competitive and aggressive. You have to give a little more guidance to people like that; you have to slow 'em down sometimes. One example is her weight training. She was doing four sessions a week of a plyometric-style weight lifting. I told her to cut it down to two or three sessions a week and include more conventional training. —*David Balsley*

THE PLAN: THE FAST TRACK

Hoof's training was designed to help her get much faster—in a hurry. Tanser boosted her intervals, building up to six-minute miles (she started at a 6:50 pace). He also had her do tempo runs each week, closer to race pace, which would be around 6:55 per mile. The idea? That after her tough intervals, race pace would feel more comfortable. Just a few weeks before race day, Hoof was able to hold her race pace for eight miles. That, Tanser felt, was a good sign. "She seemed to be really responding," he says.

While Hoof relished the physical rigors of her training, like so many other runners, she wrestled with self-doubt and anxiety. Even when she followed the program to the letter, she wondered whether she was doing enough. Tanser tried to pump her up with confidence. He gave her a mantra: "I will, I can" to repeat during her workouts.

BELOW IS HOOF'S FIRST FIVE WEEKS OF TRAINING.

WEEK 1

Monday: 4 miles easy

Tuesday: 3 x 1200 meters hard, with 1-lap recovery

Wednesday: Rest

Thu: 5 miles medium, with 1 mile easy

Friday: 4 to 5 miles easy

Saturday: 90 min. easy, with 5 x 20-sec. footwork drills

Sunday: XT

WEEK 2

Monday: 5 miles easy, with 5 footwork drills

Tuesday: 4 x 1200 meters hard, with 1-lap recovery

Wednesday: Rest

Thursday: 5 miles medium, with 1 mile easy

Friday: 6 miles easy

Saturday: 20 min. easy; 40 min. medium; 10 min. hard; 20 min. easy, with 5 strides

Sunday: 5 miles easy on trails

WEEK 3

Monday: 6 miles, with 8 strides

Tuesday: 5 x 800 meters hard, with 1-lap recovery

Wednesday: Rest

Thursday: 2 miles easy; 6 miles medium; 2 miles easy

Friday: 5 to 7 miles easy on grass

Saturday: 40 min. easy

Sunday: 70 min. XT in morning; 20 min. easy in evening

WEEK 4

Monday: 6 miles easy on trails

Tuesday: 7 x 800 meters hard, with 1-lap recovery; 2 miles hard

Wednesday: Rest

Thursday: 7 miles medium; 2 miles easy

Friday: 6 miles easy

Saturday: 50 min. easy; 15 min. hard

Sunday: 5 miles easy

WEEK 5

Monday: 6 miles easy; 4 x 20 strides

Tuesday: 3 x 1-mile repeats, with 400-meter slow jog; 10 min. hard

Wednesday: Rest

Thursday: 7 miles medium, plus 2-mile cooldown

Friday: 5 to 6 miles easy on grass

Saturday: 60 min. easy; 15 min. hard; 5 min. easy; 7 min. hard

Sunday: 3 to 4 miles easy; 10 x 100-meter strides

KEY

Easy: 8 to 8:30 min./mile

Medium: 6:45 to 7:15 min./mile

Hard: 6 to 6:30 min./mile

XT: Cross-training, such as swimming, biking, or hiking

Footwork drills: Running on sloping downhills to practice fast leg turnover

---

RACE DAY

Hoof woke up on race day, in her words, "a nervous wreck. Even though I'd done the training, I just didn't have the confidence." Tanser urged her to start at a 7:10 pace—a warmup for her—then ease into the 6:50 pace she'd need for her PR. In the first mile, going at an easy 7:30 pace, her breathing was labored. "By mile two, I remember thinking, I hope I just finish." That left 11 very difficult miles ahead.

While she fell short of her goal, finishing in 1:43:53, she earned her coach's admiration. "Minutes don't always tell the story," Tanser says. "She did the best she could on the day. For seasoned runners, there are going to be races like this. In the reality of running, this is sometimes the reality result."

BEYOND THE FINISH LINE

Hoof didn't abandon her PR hopes and plans to try again to better her half-marathon time. She has kept up her speedwork, and she's cross-training on the bike and doing more trail runs. She says she learned to focus less on finishing times and more on the training process—even though that effort may not be enough. "Hard work is not a guarantee," she says. "You can work as hard as you can, and still anything can happen on race day."

Amby Burfoot's Running Round-Up

The half-marathon requires a well-balanced combination of endurance and speed, making it the perfect distance for almost any runner. You can't run strongly to the finish unless you've done enough endurance training, and you can't improve your time much unless you add in a few tempo and intervals workouts. So the distance isn't really "half" of anything; it's more like a double dose of the good stuff.

In eastern Pennsylvania, where I live, the Lehigh Valley Road Runners have put on a popular half-marathon every spring for many years. Many of us local runners use it to motivate us in the dark, cold days of winter. I know I have. I particularly like the way I can build endurance during the frigid months, focusing on the half-marathon, and then switch to shorter, faster running in the hot summer months. It's the perfect combination. Add a fall or early winter half-marathon or marathon, and you've got enough race dates on the calendar to keep you going strong all year.

Chapter 34

Lessons Learned for Half-Marathon Wisdom

A group of *Runner's World* experts offer tips from their decades of running

A training program, like a bicycle wheel, should have many spokes. That's where the strength, balance, and foundation come from. As you build up to your first half-marathon, or perhaps a return to the half-marathon, you'll want to add more spokes to your training. You'll get fitter and you'll gain confidence. Both are crucial to half-marathon success.

This chapter pulls together an impressive amount of information from an even more impressive group of running experts—from Olympic gold medalists to some of the coaches who have advised more beginning runners than just about anyone else. Their thoughts will help you train better, eat better, and avoid injuries. But even more important, you'll be inspired by the depth of their experiences. You'll see that they have encountered obstacles similar to those you face, and that they sometimes need motivation just as much as you do. The half-marathon is a distance that will force you to dig deep and call on many resources; here's the perfect place to begin.

Running has changed a lot since the earliest hint of a running boom in the late 1960s and the first full-fledged boom of the mid-1970s. Changed, but also stayed the same, as you could only learn by running through the decades yourself. That's been true of the longtime *Runner's World* contributors featured in the pages that follow. We asked these experts, all masters runners now, to tell us about the most important lessons they've learned over the years—the crucial training knowledge they've accrued through scientific study, simple intuition, and good old trial and error.

Their success as lifelong runners shows they've learned from their mistakes. And now you can, too. While not all of their "lessons learned" are directly applicable to the half-marathon, you'll find that many of their suggestions will help you build the strong, stable foundation you need to get ready for peak half-marathon performance.

Ed Eyestone's Great Strength Workout: "Run four or five mile-repeats between 5-K and 10-K pace. You're moving at close to VO2 max pace for an extended period of time. Runners were doing this type of workout 40 years ago. And 40 years from now, they'll still be doing such long intervals, because they work."

Bill Rodgers's Newest Workout: "I've started doing Pilates because it can reveal where you're weak. After running all these years, I've suddenly discovered that I'm really tight on one side. Masters runners especially should try it."

Be Glad You're Running Now: "Thirty or 40 years ago, high mileage was everything. Back in the '70s, I remember asking a runner at the University of Texas if he'd be interested in competing in the 10-K. He said, 'No, I'm getting in only 80 miles a week. I can't race longer than 5-K.' These days, I'm losing interest in high mileage, particularly at the developmental level, because you drive people away from the sport."—*Jack Daniels*

Joan Benoit Samuelson's Training Secret: "I've always run by the seat of my pants. I've never been very scientific about my training. I run the way I feel. Now, of course, with things like heart-rate monitors, it's easier to get more scientific about it all. But to tell you the truth, if I was coming into my prime right now, I probably wouldn't do things much differently."

Trust Your Instincts: "These days, science often just validates what elite athletes have done intuitively. Like the practice of drinking only when thirsty. That's what the experts are recommending now. Why? Because they asked elite ath-

letes if they drink at every aid station, and they found out they didn't. So then they studied why not and realized that drinking according to thirst is simply a better way to do it."—*Frank Shorter*

Race Easy: "Not every race has to be an all-out effort. In the new world of running, you can go to a race and actually enjoy yourself. Make it what I call an experiential weekend, a fun travel holiday. You might run the Big Sur Marathon 30 minutes slower than you would normally run a marathon, then add a wine tasting and a spa treatment to your trip. Four months later, you can always go for a PR at another race. If you learn that lesson, you can be a runner for a longer period of time."—*Bart Yasso*

Joe Henderson's Best Reason to Run: "My college coach believed second place wasn't worth a damn. If you weren't running for first, there was no reason to run. That really limited the number of people who could be runners. These days, the only reason I run is so I can run again tomorrow."

Go Offline: "The Internet has certainly expanded the amount of training information available to runners. While I have occasionally checked out workouts of certain superstars on the Web, I view these more as entertainment because it's difficult to know the accuracy of such posts. I think there are more than a few runners who would benefit from less time on the Internet and more time on the track."—*Ed Eyestone*

Amby Burfoot's Workout Strategy: "To improve, train simply and progressively. By that I mean, do the same workouts week after week, only go a little farther or a little faster each week. Many runners take this approach with their marathon long runs. But you can do the same with interval training: Try 3 x 800 one week, 4 x 800 the next, then 5 x 800, and so on. Do this for six to eight weeks, and over that amount of time it can make a real difference in your fitness."

Frank Shorter's Favorite Workout: Six times 800 meters at faster than 5-K race pace with a very short recovery.

Bend, Don't Break: "We now know a flexible body is a more efficient body. And the best way for runners to increase their flexibility is through range-of-motion exercises in which you move isolated body parts quickly and gently through their natural range of motion, holding the position for no more than two seconds. Yoga and Pilates build on this principle."—*Jim Wharton*

Know the Pace: "I was meeting with a group I coach when a man came up and said 'I think you might know my nephew, Mike McQueenie. He's Deena Kastor's pacesetter.' Yes, I had watched him run with Deena in Chicago. Pacesetters are now commonplace among all elite runners. That's a big difference from when I was running. Back then it was illegal for women in the marathon to have pacers."—*Joan Benoit Samuelson*

Cross the Street: "After 40 years of running on one side of the road and always tilting a little bit to the left, I think it tilted me a bit and resulted in a leg-length differential. Runners can counter such effects by periodically switching to the other side of the road."—*Bill Rodgers*

Budd Coates's Reading List: "When it comes to training, nothing has been proven to work any better than the methods of Ernst van Aaken in the 1940s and Arthur Lydiard in the 1950s. For instance, core training and plyometrics sound like they are brand new, yet Lydiard was doing this stuff long before anyone else. Check out his book *Running, the Lydiard Way*."

Why You Should Walk: "When I started teaching my run/walk method back in 1973, it was intended to help people who were totally out of

shape get interested in running. But what I've discovered over the years is that inserting regular one-minute walk breaks from the beginning of a run enables even veteran runners to improve their times. When people insert walk breaks early enough and often enough in the marathon, I've seen an average 13-minute improvement. Beginners might start with a run/walk ratio of two minutes of running with one minute of walking, while experienced runners might use one-minute walk breaks for every mile covered. Walk breaks have totally surprised me in their effectiveness across the continuum of runners."—*Jeff Galloway*

Stay Fresh: "Every week, take one day off from running. That day off gives you a definite beginning and end to your training week and encourages the body to recover. A weekly break also keeps you mentally fresh."—*Ed Eyestone*

Love What You Do: "Training has to be a relatively enjoyable experience to get peak results. Otherwise, you won't be willing to put up with the discomforts that come with hard effort." —*Jack Daniels*

Experiment Indoors: "You can actually be pretty playful with treadmill training, which can result in some excellent workouts. You can speed up or slow down at will, and you can throw in 'hills' any time you want. And you're not stuck out in the middle of nowhere if you can't handle what you're doing."—*George Sheehan III*

Rest Easy: "Rest and recovery are part of training. A recovery run of three easy miles is just as important as a quality track workout, hill workout, or speed session. That's because you won't be able to perform well on your quality days if you aren't fully recovered from previous workouts." —*Bart Yasso*

Careful What You Eat: "Don't eat anything new before a big race. I once developed a craving

for apple butter the night before the Boston Marathon. Unfortunately, I also satisfied that craving. The next day, I ran almost as many miles off the course to the nearest bathroom as I did on the course between Hopkinton and Boston."
—*Amby Burfoot*

LIZ APPLEGATE'S TOP 4 EATING TIPS

1. "There's no one food that has everything you need."

2. "We used to think that having adequate glycogen [carbohydrate] stores was important only if you were running a marathon. We now know good glycogen stores help even if you're running 60 minutes. Eat 400 to 800 calories of high-carbohydrate foods two to four hours before a run."

3. "Over the years, research has shown that it's best to have variety in your diet. But most people eat the same 10 foods daily. Try rotating foods within food groups—have a banana one day and a nectarine another."

4. "Don't believe every new research study you read. You want to see scads of other studies that say the same thing before you act on it."

BENJI DURDEN'S TOP 3 LIFE LESSONS

1. Fast long runs don't result in fast marathons. "I know it from experience. Run at a comfortable pace. You don't want to exhaust yourself on your long runs."

2. Regular massage therapy helps keep injuries at bay. "I get one every other week."

3. You can run more than one marathon per year.

"If you do marathons too infrequently, you have to learn how to run them all over again every time."

Go Soft: "Mix up your running surfaces. Don't continually pound the pavement, or it will take its toll on your body. I got off the pavement in the early '90s, and, at 65, I'm still out there running without injury."—*Jim Wharton*

Run Better with Age: "Age-related decline in running performance is as much a psychological factor as a physiological one. Warren Utes didn't start running until age 58 and a decade later he was setting world records. Some say older runners like Warren are successful because they haven't worn out their legs. I think it's because they haven't worn out their minds, so they're able to motivate themselves to do the tough training necessary to perform at a high level. The mind can also figure out ways to train smarter—more quality, less quantity—which is key for healthy masters running."—*Hal Higdon*

Train Hard: "There's no substitute for hard training. Along with the drug era came the desire to look for an easy answer off the track. But the people who still beat up on everybody else in the world are the Kenyans and Ethiopians. What do they do? They train hard."—*Frank Shorter*

Welcome, Women: "It's been 40 years since my first road race—the Manchester Road Race in Connecticut. The biggest change between then and now? Back then, women weren't allowed to participate. It certainly made the sport more socially acceptable once the other half of the population could be involved."—*Bill Rodgers*

For Women Only: "During a healthy pregnancy, running is safe and beneficial. Forty years ago, most obstetricians encouraged rest, not running, for pregnant women. Although no scientific evidence had shown any harmful effects from running, many obstetricians at that time erred on the side of being overly cautious. But because no studies have ever shown detrimental effects from running during a healthy pregnancy, doctors now encourage runners with normal pregnancies to continue their routine. Just keep your doctor informed."—*Mona Shangold, M.D.*

Bart Yasso's Famous 800s: "Yasso 800s are a good way to gauge your fitness level during marathon training and help you predict your finishing time. The key is to build up to running 10 x 800 meters with a 400-meter recovery between each repeat. You need to do at least two of these sessions, three to five weeks before the marathon. If you're able to run your 800s in three minutes and 30 seconds, you're in shape to run a 3:30 marathon. For many people, the correlation is spot on. Do these workouts midweek, say on Wednesday, when you've done your long run on the weekend. If you run your 800s on totally fresh legs, you'll do them a heck of a lot faster."

Get Active: "Use active recovery to help you recover faster after a marathon. Try water workouts, strength training, cycling, or just get out there walking. You'll get back into the game faster and stay in the game longer."—*Jim Wharton*

Who's Slow Now? "As part of the *RW* Pace Team for the 1997 Dallas White Rock Marathon, I led the 4:30 group. At the time, we were nearly last. These days, finishing in 4:30 puts you right in the middle. For many, races are no longer final exams—they are parties we throw to celebrate the completion of our training."—*John "The Penguin" Bingham*

Find a Friend: "Most runners in the 1960s, '70s, and even '80s ran by themselves. Now running groups are everywhere and are very popular. I strongly believe the motivation, encouragement, and friendly competition from groups can help most runners improve performance. Find one based on your current fitness level."—*Jeff Galloway*

Information Overload: "When I started run-

Amby Burfoot's Running Round-Up

As I type this short chapter summary, I'm looking at my own name in the lines above. I didn't plan things this way; it just happened. That's precisely the point I'm trying to make with the "Down But Not Out" comment: We can all make comebacks. In fact, life is nothing but one comeback piled on top of another.

Aging makes this inevitable. I ran my fastest times in my early 20s. Others maintain peak racing fitness into their 30s or even early 40s. But eventually we all slow down. And then we face the big question: What next? If I'm getting slower, should I just quit and give up entirely?

It's a tempting thought, especially when you bump up against those occasional injuries that force you onto the bike, into the pool, or maybe even onto the sofa. But ultimately it's much less satisfying and much more dangerous, health-wise, to quit than it is to stay engaged in the lifelong fitness process. Yes, you're going to get slower this year, and next year, and the year after that. But you can keep on keeping on, and let that be its own reward.

I've found the half-marathon race distance perfect for my keeping-on. I still run marathons in my 60s, but not at a high intensity. I take them easy, and just try to reach the finish line in reasonably good shape. But 13.1 miles? That's a distance I can and still do race. It gets me excited. And that helps keep me younger even if the calendar and stopwatch insist on their objective reporting.

ning, high-tech was a wristwatch with a second hand on it. Now there are all these gadgets that tell me more about my running than I want to know. About five years ago, for example, I was doing a run around Mount St. Helens. My running partner and I were totally lost in fog. He looked at his wrist and said, 'We're climbing at a rate of nine feet per minute.' Talk about a useless piece of information. I say, keep the gadgets to a minimum."—*Don Kardong*

Down But Not Out: "Don't expect to be in top shape at all times. Everyone has down periods, either deliberate or otherwise. You can always get back in shape."—*Amby Burfoot*

[X]

The Marathon

Chapter 35

11 Rules for Marathon Success

Follow This Plan to Run a Great Race

Across the country in dozens of different cities and towns, marathon-training groups have sprung up to help runners train for the 26.2-mile distance. These groups prepare novices for their first marathons, help midpackers improve on their personal bests, and often set up special workouts for more advanced runners hoping for a big marathon improvement.

Here, Hal Higdon, a contributor to *Runner's World* magazine, who ran his 100th marathon at the 100th running of the Boston Marathon in April 1996, gathers the best information from all the varied training groups. The result is a chapter that concentrates on key principles, or truths, as Hal calls them. He came up with 11 of these truths and, as any marathon veteran will tell you, each is essential to marathon success.

Because of the emphasis on truths, this program can be followed by almost any marathoner, no matter what background. Keep the truths always in mind, and adjust the training program as seems best for your needs. The result will be a self-designed, personalized program that's a good bet to lead you to better results.

Running a marathon doesn't have to be a painful and frustrating experience. In the quarter century that has passed since the marathon boom in the late 1970s, a body of knowledge has emerged concerning how to train for a marathon, how to ensure that the completion of that marathon will be a joyful—rather than painful—experience, and how to strive for peak performance with a reasonable chance of success.

Dozens of training experts around the country have gradually assembled that knowledge and are using it to lead marathon programs for average runners. I've talked to many of these marathon coaches, including Bob Williams, who works with both advanced and beginning runners as they prepare for the Portland Marathon in Oregon; Robert Vaughan of Dallas, an exercise scientist and coach of elite runners;

and Jack Scaff, M.D., a cardiologist who founded the Honolulu Marathon Clinic in 1974, through which thousands of runners are trained every year.

These coaches know their stuff, and their programs have helped thousands of runners achieve marathon success. I analyzed their training plans and extracted 11 essential truths crucial to the success of any marathon program. Then I incorporated these truths into an 18-week plan. It's here for you to try. I believe it will help you run a great marathon from start to finish.

Before beginning this program, I suggest that you should have been running for about a year and should be able to cover 20 miles a week comfortably. It also helps if you've run one or two 10-K races. Follow the training program for beginners if you currently run 20 to 25 miles a week. If you average 25 to 30 miles per week, use the intermediate program; follow the advanced program if your average is more than 30 miles per week.

1. Long runs get you to the finish line. The

long run is considered the most important element of marathon training because it prepares you physically and mentally for the 26.2-mile distance ahead of you. You don't want, however, to jump right into a 20-mile run in the first week of training. You need to increase the distance progressively throughout your marathon preparation.

In the first week of the program, beginning runners should start with a long run of six miles, then add one mile to that distance every week. By following this schedule, you'll reach 20 miles (the longest run) three weeks before your first marathon.

Intermediate and advanced runners who can run 35 to 40 miles a week may feel like beginning with a long run of 10 miles, also adding a mile a week. These runners will then reach 20 miles in the 11th week of their training schedule and will

do a couple more 20-mile runs during the remainder of their programs.

It makes sense to schedule your long runs on the day of the week when you have the most free time—Saturdays or Sundays for most people.

2. Rest days keep you healthy. Rest days are

the second most important part of marathon training; they are essential to staying healthy. The mileage buildup required to run a good marathon creates stress. And while you need to stress your body in order to prepare it for the rigors of running the marathon, you don't want to overdo it.

"The whole purpose of training is to break the body down so that it will rebuild itself stronger than before," notes Dr. Scaff. "It's when you fail to allow time for the rebuilding phase that problems occur." The musculoskeletal system generally requires 48 hours to recover after hard work. Failure to allow your body time to recover can result in fatigue, muscle injuries, stress fractures, or upper-respiratory illness—all of which can hinder your training and ultimately limit performance.

For novices, I recommend two nonconsecutive days a week of complete rest—not days on which you jog easily or cross-train, but days when you don't work out at all. The best strategy is to bracket the weekend with rest days on Friday and Monday (assuming that you are running long during the weekend). If you need a third rest day midweek, take it.

Intermediate and advanced runners may want to do some jogging or stretching on one or both of the rest days or weave in some cross-training. But don't run hard. Even elite athletes must take rest days.

3. Cross-training lets you work while you rest. You can rest and work out at the same time by cross-training. This gives you a break from the

pounding of running while you continue to train aerobically. Cycling and swimming are excellent cross-training activities, and you can add some stretching and strength training, too.

4. Pace work is critical to race success. "Anybody can run 26 miles if he runs the right pace," says Vaughan. "But if you try to run too fast, you'll crash. If you run slowly enough at the start, you'll make it." Whether your pace is six-minute miles (2:37 finish) or 10-minute miles (4:22 finish), you need to know how that pace feels to achieve it.

One way to fine-tune your pace is to do some training at marathon race pace. Picking that pace, however, takes skill. Vaughan offers two formulas for predicting your marathon time. Either multiply your best recent 10-K time by 4.65, or multiply your half-marathon time by 2 and add 10 percent of that total.

5. Speed training can help you reach a personal record. If you're a first-time marathoner, you don't need to do any speed training. Building up your mileage and running long runs is enough of a stress to your body; adding speedwork, which is a different physical stress, may lead to injury.

When you're aiming, however, for a second marathon, or if you've reached a plateau in your performance and want to improve, speed training can provide that "something extra" that helps you to a breakthrough. Once a week, schedule an interval workout, hill repeats, or a fartlek.

It's also a good idea to do a tempo run once a week. This is a run during the middle of which you run 20 to 30 minutes at a little faster than marathon race pace—fast enough so that you are breathing somewhat hard but not so fast that you're out of breath. Advanced runners can schedule a tempo run on Tuesday and speed training on Thursday with an easy day of running in between.

Cross-training time

For beginners, schedule a cross-training session on the weekend, on the day that you are not doing your long run. For intermediate runners, schedule your cross-training on the day after your long run. Keep your effort in this workout moderate so that you don't compromise your long run.

6. Plain running days are the staple of your program. Yes, there's still room in your training program for days of just plain running. One day a week, do a run that's approximately half the distance of your long run for that week, and run it at the same pace you would your long run. Beginners should schedule this in the middle of the week (I've chosen Wednesday). Reserve the day before and the day after this medium-long workout for easy runs covering short distances. If you want to do some extra stretching or strength training, schedule it on these easy days.

Intermediate and advanced runners also need to reserve a few days for easy runs; schedule them in between your hard workouts (the long run, tempo run, and speedwork).

7. Weekly mileage doesn't have to be mega-mileage. Total weekly mileage for novice runners should be about double the length of the long run. For example, in a week when your long run is 15 miles, your total mileage should be about 30. Intermediate and advanced runners will, of course, have a higher weekly total, but it should not exceed triple the length of the long run (such as 45 miles, given a long run of 15).

8. Stepbacks help you step up your training. Taking rest days is not enough to guard against the

Keep your runs fresh

Total weekly mileage for advanced runners shouldn't exceed more than triple the length of their long run, as this can lead to overtraining. Signs of this include fatigue, "dead" legs, and a lack of enjoyment of running. If you notice these symptoms, you may want to take a few days of rest and then resume your training plan.

dangers of overtraining. Most successful marathon programs also include rest weeks. No, this doesn't mean that you take a week off (although if you need to for some reason, that's okay, too). During a rest week, you cut back on your weekend long run.

Once every third week, cut the distance of your long run by approximately one-third. If your schedule calls for an eight-mile long run, cut it back to five. The following week, resume your progression by doing nine miles on your long run. The last stepback would occur four weeks before the marathon.

Even advanced runners need to do a stepback every few weeks for a physical and mental break from the intensity of marathon training. During these weeks, you'll relax and store your strength for a push ahead to the next level of training.

9. Racing builds experience. Doing some racing during your marathon preparation is particularly important for novice runners. "Running occasional races will help you get used to the race experience: warming up, what it feels like running in a crowd, how to take liquids, when and what to eat, and whether or not your shoes will cause blisters," says Vaughan. "It's always best to make your mistakes in less important races so that you won't make any on marathon day."

Like most coaches, Vaughan warns against racing too often during the marathon buildup period. "Once every third or fourth week seems to be the limit," he says, "otherwise, you risk tearing yourself down."

Try to schedule a 10-K race two weeks before your marathon. From this race effort, you'll have a good sense of your level of readiness for the marathon and should be able to estimate your marathon pace.

At earlier points in your training schedule, you might want to try other distances: 5-K, 15-K, 10 miles, or the half-marathon. On the weeks that you race, cut back on your mileage, and eliminate your long run.

10. The taper is the time to recover and refuel for peak performance. "Too many runners want to train right up to the marathon," says Al DiMicco, who for 30 years has directed a training clinic for the Vulcan Marathon in Birmingham, Alabama, "but you need to let your body recover after all the hard training." DiMicco recommends a 50 percent cutback in mileage during the last two weeks, with very little running the final two or three days. This rest not only permits any damaged muscles to heal but also promotes maximum storage of glycogen (a complex carbohydrate that your body uses for quick energy) within your muscles.

Though mileage drops during the taper, the speed at which you run that mileage should not. The taper period is a good time to practice marathon race pace but at much shorter distances. One way to cut mileage is to convert easy days into days of complete rest. You may want to run some the day before the marathon to reduce nervousness and loosen up, but a few easy miles is the most you should do. The next day, you'll arrive at the starting line rested and ready to go.

Reap what you sow

Say what you will about it, but running 26 miles is one activity in which you get what you pay for. Runners willing to train properly and thoroughly will find that the marathon can be an experience that provides much more joy than pain.

11. Motivation holds it all together. Bill Wenmark of Minnesota has coached more than a thousand runners to finish the Twin Cities and Grandma's marathons. Described as someone who "could motivate a penguin to fly," he takes no credit for supplying motivation to the marathoners that he coaches. "The motivation has to come from within," he says. He feels that people sometimes underestimate the effort required to go 26 miles. Finishing a marathon requires courage, perseverance, and commitment, Wenmark says.

"If running marathons were easy, everybody would be doing it, but they're not," he adds. "You have to be committed to your training. If you're not focused on success, you won't be successful. You'll never succeed if you're not willing to prepare. If you want to succeed in the marathon, you need to be ready to pay the price."

THREE LEVELS OF SCHEDULES

Following are sample marathon-training schedules for beginning, intermediate, and advanced marathoners. Based on the principles and workouts described in this chapter, the schedules give recommended mileage for each day of the week except those days reserved for cross-training (designated "X-train").

Keep in mind that these schedules allow flexibility. If you're feeling fatigue on a particular day, shorten your run or don't run at all. Then resume training according to the schedule; don't try to make up for missed miles. You'll still run a great marathon.

Amby Burfoot's Running Round-Up

In my own marathon training I've abused most of Hal's truths and paid a heavy price for it. Eventually, though, I learned a couple of additional principles: (1) There are no shortcuts, and (2) Less is better than more. The crucial ingredient in a successful marathon is to arrive at the starting line strong, healthy, and well-rested.

The best way to do this, I've found, is through ample use of Higdon truth number 8—the stepback. Hal explains how to reduce the length of your long run every third week. When I'm training particularly hard, I'll reduce the mileage of an entire week of training, usually one week out of every month. In a three-month marathon-training program, I might have two stepback weeks and the taper week before the marathon.

Stepbacks work because they force you to take rest as part of the training. You plan for rest, and you make sure that you get it. The wrong way to do a stepback is by getting injured or catching a cold. Both of these happen often during marathon training, and when they do, you have no control over the outcomes. When you plan stepbacks, on the other hand, you know when you're going to begin resting and when you're going to train again. What's more, it's all part of a plan, which is just the way it's supposed to be.

Beginner

(20-25 miles per week)

	MONDAY	TUESDAY	WEDNESDAY	THURSDAY	FRIDAY	SATURDAY	SUNDAY
Week #1							
Type of Work	Rest	Easy	Medium	Easy	Rest	X-train	Long
Distance or Time	0 mi.	3 mi.	3 mi.	3 mi.	0 mi.	1 hr.	6 mi.
Week #2							
Type of Work	Rest	Easy	Medium	Easy	Rest	X-train	Long
Distance or Time	0 mi.	3 mi.	3 mi.	3 mi.	0 mi.	1 hr.	7 mi.
Week #3							
Type of Work	Rest	Easy	Medium	Easy	Rest	X-train	Long
Distance or Time	0 mi.	3 mi.	4 mi.	3 mi.	0 mi.	1 hr.	5 mi.
Week #4							
Type of Work	Rest	Easy	Medium	Easy	Rest	X-train	Long
Distance or Time	0 mi.	3 mi.	4 mi.	3 mi.	0 mi.	1 hr.	9 mi.
Week #5							
Type of Work	Rest	Easy	Medium	Easy	Rest	X-train	Long
Distance or Time	0 mi.	3 mi.	5 mi.	3 mi.	0 mi.	1 hr.	10 mi.
Week #6							
Type of Work	Rest	Easy	Medium	Easy	Rest	X-train	Race
Distance or Time	0 mi.	3 mi.	5 mi.	3 mi.	0 mi.	1 hr.	10-K or 15-K
Week #7							
Type of Work	Rest	Easy	Medium	Easy	Rest	X-train	Long
Distance or Time	0 mi.	3 mi.	6 mi.	3 mi.	0 mi.	1 hr.	12 mi.
Week #8							
Type of Work	Rest	Easy	Medium	Easy	Rest	X-train	Long
Distance or Time	0 mi.	3 mi.	6 mi.	4 mi.	0 mi.	1 hr.	13 mi.
Week #9							
Type of Work	Rest	Easy	Medium	Easy	Rest	X-train	Long
Distance or Time	0 mi.	3 mi.	7 mi.	4 mi.	0 mi.	1 hr.	10 mi.

	MONDAY	TUESDAY	WEDNESDAY	THURSDAY	FRIDAY	SATURDAY	SUNDAY
Week #10							
Type of Work	Rest	Easy	Medium	Easy	Rest	X-train	Long
Distance or Time	0 mi.	3 mi.	7 mi.	4 mi.	0 mi.	1 hr.	15 mi.
Week #11							
Type of Work	Rest	Easy	Medium	Easy	Rest	X-train	Long
Distance or Time	0 mi.	4 mi.	8 mi.	4 mi.	0 mi.	1 hr.	16 mi.
Week #12							
Type of Work	Rest	Easy	Medium	Easy	Rest	X-train	Race
Distance or Time	0 mi.	4 mi.	8 mi.	5 mi.	0 mi.	1 hr.	20-K or 25-K
Week #13							
Type of Work	Rest	Easy	Medium	Easy	Rest	X-train	Long
Distance or Time	0 mi.	4 mi.	9 mi.	5 mi.	0 mi.	1 hr.	18 mi.
Week #14							
Type of Work	Rest	Easy	Medium	Easy	Rest	X-train	Long
Distance or Time	0 mi.	5 mi.	9 mi.	5 mi.	0 mi.	1 hr.	14 mi.
Week #15							
Type of Work	Rest	Easy	Medium	Easy	Rest	X-train	Long
Distance or Time	0 mi.	5 mi.	10 mi.	5 mi.	0 mi.	1 hr.	20 mi.
Week #16							
Type of Work	Rest	Easy	Medium	Easy	Rest	X-train	Race
Distance or Time	0 mi.	5 mi.	8 mi.	5 mi.	0 mi.	45 min.	10-K
Week #17							
Type of Work	Rest	Easy	Medium	Easy	Rest	X-train	Long
Distance or Time	0 mi.	4 mi.	6 mi.	4 mi.	0 mi.	30 min.	8 mi.
Week #18							
Type of Work	Rest	Easy	Easy	Rest	Rest	Easy	Marathon
Distance or Time	0 mi.	3 mi.	4 mi.	0 mi.	0 mi.	1-3 mi.	26.2 mi.

Intermediate

(25-30 miles per week)

	MONDAY	TUESDAY	WEDNESDAY	THURSDAY	FRIDAY	SATURDAY	SUNDAY
Week #1							
Type of Work	X-train	Easy	Tempo	Easy	Rest	Pace	Long
Distance or Time	1 hr.	3 mi.	5 mi.	3 mi.	0 mi.	5 mi.	10 mi.
Week #2							
Type of Work	X-train	Easy	Tempo	Easy	Rest	Pace	Long
Distance or Time	1 hr.	3 mi.	5 mi.	3 mi.	0 mi.	5 mi.	11 mi.
Week #3							
Type of Work	X-train	Easy	Tempo	Easy	Rest	Pace	Long
Distance or Time	1 hr.	3 mi.	6 mi.	3 mi.	0 mi.	6 mi.	8 mi.
Week #4							
Type of Work	X-train	Easy	Tempo	Easy	Rest	Pace	Long
Distance or Time	1 hr.	3 mi.	6 mi.	3 mi.	0 mi.	6 mi.	13 mi.
Week #5							
Type of Work	X-train	Easy	Tempo	Easy	Rest	Pace	Long
Distance or Time	1 hr.	3 mi.	7 mi.	3 mi.	0 mi.	7 mi.	14 mi.
Week #6							
Type of Work	X-train	Easy	Tempo	Easy	Rest	Pace	Race
Distance or Time	1 hr.	3 mi.	7 mi.	3 mi.	0 mi.	7 mi.	10-K or 15-K
Week #7							
Type of Work	X-train	Easy	Tempo	Easy	Rest	Pace	Long
Distance or Time	1 hr.	3 mi.	8 mi.	3 mi.	0 mi.	8 mi.	16 mi.
Week #8							
Type of Work	X-train	Easy	Tempo	Easy	Rest	Pace	Long
Distance or Time	1 hr.	4 mi.	8 mi.	4 mi.	0 mi.	8 mi.	17 mi.

Note: Tempo runs are workouts that include 20 to 30 minutes of faster-paced running in the middle of the workout; you do not run all your mileage at tempo pace on these days. After a brief warmup, you should try to do pace runs at your marathon goal pace.

	MONDAY	TUESDAY	WEDNESDAY	THURSDAY	FRIDAY	SATURDAY	SUNDAY
Week #9							
Type of Work	X-train	Easy	Tempo	Easy	Rest	Pace	Long
Distance or Time	1 hr.	4 mi.	9 mi.	4 mi.	0 mi.	9 mi.	12 mi.
Week #10							
Type of Work	X-train	Easy	Tempo	Easy	Rest	Pace	Long
Distance or Time	1 hr.	4 mi.	9 mi.	4 mi.	0 mi.	9 mi.	19 mi.
Week #11							
Type of Work	X-train	Easy	Tempo	Easy	Rest	Pace	Long
Distance or Time	1 hr.	4 mi.	10 mi.	4 mi.	0 mi.	10 mi.	20 mi.
Week #12							
Type of Work	X-train	Easy	Tempo	Easy	Rest	Pace	Race
Distance or Time	1 hr.	5 mi.	6 mi.	5 mi.	0 mi.	6 mi.	20-K
Week #13							
Type of Work	X-train	Easy	Tempo	Easy	Rest	Pace	Long
Distance or Time	1 hr.	5 mi.	10 mi.	5 mi.	0 mi.	10 mi.	20 mi.
Week #14							
Type of Work	X-train	Easy	Tempo	Easy	Rest	Pace	Long
Distance or Time	1 hr.	5 mi.	6 mi.	5 mi.	0 mi.	6 mi.	12 mi.
Week #15							
Type of Work	X-train	Easy	Tempo	Easy	Rest	Pace	Long
Distance or Time	1 hr.	5 mi.	10 mi.	6 mi.	0 mi.	10 mi.	20 mi.
Week #16							
Type of Work	X-train	Easy	Tempo	Easy	Rest	Pace	Race
Distance or Time	1 hr.	5 mi.	8 mi.	5 mi.	0 mi.	4 mi.	10-K
Week #17							
Type of Work	X-train	Easy	Tempo	Easy	Rest	Pace	Long
Distance or Time	45 min.	4 mi.	6 mi.	4 mi.	0 mi.	4 mi.	8 mi.
Week #18							
Type of Work	X-train	Easy	Tempo	Rest	Rest	Easy	Marathon
Distance or Time	30 min.	3 mi.	4 mi.	0 mi.	0 mi.	1-3 mi.	26.2 mi.

Advanced

(more than 30 miles per week)

	MONDAY	TUESDAY	WEDNESDAY	THURSDAY	FRIDAY	SATURDAY	SUNDAY
Week #1							
Type of Work	Easy	Tempo	Easy	Speedwork	Easy	Pace	Long
Distance or Time	3 mi.	5 mi.	3 mi.	—	3 mi.	5 mi.	10 mi.
Week #2							
Type of Work	Easy	Tempo	Easy	Speedwork	Easy	Pace	Long
Distance or Time	3 mi.	5 mi.	3 mi.	—	3 mi.	5 mi.	11 mi.
Week #3							
Type of Work	Easy	Tempo	Easy	Speedwork	Easy	Pace	Long
Distance or Time	3 mi.	4 mi.	3 mi.	—	3 mi.	6 mi.	8 mi.
Week #4							
Type of Work	Easy	Tempo	Easy	Speedwork	Easy	Pace	Long
Distance or Time	3 mi.	6 mi.	3 mi.	—	3 mi.	6 mi.	13 mi.
Week #5							
Type of Work	Easy	Tempo	Easy	Speedwork	Easy	Pace	Long
Distance or Time	3 mi.	7 mi.	3 mi.	—	3 mi.	7 mi.	14 mi.
Week #6							
Type of Work	Easy	Tempo	Easy	Speedwork	Easy	Rest	Race
Distance or Time	3 mi.	5 mi.	3 mi.	—	3 mi.	0 mi.	10-K or 15-K
Week #7							
Type of Work	Easy	Tempo	Easy	Speedwork	Easy	Pace	Long
Distance or Time	3 mi.	8 mi.	3 mi.	—	3 mi.	8 mi.	16 mi.
Week #8							
Type of Work	Easy	Tempo	Easy	Speedwork	Easy	Pace	Long
Distance or Time	4 mi.	8 mi.	4 mi.	—	4 mi.	8 mi.	17 mi.

Note: Tempo runs are workouts that include 20 to 30 minutes of faster-paced running in the middle of the workout; you do not run all your mileage at tempo pace on these days. After a brief warmup, you should try to do pace runs at your marathon goal pace.

	MONDAY	TUESDAY	WEDNESDAY	THURSDAY	FRIDAY	SATURDAY	SUNDAY
Week #9							
Type of Work	Easy	Tempo	Easy	Speedwork	Easy	Easy	Long
Distance or Time	4 mi.	6 mi.	4 mi.	—	4 mi.	9 mi.	12 mi.
Week #10							
Type of Work	Easy	Tempo	Easy	Speedwork	Easy	Easy	Long
Distance or Time	4 mi.	9 mi.	4 mi.	—	4 mi.	9 mi.	19 mi.
Week #11							
Type of Work	Easy	Tempo	Easy	Speedwork	Rest	Pace	Long
Distance or Time	4 mi.	10 mi.	4 mi.	—	0 mi.	10 mi.	20 mi.
Week #12							
Type of Work	Easy	Tempo	Easy	Speedwork	Easy	Rest	Race
Distance or Time	5 mi.	6 mi.	5 mi.	—	5 mi.	0 mi.	20-K
Week #13							
Type of Work	Easy	Tempo	Easy	Speedwork	Rest	Pace	Long
Distance or Time	5 mi.	10 mi.	5 mi.	—	0 mi.	10 mi.	20 mi.
Week #14							
Type of Work	Easy	Tempo	Easy	Speedwork	Easy	Easy	Long
Distance or Time	5 mi.	6 mi.	5 mi.	—	5 mi.	6 mi.	12 mi.
Week #15							
Type of Work	Easy	Tempo	Easy	Speedwork	Rest	Pace	Long
Distance or Time	5 mi.	10 mi.	5 mi.	—	0 mi.	10 mi.	20 mi.
Week #16							
Type of Work	Easy	Tempo	Easy	Speedwork	Easy	Rest	Race
Distance or Time	5 mi.	8 mi.	5 mi.	—	4 mi.	0 mi.	10-K
Week #17							
Type of Work	Easy	Tempo	Easy	Speedwork	Easy	Easy	Long
Distance or Time	4 mi.	6 mi.	4 mi.	—	3 mi.	5 mi.	8 mi.
Week #18							
Type of Work	Easy	Tempo	Easy	Rest	Rest	Easy	Marathon
Distance or Time	3 mi.	4 mi.	3 mi.	0 mi.	0 mi.	1-3 mi.	26.2 mi.

Chapter 36

Incredible but True: Yasso 800s

This Simple Marathon Workout Really Works

During my 25 years at *Runner's World* magazine, I have probably written hundreds of articles, some of them so encyclopedic that they could practically have stood alone like a book. The one that follows is the shortest I have ever written—and also my favorite.

I still remember the absolute delight that I felt when Bart Yasso first explained his "Yasso 800s" to me. I had been running and hanging around runners for a long time. I thought I knew, or had heard, just about everything, including plenty of crackpot ideas. But I had never heard of Yasso 800s.

Naturally, I had to put Bart's idea to the test. I'm a skeptic at heart; I don't accept anything until it has met my standards for scrutiny. Yasso 800s passed with flying colors. They have become one of the classic workouts of marathon training. I believe they're going to remain that for a long, long time.

When physicists discover a new subatomic particle, they claim the right to name it. Same with astronomers. Locate a new star out there in the way beyond, and you can name it anything you want: Clarence, Sarah, Mork, or even Mindy. I think runners, coaches, and writers should be able to do the same. And I'm going to take this opportunity to invoke the privilege.

A few years back, I discovered an amazing, new marathon workout. Amazing because it's the simplest marathon workout that I had ever heard of. (And simplicity in marathon training, as in physics and astronomy, is much to be prized.) Amazing because I'm convinced that it actually works.

In truth, I didn't find this workout. It found me, through the person of Bart Yasso, the race coordinator at *Runner's World* magazine, who has run more than 50 marathons on four continents. But Bart's not much of a proselytizer, while I sometimes am, so I'm going to seize this chance to name the workout. I'm going to call it Yasso 800s.

BART ENLIGHTENS ME

Bart and I were at the Portland Marathon when he told me about his workout. He was training for a marathon later in the fall, so two days before Portland he went to a nearby track and ran Yasso 800s. "I'm trying to build up to 10 repeats of 800s in the same time as my marathon goal time," he told me.

Huh? Half-miles in 3 to 4 hours? I didn't get it. Bart saw that he would have to do more explaining. "I've been doing this particular workout for about 15 years," he continued, "and it always seems to work for me. If I can get my 800s down to 2 minutes, 50 seconds, I'm in 2:50 marathon shape. If I can get down to 2:40 (minutes), I can run a 2:40 marathon. I'm shooting for a 2:37 marathon right now, so I'm running my 800s in 2:37."

Suddenly, things started to make sense. But would the same workout apply to a three-hour marathoner? A four-hour marathoner? A five-hour marathoner? It didn't seem very likely.

PUTTING IT TO THE TEST

Over the next couple of weeks, I decided it was time to check it out. I played around with lots of mathematical equations and talked to about 100 runners of widely differing abilities (from a 2:09 marathoner to several well over 4 hours), and darn if the Yasso 800s didn't hold up all the way down the line.

Now, this is a remarkable thing. Anyone who has been running for a few years and, in particular, trying to improve his marathon time, knows that training theory can get quite complex. You have pace, you have lactate threshold, you have cruise intervals, you have tempo training, you have enough gibberish to launch a new line of dictionaries.

Following a classic workout like Yasso 800s could help you in training for a marathon.

And now you have an easier way: You have Yasso 800s. Want to run a 3:30 marathon? Then train to run a bunch of 800s in 3:30 each. Between the 800s, jog for the same number of minutes that it took you to run your repeats. Training doesn't get any simpler than this, not on this planet or anywhere else in the solar system.

TRIED AND TESTED

Bart begins running his Yasso 800s a couple of months before his goal marathon. In the first week he does four, all in one workout. In each subsequent week he adds one more until he reaches 10. The last workout of Yasso 800s should be completed at least 10 days before your marathon, and 14 to 17 days would probably be better.

The rest of the time, you should just do your normal marathon training, paying special attention to weekend long runs. Give yourself plenty of easy runs and maybe a day or two off during the week.

But don't skip the Yasso 800s. This is the workout that's going to get you to the finish on time.

Amby Burfoot's Running Round-Up

I was so enthusiastic about Yasso 800s that I wrote about them before I had a chance to use them in my own training. But believe me, I began using them the next time I trained for a marathon, and I have used them for every marathon since.

Okay, so I admit, I cheat a little. The truth is, the most that I've ever done is nine. And I often reach only as high as seven or eight Yasso 800s. The fault isn't in the workout, though. The fault is in myself, in that I don't train hard enough for most of my marathons these days.

Even at just seven or eight repeats, however, I find Yasso 800s to be a great benefit to my marathon training. Basically, they build my confidence. I know that if I run them in the appointed time, my marathon goal time lies within my grasp. And you only need to do one Yasso workout a week. A form of tempo training, Yasso 800s provide a hard, solid, somewhat fast workout but don't push you over the brink of fatigue. (If they do, you're aiming for too fast a time, and you should recalibrate.) They allow you to recover and run another good workout in two days.

Indeed, Yasso 800s and long runs now form the backbone of my marathon training. I do a Yasso workout in the middle of the week, a long run on the weekend, and fill in the rest of my training as best I can. A marathon training schedule couldn't be simpler.

Chapter 37

The Perfect Marathon Taper

A Close Look at the Two Weeks Before Your Marathon

Preparing for a marathon is at the same time both simple and complex. The simple part is the training. If you follow any reasonable schedule for several months, you'll probably get yourself in shape for the distance.

Putting all the other pieces in place, on the other hand, often amounts to a considerable challenge. You have to eat right, get enough sleep, avoid injuries and colds, pick a good marathon, travel perhaps to a strange city, and then negotiate all the ins and outs of number pickup, meals, getting to the start on time, and so on. Marathon morning, by itself, is often a graduate-level course in logistics and deployment.

With all these things to consider, it helps to have a plan and a checklist. That's the purpose of this chapter by Gordon Bakoulis. Here he describes everything that you have to think of and how to go about handling it. With this plan, your marathon success is practically guaranteed.

The marathon is a gamble. Over its vast distance and time, anything can happen. And you can't control the weather or the course. So the object of the game is to focus on those things that you can control. And we're not just talking about long runs and pasta. The well-prepared marathoner looks after every detail of proper physical and mental training, nutrition, hydration, clothing, and equipment.

In the last two weeks before your marathon, you should focus on these matters even more as you fine-tune your training and your diet and put all the last-minute details of your race in order. In general, you shouldn't introduce new elements into your training or—if possible—into your life during these two weeks.

To help you in your final preparation for the marathon, here's a daily checklist of things that you should do in the last two weeks prior to your race. Grab a calendar and a pencil, and get ready for your best-planned marathon ever.

If you have done the training and can check off every item listed here (or most of them), you're virtually guaranteed success on marathon day. You've taken control of everything you can; the rest is up to fate. With reasonably good weather and a decent course, you may have the race of your life.

SATURDAY, DAY 15

Training: This is the day before your last long run, so you want to run lightly. Either take a day off, or jog for 30 to 45 minutes easy. Stretch in the evening.

Mental preparation: Mentally prepare yourself for your last long run. Remind yourself that the hard work is nearly over but that you want this final long training effort to count. Do something relaxing and inspiring, such as listening to your favorite music.

Diet: Eat a high-carbohydrate dinner to top off your stores of glycogen (a complex carbohydrate that your body uses for quick energy), and drink plenty of nonalcoholic beverages without caffeine.

SUNDAY, DAY 14

Training: This last long run should not be your longest. (Most experts suggest doing that no later than three to four weeks before your race.) Run at a comfortable pace, saving your best effort for the race. Include surges only if you have done so previously in training. A good last long run will give you a tremendous mental boost. But don't let a subpar effort discourage you. Remember that the race is what counts.

Mental preparation: Plan some visualization exercises for the next two weeks to help you relax and build your confidence. Find a quiet place, close your eyes, and relax. Imagine yourself running well at various points in the race.

Diet: Weigh yourself before and after your long run and drink enough to make up for any lost pounds. Or drink until your urine is plentiful and clear. Also, you should replace carbohydrates within two hours after your run, when your muscles are most receptive.

Other details: This is your last chance to experiment with the food or drinks that you may eat before and after the marathon. You can test, for example, whether a bagel eaten an hour before a long run sits well in your stomach. If you think that you might take a sports drink during the race, find out which beverage will be available on the course, fill up a few water bottles with it, and plant them along the course of your long run.

MONDAY, DAY 13

Training: Run or do some form of cross-training (if you have been cross-training) for 30 to 45 minutes, or take a day off to recover from your long run.

Mental preparation: Shift gears to think "countdown" from here until your marathon. Rather than building up your training, you're backing off. Visualize the race start: standing on the line feeling relaxed, confident, and eager to run.

Diet: Evaluate how you handled yesterday's food and fluid intake. Eat extra carbohydrates if you're hungry, and drink more if your urine is still sparse or dark. It can take 24 to 48 hours after a long run to restore fluid and glycogen stores.

TUESDAY, DAY 12

Training: Run for 45 to 60 minutes. After the first 20 minutes, do eight 30-second hard efforts with 30-second recoveries between each. This workout should shake your legs out but not drain you. Include the pickups if you have been doing intervals throughout your training.

Mental preparation: Visualize the first five miles of the race. You're holding back, letting other runners go because you know you'll pass them later. You feel fresh, alert, even able to chat with those around you.

Travel: If you're traveling a long distance to your marathon, call your airline and hotel to reconfirm your reservations.

WEDNESDAY, DAY 11

Training: If you usually do a midweek semi-long run, run 60 to 90 minutes today at training pace. Otherwise jog for 30 to 45 minutes.

Equipment: This is a good time to make a list of clothing and equipment that you'll need to take with you to the marathon, such as petroleum jelly, tape, extra shoelaces, a key holder (attaches to your shoe), plastic garbage bags to wear at the start if it rains, containers for water and food, and clothing for before, during, and after the marathon. Purchase any items you need now. Don't count on being able to buy them once you get to the race.

THURSDAY, DAY 10

Training: You should do your last hard speed workout today. Do three- to five-minute intervals 10 to 30 seconds faster than your planned mara-

Get the right gear

If you haven't bought the shoes that you plan to wear in the race, do so now. If your current pair has more than 400 miles on it or is worn or frayed in any way, you should replace it. Train in your new shoes during these next two weeks. Never race in brand-new shoes and don't change models, either. Stick to the shoes that you've been wearing throughout your training.

thon pace, with 30-second to two-minute recovery jogs.

Mental preparation: Congratulate yourself on another hard workout well done. Visualize miles five to nine of the marathon. You're settled in, running comfortably, recording even splits, and making sure you take on plenty of water. You feel well-trained and rested and know that you're going to have a great marathon.

Diet: Plan some of your tried-and-true high-carbohydrate meals for the next 10 days. Don't try unfamiliar foods, but don't eat the same thing every day (even pasta). Choose from a variety of high-carbohydrate foods such as potatoes, certain vegetables, fruit, bread, rice, and other grains. And don't neglect protein. Figure low-fat meat, poultry, fish, legumes, egg whites, and low-fat dairy products into your diet as well.

FRIDAY, DAY 9

Training: Take a day off, or cross-train for no more than 45 minutes. Remember, nothing new now.

Equipment: Go over your marathon shopping list and make sure that you have everything you need.

Travel: Make sure that you know exactly where your airline tickets are, and check on your passport or any other travel documents you'll need.

SATURDAY, DAY 8

Training: Many marathoners do a semi-long run (no longer than two hours) or a race of 10-K or less a week before their marathon. Either way, this is your last hard effort. The semi-long run keeps you in a pattern of going long without overtaxing yourself close to race day. You should finish feeling refreshed, not drained. Afterward, you may want to schedule a massage to work out any kinks and help move lactic acid out of your legs.

Mental preparation: Visualize miles 10 to 13 of the marathon. You're still feeling great, although you're starting to work yourself a little harder. You're holding a steady pace. No one's passing you, and you're looking forward to the half-marathon point.

Diet: Are you obsessing about carbo loading? Contrary to popular belief, if you have followed a high-carbohydrate training diet, you don't need to change your pattern very much this week. You may want to increase your carbohydrate intake by roughly 10 percent in the few days before the race by eating extra servings of bread, fruit, pasta, or rice. Vary your diet, but don't add unfamiliar foods.

SUNDAY, DAY 7

Training: Run easy or cross-train for 30 to 45 minutes.
Mental preparation: Listening to music or inspi-

rational words before the start of a marathon can get you psyched. If you think it may help you, prepare some tapes to bring along to the race.
Diet: Continue to follow your high-carbohydrate, low-fat diet and make sure that you're drinking plenty of fluids.
Equipment: If you're traveling to your marathon, make a packing list and start gathering the clothes and other items that you're going to need.

MONDAY, DAY 6

Training: Run for 45 minutes. After the first 20 minutes, do 8 to 10 pickups of one minute each with one-minute recoveries between. Stretch thoroughly afterward.
Mental preparation: Visualize miles 14 to 17. You are working hard, running steadily, feeling calm and confident. You have taken plenty of water, and your muscles are relaxed and loose. You're on pace for a personal record.
Travel: If you're flying to your race and have to cross time zones, plan, if possible, to arrive a few days before the marathon so that you have time to adjust to the new environment. The air in planes is especially dry, so drink extra fluids. And eat lightly; airline food is generally high in fat. Or, better yet, bring your own low-fat, high-carbohydrate snacks. Once you reach your destination, get on the new time schedule immediately.

TUESDAY, DAY 5

Training: Jog for 30 to 45 minutes.
Mental preparation: You may feel restless at this point and be tempted to add extra last-minute miles. Don't! Extra training now will hurt rather

than help your performance by tiring you and preventing your legs from saturating with glycogen. Relax once you get to the race site, but don't spend days lying around your hotel room. Just avoid excessive walking and standing, and get plenty of sleep.

Diet: Don't worry if you gain a few pounds between now and the race. It's extra water and carbohydrates that you'll need for the marathon.

Equipment: Check race-day forecasts, and start to plan your outfit. Make a list of any items that you have forgotten and need to buy.

WEDNESDAY, DAY 4

Training: Jog or cross-train for 30 minutes. If you like, do four to five pickups of 30 seconds each after the first 15 minutes of running.

Mental preparation: Visualize miles 18 to 21. This is a tough segment for many people. You have been running for at least two hours, yet you still can't smell the finish. See yourself digging down, working hard, holding your own, and starting to pass others.

Other details: If friends or family have come to watch you race, make arrangements to meet them near the finish.

THURSDAY, DAY 3

Training: Take the day off, or jog for 30 minutes. Remember, the less you run now, the more stamina you'll have on race day.

Mental preparation: You're likely to feel keyed up and irritable in these final days. Do what feels right for you: Spend time alone, hang out with a group, or visit with one or two friends or family members.

Diet: Your carbohydrate intake should be at least 65 percent of total calories. You should feel comfortable after each meal, not unpleasantly stuffed.

Other details: It may sound overly cautious, but you should plan to have two working alarm clocks. You never know when one will fail. Don't rely solely on a friend or a hotel wake-up call, either.

FRIDAY, DAY 2

Training: Jog for no more than 20 minutes. Some advanced runners throw in a few light pickups to remind themselves that they still have leg speed. This isn't necessary for most people.

Mental preparation: Visualize miles 22 to 26. These miles are usually the toughest, but you'll be ready because you have trained hard and raced smart. Imagine yourself running strong and steady toward the finish, passing all those who started too fast.

Diet: The food you eat today will help you more in the race than the food that you'll eat tomorrow. Keep up your pattern of ample carbohydrates and fluids. And especially now, don't try anything new or exotic.

Equipment: Race-day weather forecasts should be detailed and accurate at this point (although surprises can happen).

Plan your race-day outfit, and if you need any last-minute items, visit the marathon expo. Pick up your race packet as early as possible to avoid the last-minute rush, and carefully read all the instructions.

Sleep: A good night's sleep matters more tonight than the night before the race. If you can't sleep, don't worry about it—lying down for your usual sleep period is still beneficial.

Prepare for lift-off

Make fail-safe plans to get to the start and meet someone at the finish. Have a backup plan for every possible disaster such as your car failing to start, missing the bus, sleeping through your alarm, or breaking a shoelace. Go to sleep confident that nothing stands between you and getting to the starting line feeling calm, strong, and ready to go.

SATURDAY, DAY 1

Training: If you run at all, jog for no more than 30 minutes. Many runners like to run the day before a marathon to get any kinks out. Just take it easy, no matter how good you feel.

Mental preparation: Visualize the finish. You have made it, and you're exhausted but triumphant as you run the final few hundred yards feeling strong and steady. See yourself raising your hands as you cross the line to the cheers of thousands of spectators.

Diet: Try to make one of today's meals a special event with family and friends who will relax with you and share your excitement. Contrary to popular belief, what you eat today will have little effect on your marathon as long as you stick to the usual—plenty of carbohydrates and beverages. Eat dinner early so that you can get a good night's sleep.

Equipment: Lay out everything that you plan to wear or bring to the start: racing singlet and shorts, tights and a short- or long-sleeved shirt if appropriate, mittens or gloves, hat, headband, bandanna, sweats, rainsuit, whatever you will need. Pack a separate set of warm, dry clothes for the finish. Your equipment should include your bag, running number, extra shoelaces and safety pins, bus ticket to the start, car key, beverages, containers, food for before and after, money, petroleum jelly (to prevent chafing and protect exposed areas from wind and cold), sunscreen, music tapes, a headset, and a plastic garbage bag if it's raining.

Sleep: Marathon-related anxiety dreams such as missing the start, losing your shoes, or running the wrong course are a common occurrence. So don't worry if you don't sleep well. If you're generally well-rested, one night's poor sleep won't hurt you.

MARATHON DAY

Diet: Wake up at least 2 hours before the start. Give yourself enough time to eat something light but high in carbohydrates. Drink water or a sports drink, stretch, and get to the starting line with time to spare.

Mental preparation: Mentally, you want to achieve a state of optimal arousal. That means that you want to be eager and excited but not crippled by nervousness. Think back to other races to recall this feeling. If you feel too keyed up, sit or lie down, close your eyes, and breathe deeply. Visualize the race or simply think peaceful, happy thoughts. On the other hand, if you're not "up" enough, walk or jog and talk to other runners, but don't tire yourself.

Equipment: Keep warm and comfortable until the last possible minute before the race. Many runners wear old sweats to the start and discard them just before the gun. Otherwise, standing around in the cold can cramp your muscles. Make sure to apply petroleum jelly to areas likely to chafe, such as underarms, nipples, and inner thighs. Mark your bag so that you can find it easily at the finish. During the race, lose layers if you feel too warm, or you'll lose precious fluids through perspiration. Keep extremities covered if it's cold.

Warmup: It's not necessary to warm up extensively prior to a marathon, but do try to do some walking and a few minutes of jogging to loosen your legs and raise your body temperature, otherwise you could be caught cold.

Racing: Running a successful marathon is an exercise in holding back. Ideally, the hard work shouldn't begin until 20 miles. Then your training and willpower will get you to the finish. During the race, remain calm and focused. Note your splits, and take encouragement from a steady pace early on, even if others are passing you. Break the race into segments, and work through each part rather than attack the full 26.2 miles.

Other details: Don't eat or drink anything on the course that you haven't tried previously in training. If you do, you may suffer digestive woes. Take water early and often. If you feel cramps or stomach upset en route, walk until the problem lessens.

Finish: When you come through the finish line, keep walking around and take on some fluids right away. Pat yourself on the back—you made it. Find your friends or family, and go celebrate.

Amby Burfoot's Running Round-Up

The last two weeks before a marathon are often an unsettling time. You begin to train less but think about the race more. You get cranky. You lose sleep. You start to feel aches and pains in your legs at the precise time when they should be feeling their best. After all, you're tapering off and giving them a break after weeks or months of hard training.

This chapter tells you how to deal with almost everything but the strange and disconcerting feelings a marathoner often experiences before his race. Suddenly, all self-confidence vanishes. He begins to wonder if he hasn't bitten off too much.

The closer the race gets, the worse he feels and the more he obsesses over his many doubts.

I can only tell you one thing: The doubts will pass, and race-day magic will take over. Race-day magic is the heady phenomenon that makes virtually all marathoners feel better during the race than they ever imagined possible. It's the magic that helps you run farther and faster than you thought you could.

And you'll never have the chance to enjoy it unless you get to the starting line. So don't let the doubts deter you. Just stick to your plan and reap the rewards.

Chapter 38

The Thinking Runner's Marathon Plan

Training for and running a marathon requires more than strong legs. You'll need some smarts as well.

Jeff Galloway likes to say that the marathon is a good training motivator because it scares people. The distance is so improbably long, no one can fully train for a 26-miler, and the stories about things that go wrong are pervasive.

All of us have heard the stories, and we all fear that we'll be next in line.

This marathon fright is what makes people get so nervous as the big day and big hour grow closer. Runners figure that they've got to do everything absolutely right, or they'll pay the consequences. (In reality, there's more wiggle room than most marathoners realize.) Here, a group of veteran marathoners who are also scientific experts deliver their proven tips for first training correctly and then marathon race-day success.

TRAINING

1. Run just enough. "Stay healthy" is the most important piece of training advice, and the most often ignored. It does you no good to train hard and then get sick or injured. Better to be slightly undertrained, but feeling strong and eager, than to be overtrained. The trick, of course, is finding that fine line between the two.

2. Build your training slowly. Increase weekly mileage by just 10 percent per week. Extend long runs by just one mile at a time up to

10 miles, then by two miles at a time if you want. Take recovery weeks as well as recovery days. Here's what eight weeks of training might look like, in terms of miles per week: 20-22-24-20-26-28-30-20.

3. Recover, recover, recover. You don't have to train hard seven days a week. You have to train smart three or four days a week. This was proven in a 1994 study at the University of Northern Iowa, where four-time-a-week runners performed just as well in a marathon as those training six times a week and covering 20 percent more total miles. A similar approach is now endorsed by the Furman FIRST marathon program, where 70 percent of veterans have improved their times on three runs a week.

4. Do your long runs. This is a no-brainer. The newer you are to marathoning, and the slower, the more important your long runs. You simply have to get accustomed to being on your feet for three, four, or more hours. There's no magic length. Most experts recommend stopping at two and a half to three hours; Jeff Galloway advises going farther, but including walk breaks. All systems work, as long as you get to the starting line healthy and strong.

5. Practice your marathon pace. Ann Alyanak, a coach at the University of Dayton, took 10 minutes off her PR at the 2007 Boston Marathon, finishing in 2:38. The key, she believes, was the addition of "progressive marathon-pace" (MP) long runs to her program. Alyanak would do a two-mile warmup, then six miles at MP + 40 seconds, six more at MP + 20, and her final six at MP. "I was able to run negative splits in Boston," she says.

6. Extend your tempo-run distance. Tempo runs were born as four-mile efforts, propounded by coaching genius Jack Daniels, Ph.D. Then another genius coach, Joe Vigil, Ph.D., began asking Deena Kastor to hold the tempo pace longer—eventually up to 12 miles. He got Meb Keflezighi to 15. Result? Two Olympic Marathon medals. Gradually extend your tempo runs, slowing by a few seconds per mile from your four-mile pace. "The longer the tempo run workout you can sustain, the greater the dividends down the road," says Vigil.

7. Run mile repeats. In a fascinating article in *Marathon & Beyond* in 2002, veteran marathoner Dan Horvath plotted various workouts against his subsequent results in 30 marathons over a 12-year period. The most effective workout? Mile repeats. Horvath would typically run 6 x 1-mile at his 10-K race pace, once a week. It turned out that the faster his mile repeats prior to a given marathon, the faster his marathon time. Mile repeats are a modified form of tempo training.

8. Try Yasso 800s. This deceptively simple workout has been used effectively by thousands of runners over the past decade. The goal, after several months of working up to it, is to run 10 x 800 meters in the same minutes:seconds as your goal time (in hours:minutes). If you want to run a 3:40 marathon, for example, you run your Yasso 800s in 3 minutes, 40 seconds. This workout isn't based on physiology; it's just a very tough effort that's got a mathematical appeal to it.

9. Eat your carbs . . . To stay healthy and recover well, you need to fuel your body efficiently. First, consume some carbs—gel, sports drink, and so on—during long, hard workouts to keep running strong. Second, eat and/or drink a good helping of carbs as quickly as possible after workouts. This will replenish the glycogen (energy supply) in your depleted leg muscles. Add a little protein for muscle repair.

10. . . . and pay attention to iron. Running increases iron loss through sweating and pounding. You don't have to be a meat-eater to run a strong marathon, but you do have to consume enough iron. Cooking in an iron skillet helps, as does consuming iron-rich foods with vitamin C, which increases the body's iron absorption.

11. Sidestep injuries. I asked exercise physiologist, author, and two-time U.S. Olympic marathoner (1984, 1988) Peter Pfitzinger what he would do differently if he were 22 years old today. He said that he'd rest and/or cross-train for several days a week at the first hint of a problem. And that he'd include core training in his regimen. "I'm convinced that core stability helps runners maintain good running form and pace late in a race," says Pfitzinger, now the CEO of the New Zealand Academy of Sport North.

12. Taper for two to three weeks. Many runners hate to taper. We are cursed with a sort of sublime obsessiveness—a big help when you're increasing your efforts, but an albatross when you're supposed to be cutting back. A study from Ball State University showed a particular gain in Type IIa muscle fiber strength—the so-called fast, aerobic muscles that can adapt to improve your performance—after a three-week taper. Of course, this isn't true for everyone. Ryan Hall ran a 2:08:24 London Marathon just three weeks after doing a fast-finishing 26-mile workout. Everyone responds differently to training. Still, it's generally considered that a taper increases your chance of 26.2-mile success.

RACE DAY

1. Don't do anything new. Race day is not the time for new shoes, new food or drinks, new clothing, or anything else you haven't done on several training runs. Stick with a routine that works for you. "I learned the hard way that when you try something new on race day, you often end up regretting it," says Russ Pate, who has a Ph.D. in exercise physiology and qualified for three U.S. Marathon Trials in '72, '76, and '80. "I eventually developed a routine that I followed ritualistically before all my races."

2. Eat first thing. Too many marathoners skip breakfast on race day, opting for just a cup of coffee and/or some sports drink. You need more than that. "From the time you go to bed until the start of the race is usually eight to 10 hours," says Ken Sparks, who has a Ph.D. in exercise physiology and ran a personal best 2:28 at age 46. "In that time, your liver glycogen—which is stored carbohydrate—gets depleted. If you don't have a simple, high-carb breakfast, you're going to be in trouble at 20 miles." Bananas, bagels, or energy bars are good picks.

3. Don't overdress. Marathons often start in the cool of early morning, and it's easy to overestimate the amount of clothing you'll need. As a rule of thumb, it will probably feel 10 or more degrees warmer once you get going, and temps will rise as the day goes on. If you wear too much clothing, you're carrying extra weight and you will sweat more than you want, possibly increasing your body temperature and risk of dehydration. "If you overdress, you create a microclimate around the skin that induces sweating," says Mel Williams, Ph.D., an exercise physiologist, author of *The Ergogenics Edge*, and veteran marathoner. "The best clothing allows for some heat loss, but not so much that you become uncomfortably cold."

4. Prevent chafing. "During a marathon, every moving body part that can chafe will chafe," says Williams. And nothing is more irritating and painful than skin rubbed raw. To prevent this, make sure your shoes, socks, and clothing have no raised seams that will rub against the skin. Also, use Vaseline, BodyGlide, or something similar in key locations, including your armpits, nipples, and inner thighs.

5. Wear sunscreen. Marathoners sometimes don't think about the fact that they're in the sun long enough to get sunburned. This is particularly true if you finish in four or five hours, which takes you into the high-sun time of the day, or if you run the Boston Marathon, which starts at 10:00 on a course with little shade. "I used to run with a cap on my head, but then I decided that the cap was holding in too much heat," remembers Williams. "So one year, I ran without the cap. My bald head got sunburned so badly, it turned into one of my most painful races. Now I put a nongreasy sunblock on my head, my shoulders, and my lips."

6. Pin your race number on your shorts. That way you can fiddle all you want with your upper-body apparel. If the temperature rises, you can peel off the long-sleeve shirt that kept you toasty for the first three miles. If the wind kicks up, reach for the shirt that's wrapped around your waist. "When you put your number on your shorts, you can add or subtract layers as needed to adjust to changing conditions," says Greg Crowther, a 2:22-marathoner with a Ph.D. in physiology and biophysics. "On a hot day, you could even exchange a sweaty shirt for a dry one. The easier you can vary your torso covering, the better."

7. Go for the jolt. Twenty years ago, researchers thought that caffeine helped runners burn more fat, thereby sparing precious glycogen. That theory has been mostly disproved, but caffeine does make the marathon feel easier. "I did a caffeine-endurance study with some researchers at Yale, and we didn't find any difference in fat burning," says Hal Goforth, who has run the past 28 Boston Marathons in a row and has a Ph.D. in kinesiology and a marathon PR of 2:28. "But the exercisers on caffeine had higher levels of beta-endorphins and a lower perceived effort." So drink your normal amount of coffee before the race. Or, if you want to be more scientific about it, Goforth suggests taking caffeine tablets 60 to 90 minutes before the marathon at a dose of three milligrams per pound of your body weight.

8. Top off your tank. Most marathoners know enough to stay well hydrated in the days before their race. It's tough to superhydrate, however, because your kidneys have time to release any excess water you consume. But in the final minutes to half hour before the start, you can trick your kidneys by sneaking in a late drink. (Your kidneys will mostly shut down once you start running hard.) "I carry my Gatorade to the starting line and keep sipping it as long as my stomach feels comfortable," says Williams, who also eats pretzels before the marathon, figuring the extra salt will help him retain the fluids he consumes.

9. Keep your warmup short. It makes sense to not warm up much before a marathon. After all, you want to save energy. But you'll actually run more efficiently if you first loosen up your leg muscles. "I do a warmup just to the point of a very light sweat," says Kitty Consolo, who has a Ph.D. in exercise physiology and a marathon best of 2:42. "I also use my warmup to gauge the weather, to see how I'll need to adjust my pace to the conditions."

10. Run at an even pace. This is possibly the oldest and most important of marathon strategies. "Both the laboratory data and experiences of countless marathoners show that even-pace running is the optimal approach," says Pate. "In my best marathons, I almost felt that I was running too slowly the first five to 10 miles." Exercise physiologist Phil Sparling, Ph.D., concurs. "You have to run so slow that it feels like you're holding yourself back," says Sparling. "Later it feels so good when you're going strong and passing people."

11. Fix it sooner, not later. You might notice that your shoelace is beginning to come untied. Or you're starting to chafe in that one particular spot. Or a pebble has taken up residence in your left shoe. These things don't go away on their own.

And the sooner you deal with them, the better you'll fare over the distance. "It's like the old saying, 'An ounce of prevention is worth a pound of cure,'" says Crowther. "Only in the marathon, it's more like an ounce of cure early is better than a pound of pain later."

12. Drink early—and late. When you're aiming for a fast marathon time—say a sub-three-hour—every ounce of fluid you consume helps maintain the blood flow to your skin (for cooling) and to your heart and muscles. Since running hard slows the absorption of fluids from your stomach, you need to begin drinking early to have the fluids become available later. That said, Crowther says drinking at the 24-mile mark also helps. "There might not be time to absorb all the water and sugars, but some can get into your system, and this will help you in that last tough mile." (Important note: If you expect to run four hours or slower, be careful not to overdrink and develop hyponatremia. Drink when you are thirsty, and stop drinking if your stomach becomes uncomfortably full of fluids.)

13. Use some gel. Sports drinks contain carbohydrates and other good stuff, but gels provide a more concentrated source of carbs that can prove especially helpful in the last half of the marathon. Williams carries four gel packs, and takes them at miles 10, 14, 18, and 22. "I'm trying to get about 60 grams of carbohydrates per hour," says Williams. "That's about the maximum the body can handle."

14. Draft off someone. Hey, it works for Lance Armstrong and other Tour de France winners. The drafting effect isn't as strong in running, but it's still there. "I always tried to tuck in behind someone in my marathons, because it's so much more efficient to follow," says Sparks. "I'd often pick one of the first women. They'd usually run a strong, even pace." Just be polite about it and don't follow too closely, or better yet, agree to take turns leading so you're working together with this person. Alternative: Find a marathon that offers pace groups, and join the peloton, just like Lance.

15. Don't charge the hills. The goal in marathon running is to maximize your efficiency over 26.2 miles. That's why drafting works. And it's why running hard up the hills doesn't work. "From an energy-output perspective, you gain more speed by putting your effort into the flats than the hills," says Crowther. "When you're on the hills, just relax. Don't worry about those people who are passing you. You'll get them back later."

Amby Burfoot's Running Round-Up

Over 40 years of marathon training and racing, I've learned two things that I consider critically important that bear repeating. The first: Don't get as fit as you can; get as healthy as you can. And second: Run with confidence.

The first refers to many runners' quest for the ultimate marathon training program. They believe they need to get in lots of miles, lots of long runs, and lots of tempo runs. It's an intimidating prospect, and it has a negative side effect worth avoiding. All that training can temporarily reduce your immunity, and you might catch a cold just at the point where you should be tapering off and get-ting stronger. That's why I advise many mara-thoners to do less training, not more, and to focus on their overall health as well as their perfect training program.

Second, the marathon is 50 percent physical and 90 percent mental. You have to do the training to succeed, but you also have to have confidence in yourself and your training if you are to run a smart race (with an even-pace strategy, or even negative splits). Without such confidence, the sheer immen-sity of the marathon can prove overwhelming. So, believe in yourself. If you've done 75 percent of the training, you're 100 percent ready.

Chapter 39

Will the Marathon Kill You?

The studies have been done, the results are in. Here's what you need to know.

Ever since Pheidippides, the marathon has sometimes gotten a bad reputation. The original Greek distance runner supposedly dropped dead at the end of his heroic run from Marathon to Athens ("Rejoice, we conquer."), and all marathon runners since him have worried about the same. Things didn't get any better in 1984 when Jim Fixx, a famous running convert, book author, and marathoner, died from a heart attack while running down a country road in Vermont.

People whispered that running could kill you. And that the longer the distance you ran, the more likely your demise. The marathon? It was 26.2 miles long—way too far to be a healthy activity.

Fortunately, a handful of running physicians and research-scientists-turned-runners began to collect data about runners and their health outcomes. Several years ago, I gathered all the information together in one article, so runners could clearly see the (minor) risks and (major) health benefits of their sport. Including the marathon.

Most days on my noontime run, I don't worry about dying. My daily run offers so many pleasant distractions. I can check out my neighbors' gardens. Work through personal problems, consider a marathon, or simply enjoy the satisfaction of another workout in the bank.

Still, a somber thought does intrude from time to time. I might remember the Saturday phone call I got almost 25 years ago, when I learned from a CBS Radio reporter that Jim Fixx, whose best-selling 1977 book had done much to popularize running, had died during a routine training run.

And then there was that tense moment in November of 2007 when news broke that Ryan Shay died near the five-mile mark of the USA Men's Olympic Marathon Trials in Central Park. Shay, just 28, was the first world-class marathoner to die from a heart attack while competing.

That fall was a tough time for those of us who believe running makes us healthier. The day after Shay's death, Matthew Hardy, 50, died of an apparent heart attack shortly after finishing the ING New York City Marathon in 4:48:21. A month earlier, Chad Schieber, 35, who'd been diagnosed with a heart defect (mitral valve prolapse), had died in the unusually hot Chicago Marathon. These stories often get more attention than those of the race winners. And they always raise the question: If running is so damn healthy, why do runners keep dropping dead in their tracks? Statistically speaking, a handful of runners will die in a marathon every year—the vast majority from heart attacks (the others from heatstroke or hyponatremia). Is running—as the alarmists and cynics often suggest—a dangerous activity?

To find out, I visited the world's leading heart and exercise experts, reviewed stacks of medical research about exercise and death risks, and consulted with the statisticians who work in this field. I learned the reassuring truth that running and other vigorous exercise do dramatically lower mortality risks. But I also learned that there are surprising paradoxes, and no guarantees. Every workout is a bit of a crapshoot. Fortunately, if you run smart and fully informed, you should be able to keep going for a long, long time.

EXERCISE MATTERS

Fitness researcher Steven Blair, 69, doesn't look like most of the lifelong runners I know. He's as round as a beach ball, with a trim gray beard. Blair figures he has run 70,000 miles in the past 40 years, including 18 marathons, with a best of 3:28 at Napa Valley. But the miles haven't chased away the weight. He's gained 30 pounds through his midlife years, largely around the waist, and now carries 195 pounds on a 5'5" frame. He knows this is disconcerting to new acquaintances who expect a pencil-thin fitness fanatic. He often describes himself as "short, fat, and bald," in part because he has a self-deprecating sense of humor and in part to emphasize that not everyone is born lean and mean.

Blair, who holds a doctorate in physical education, worked for 22 years at the groundbreaking Cooper Aerobics Center in Dallas, first as a researcher but eventually as CEO. He was the guy who did the work that helped Kenneth H. Cooper spread the word about the health benefits of exercise. Now a professor in the Arnold School of Public Health at the University of South Carolina, Blair continues his research while arguing at every opportunity that America's public health could be improved, and its medical bills reduced, if everyone would just get up and get moving for 30 minutes a day. He's got the studies to prove it, too—hundreds of them. Blair has also held leadership positions on committees of the American Heart Association and the American College of Sports Medicine. "Steve's probably our most famous faculty member," another University of South Carolina professor told me.

An exercise epidemiologist looks for connections between exercise habits and health outcomes, such as heart disease, stroke, diabetes, and high blood pressure. Most epidemiologists resort to questionnaires to quantify human behavior, a dicey prospect. All of Blair's subjects, in contrast, have actually visited the Cooper Clinic and taken a treadmill stress test, running to exhaustion. Years and even decades later, the same subjects are polled to determine their health. Some will be fit as a fiddle, some won't. Some will have died. Epidemiologists love dead people. You just can't find a medical condition more clearly defined than death. "I give Ken Cooper a lot of credit," Blair says. "He realized from the very beginning that we had to put our treadmill tests into a database, so we could follow these people and see what happens to them."

Over the past 30 years, more than 80,000 subjects, male and female, have been poked, prodded, and treadmill-tested at the Cooper Center. Every year, Blair and colleagues issue a handful of new reports that slice and dice the data, officially known as the Aerobics Center Longitudinal Study (ACLS). The results are eye-popping. In general, the most-fit subjects have heart-disease death rates 50 percent lower than the least fit. They're also much less likely to have strokes, or to develop diabetes or high blood pressure. They have a lower incidence of many cancers. And now, in the latest and most startling development, they are showing lower risk for senile dementia and diseases like Alzheimer's.

It's crucial to note that these "most fit" individuals are not super athletes. They're not the winners of the Boston and New York City marathons. Most exercise the equivalent of 15 to 25 miles of running per week at about 10 minutes per mile. Other studies have produced results that reinforce the ACLS research. Exercise doesn't just feel good and provide a mental break from our overstressed lives; it also produces measurable health benefits. "Our data probably show the strongest association between fitness and various health outcomes," says Blair. "That's because our treadmill tests come closer to the truth about someone's fitness than questionnaire studies."

Reams of research have shown that excess body fat increases mortality rates, but Blair is banking on his morning runs to protect him. His own findings offer much hope. Evidence from the ACLS indicates that the fit-but-fat are nearly as healthy as the fit-of-normal-weight. In other words, regular exercise offsets many of the dangers of being overweight. For that reason, Blair believes American public-health leaders should stop screeching from the rooftops about obesity and instead switch their message to the benefits of exercise. "When you look at me, you can tell I'm surprised and delighted by the fit-fat finding," says Blair. "But the point is, we're losing the obesity battle. So let's try something else. Let's focus on fitness."

THE HEART-HEALTH CONNECTION

In their studies, Steve Blair and all modern exercise epidemiologists have built on the work of Jeremy Morris and Ralph Paffenbarger, the pioneering giants in the field. More recently, Paul Williams has expanded our knowledge of serious exercisers by using *Runner's World* readers to build his database. Williams's National Runners Health Study was launched in these pages in 1991. While all the studies have reached similar conclusions—regular exercise provides significant health benefits—each has made interesting and unique contributions of its own.

Great Britain's Morris spent the WWII years as an army doctor in India and Burma. His first big exercise study ("Coronary heart disease and the physical activity of work," *The Lancet*, 1953) investigated the different heart-health outcomes of London transport workers: the bus drivers who sat on their arses all day versus the ticket-takers who walked up 600 stairs a day on London's double-decker buses. Result: The ticket-takers suffered 30 percent fewer heart attacks, and their attacks were less severe.

Later, in his 27-year career as England's director of the Medical Research Council's Social Medicine Unit, Morris realized that physical activity had disappeared from most jobs. Everyone sat at a desk all day long. He decided to begin looking at "leisure-time exercise" and its impact on heart health. He followed 17,000 male civil servants between the ages of 40 and 64, and discovered that those who frequently burned about 450 calories per hour in exercise (roughly equivalent to an easy four-mile run) had only one-third the heart attacks of those who had little or no exercise. He concluded that "vigorous exercise is a natural defense of the body, with a protective effect on the aging heart against ischemia and its consequences." In 1996, Morris received the International Olympic Committee's first award for excellence in sport sciences—an honor he shared with Ralph Paffenbarger.

Paffenbarger grew up in Columbus, Ohio, and received a bachelor's degree from Ohio State before taking a doctorate in public health at Johns Hopkins in 1954. He later taught at Berkeley, Stanford, and Harvard, concentrating on the relationships between exercise and health. In his early work with San Francisco longshoremen, Paffenbarger showed that those with the most arduous jobs, the cargo handlers, had heart-attack death rates significantly lower than those with desk jobs.

In 1960, Paff, as he was widely known, helped create the influential Harvard Alumni Study, which produced and continues to yield valuable information about physical activity and health. Among its most important findings: that student sports participation at the collegiate level yields no long-term health benefits, but adult exercise does. Paff also found that while health benefits begin to

slow beyond 1,000 exercise calories burned per week (approximately 10 miles of running), the benefit curve doesn't flatten. You still get more benefit at 20 miles per week and beyond, particularly if you do some harder workouts.

Paff was so impressed by his own findings that, after a previously sedentary life, he took up running in 1967 at age 45. In the next 25 years, he ran 151 marathons and ultras, including 22 Boston Marathons (5:05 his first; 2:44 his best). In 1977, he became, at age 54, the oldest-yet finisher of the Western States 100-miler, in 28:36, persuading Western States organizers to extend the cut-off time to 30 hours. One of the great unsung heroes of the running boom, Paff died on July 9, 2007, at age 84.

Most epidemiologists struggle to find subjects who burn more than 2,000 calories a week in exercise. Paul Williams, Ph.D., has made his mark by exploring the health outcomes of serious runners, some of whom exceed two or three times that amount in their weekly training. From his results, he insists on a simple but important message: More is better. Other exercise epidemiologists don't disagree; they just think Williams is mostly irrelevant, since so few Americans are willing to exercise as much as *Runner's World* readers. These scientists point out that the biggest public-health benefits come from getting more people to simply walk a few miles a week.

This doesn't discourage Williams. In one 1997 study of 8,283 male runners, he compared those running more than 50 miles a week with those running less than 10. The high-mileage guys were 2.5 times as likely to have heart-protective levels of HDL, the "good" cholesterol, and 50 percent less likely to suffer from high blood pressure. In 2008 Williams updated his information on running mileage and high blood pressure, now using data from more than 24,000 male runners. He looked at runners doing more than 25 miles a week versus those doing less than five. Depending on age, the higher-mileage runners had a 57 to 80 percent lower rate of high blood pressure, a major contributor to disease and death.

THE RUNNING EFFECT

"I feel a little awkward about meeting John Fixx," says heart specialist Paul Thompson, M.D. "His father made me famous." By the time of Jim Fixx's death at age 52 in 1984, Thompson had graduated from medical school, done some advanced studies at Stanford, and published two papers on heart-attack deaths in runners. That made him the go-to expert for hundreds of TV, radio, and newspaper reporters chasing down the Fixx story. Over the years, Thompson has remained everyone's favorite expert for insights on exercise and heart disease. He has also worked as a TV commentator at the Seoul Olympics and the New York City Marathon, and his name turns up frequently in publications like *The New England Journal of Medicine*.

Thompson, 61, has had a lifelong fascination with the workings of the heart, in particular its response to exercise. "Sometimes I wish I could read heart studies all day long instead of attending to administration details," he says. "Think about the overweight guy who's totally out of shape until he begins exercising. A couple of months later, he's a different person. The heart is so amazing, and so damned good at what it does."

Thompson runs with the quick, light stride of the veteran marathoner, and has already covered eight miles in the early morning. "It's the one time of day I get to focus on myself," he says. "This makes me a much better person when I get to work and have to focus on staff and patients."

I ask Thompson why some runners keel over and die from heart attacks. He explains, first, that the young ones, mostly under 30 or 35, generally have structural defects in their hearts, such as the heart scarring that apparently led to Ryan Shay's death. These include a bewildering variety of rare conditions, and one—hypertrophic cardiomyopathy—that gets mentioned much more than the others for two reasons. First, it's the most common cause of sudden heart death in young athletes. Second, it results from an enlarged heart. This leads to widespread confusion, because endurance athletes like marathoners also have enlarged hearts. But the two are completely different. The marathoner's heart is large, healthy, and efficient; it's like a car that gets 40 miles per gallon. The hypertrophic cardiomyopathy heart is misshapen, malfunctioning, and dangerous; it results from a physical defect, not from hard endurance training.

When an over-35 exerciser dies on the run, Thompson continues, the cause is almost always artery disease—that is, cholesterol deposits that rupture and provoke a heart attack. He describes it like this: Imagine a garden hose with a modest flow of water moving through it. That's your arteries when you're resting. When you begin to run faster, the flow of blood increases dramatically. The hose begins to twist and flail. You've felt this with your own garden hose, or noticed how firemen must brace themselves to control a high-pressure hose. "So your arteries are flexing and bending," says Thompson. "Now if you've got a cholesterol deposit in the artery, the movement can crack the deposit open. Your blood mixes with the cholesterol to form a clot that blocks the artery. A few minutes later, you've bought the farm."

In Thompson's classic 1982 study of runners' heart-attack deaths in the state of Rhode Island, he found that a runner's relative risk of dying during a workout was about seven times that of dying in front of the TV. It amounted to one death for every 396,000 hours of running, almost exactly the same rate found decades later in several marathon studies. This doesn't mean that running caused the deaths. It would be more accurate to say that artery disease caused the deaths, and running was merely the trigger. Here's why: Another Rhode Island study showed that the blizzard of February 1978 touched off a mini-epidemic of snow-shoveling deaths. A week later, however, heart-attack deaths dropped below normal levels. In other words, after all the people with advanced artery disease had died, there were few diseased hearts left.

Like other heart experts, Thompson notes that regular exercise offers no sure protection from heart disease. Three hundred and twenty-five thousand Americans suffer an outside-a-hospital heart attack every year, often without warning, and 40 percent of these events end in sudden death. "Exercise is not a savior," Thompson says. "The risks are very low, the benefits are real, and the benefits outweigh the risks. But there are no guarantees."

An exercise death can happen even to fit runners with low cholesterol who've passed a stress test in the past 48 hours. But that fact doesn't change the advice for healthy living. "If you want to live a long, vigorous life, you should do an hour of moderate exercise a day," says Thompson. "If your only goal is to survive the next hour of your life, you should get into bed—alone."

DEATHS DURING MARATHONS

In the mid-1970s a California pathologist named Thomas J. Bassler, M.D., advanced the alluring theory that marathon runners might develop a sort of immunity from heart disease. He likened marathoners to the Masai warriors of Kenya and the Tarahumara Indians of Mexico—groups with little or no heart disease. "Marathon runners have much in common with these primitive populations," Bassler wrote. Runners everywhere repeated Bassler's tale to friends and skeptics alike. Then a trickle of case studies proved Bassler wrong, and the party was over.

Since the mid-1970s, three independent groups have collected data on heart-attack deaths during marathons. When the results are pooled together, we're looking at more than 4.5 million marathoners over the past 30 years. Of these, 41 runners died of heart attacks, a rate of one in every 110,476 marathoners. However, the two best of the three marathon studies have produced death rates somewhat higher than this average.

Family doctor and University of Minnesota Medical School professor Bill Roberts, M.D., has been medical director of the Twin Cities Marathon since 1985. Along with Barry Maron, M.D., a sudden-cardiac-death specialist also from Minneapolis, Roberts has gathered death statistics on both the Twin Cities and Marine Corps marathons going back to 1976. During that time, the combined marathons have had 525,700 finishers and seven cardiac deaths, an average of one death per 75,000 runners. Roberts and Maron have also found that this rate is declining, no doubt due to the increased availability of portable defibrillators. At Twin Cities, Roberts has established a goal of reaching any fallen runner with a defibrillator within five minutes. "If you're going to have a heart attack, a marathon is a great place to have one," he says. "Your chance of surviving is about 50 to 75 percent, versus 5 to 15 percent anywhere else on the streets."

In London, cardiologist Daniel Tunstall Pedoe served as London Marathon medical director from the inaugural 1981 marathon, which he ran in 3:19, through the 2007 event. Pedoe has studied marathoner deaths during all 27 London Marathons. Almost 712,000 runners have completed the race, with eight dying from heart attacks, a rate of one in every 89,000. The eight London deaths included five attributed to artery disease (cholesterol deposits) and three to structural heart abnormalities such as those that killed Ryan Shay and Chad Schieber. The deaths have occurred all along the course and in the finish chute. "Marathon running has a comparatively low, but not negligible, risk, and it's not surprising that people are frightened when they hear about a marathon death," says Pedoe. "That's why we have to keep educating everyone about the lifetime benefits of exercise."

At the end of 2007, barely a month after the deaths of Chad Schieber, Ryan Shay, and Matthew Hardy, the *British Medical Journal* published the biggest-by-far study of deaths during marathons. It was less definitive than the other two, however, since it relied on a search of newspaper articles to determine marathon-related deaths. Nonetheless, the *BMJ* study, conducted by Donald Redelmeier, M.D., from the Department of Medicine at the University of Toronto, surveyed 750 separate marathon days that were taken from 26 marathons over 30 years. The total number of runners in these races was 3,292,268, and Redelmeier found newspaper articles noting 26 heart-attack deaths. Hence, his ratio is one death in 126,000 runners. Redelmeier's most striking finding was that nearly half of all deaths occurred in the last mile of the race, or after the finish. This conclusion led Redelmeier to advise runners not to sprint at the end. In fact, in his one marathon, he deliberately jogged over the finish in 4:17. "I just tried to finish with a smile," he says.

Overall, Redelmeier concluded: "Clinicians interested in preventing sudden cardiac death

might be surprised by the low risk associated with marathon running. [It's about] the same as the baseline hourly risk of death for a middle-aged man."

THE HEART ATTACK HEARD 'ROUND THE WORLD

John Fixx was just 8 or 9 when he started running with his not-yet-famous father in the late 1960s, and a fourth-grader when he ran his first road race, the Greenwich (Connecticut) Memorial Day Five-Mile. "I enjoyed running from the very beginning," says Fixx, now 47. "At first it gave me a chance to spend time with my father, a typically busy New York editor. Later it kept me in good shape for all the other sports I liked."

In college, in the heady period following the 1977 publication of his dad's unexpected bestseller, *The Complete Book of Running*, Fixx ran on the cross-country and track teams at Wesleyan University, and continued racing after graduation, achieving bests of 54:10 for 10 miles and 2:51 for the marathon.

A year out of college, Fixx was visiting a family friend, Todd Benoit, in Greenwich when the news arrived: His father had died that afternoon while running in Vermont. Other family members were scattered across the country; it fell to John to organize the funeral. He took time out only for an evening run with his friend. "The news about Dad's death was just devastating," he says. "But going out for a run also seemed like the right way to honor him. I remembered that he used to say, 'I don't know if running adds years to your life, but it definitely adds life to your years.'"

Fixx and Benoit ran again the next day. This time they passed a country-club patio crowded with overweight golfers swilling beers after their 18 holes. The golfers couldn't have known who was running past, but neither could they restrain themselves. "Hey, you idiots," they called out. "Don't you know that running will kill you?"

A family-ordered autopsy showed that Jim Fixx had significant blockage in all three coronary arteries. The Vermont state chief medical examiner briefed the family and said that his heart muscle, strengthened by running, had probably extended his life by 8 to 10 years. (Before beginning to run in 1968, Jim Fixx smoked and weighed well over 200 pounds. His own father had suffered a first heart attack at 37, and died at 41.) In retrospect, family members pieced together a number of warning signs. One night shortly before his death, Jim had awakened in a cold sweat, barely able to breathe. On a run with John, he had to stop uncharacteristically after a half-mile. He complained that allergies or something were leaving him breathless and he had tightness in his upper arm. He said he might go to the doctor if the allergies persisted. "He was a typical Yankee, a private guy who didn't like to bother others with his problems," says John. "After he died, my three siblings and I said that we would always check in with each other."

"Family history is such a strong risk factor, you can never ignore it," Paul Thompson says. "And people need to understand that the warning signals aren't always a classic chest tightness or pain down the left arm. You can have pain in the right arm. You can have what feels like indigestion. I tell people: If you notice something very quick and transitory—bing! bing!—you've got nothing to worry about. But if you have a persistent sense of discomfort or breathlessness, you need to see your doctor right away. When in doubt, check it out."

Three months after his father's death, John

Fixx accepted Ken Cooper's invitation for a complete stress test and workup at the Cooper Clinic in Dallas. "I was 23. I thought I could eat and drink anything," he says. "I didn't break Dr. Cooper's treadmill record, but I might have broken the record for sugar consumption." He has returned to the clinic three more times, and also sees a Connecticut cardiologist for a stress test every two years. After his last test, the good news was that a cardiac calcium scan gave him a zero score, indicating no calcified cholesterol deposits in his heart arteries. The bad news: He was a few pounds heavier, and couldn't run as long on the treadmill.

Since then, Fixx says he has worked a little harder to maintain his 20 to 25 miles a week of running, along with a regular blend of tennis, golf, soccer, and kayaking. But he admits that he should probably pay more attention to calorie control. He's now just four years younger than his father's age on his last run; he's six years older than the time of his grandfather's death. I ask if he's scared that he'll die young, maybe while running.

"My wife is probably more scared than I am," he says. "I want to live a long time. Running feels like the best 45-minute investment I make in a day. It's enjoyable, it makes me feel better, and it's probably paying dividends way into the future. Running is a really easy choice."

ADD LIFE TO YOUR YEARS

Most days, on my noontime run, I still don't worry about dying. But now I do find myself thinking more about my heart. Seeking reassurance, I try a Web-based cardiac risk calculator. It uses results from the famed Framingham Heart Study, and tells me—after analyzing my total cholesterol of

170, my HDL of 35, and my blood pressure at 120/80—that I have a 10 percent chance of dying from heart disease in the next decade. Ten percent! That sounds high. I react like a marathoner trying to qualify for Boston. I wonder, What can I do to get better?

So I check in again with cardiologist Paul Thompson. "We're not magicians," he says. "And heart disease is a really complex, unpredictable disease."

Thompson gives me a short list of strategies: Eat a mostly vegetarian diet, consume more fish (or a fish-oil supplement) rich in omega-3 fatty acids, take a daily baby aspirin (81 milligrams), and consider a low-dose statin to lower total cholesterol.

For a day or two, I'm depressed that I can't do more to lower my risk. Then Jim Fixx's words come ringing back to me: "Running might not add years to your life, but it definitely adds life to your years." Another maxim follows: We live too short, and die too long. That's the snappy title that irrepressible Walter Bortz II, M.D., gave one of his books. Bortz ran the 2008 ING New York City Marathon at age 78.

With a little more reflection, I realize I'm chasing a false prophet. Long life alone means little. An active, challenge-filled life, that's what I want. I need just one more nugget—Dr. George Sheehan's timeless "Listen to your body"—to form my own new mantra: Listen and live. When my body says "Go for it," I'll run like crazy. When it says "Rest," I'll slow down. When it says "Stop," I hope to pay particular attention.

I'm looking forward to my next run.

Amby Burfoot's Running Round-Up

Life is a risky undertaking: When you get out of bed in the morning, your chances of suffering from a heart attack rise, as do the chances for an accidental fall or choking on your breakfast. You'd be a lot better off, in the short term, if you never got out of bed. In the long term, however, staying in bed is a very unhealthy activity: It leads to muscle deterioration and disease.

We now know that the same observation can be made about going out for a run: It's a risky business. You could have a heart attack, you could sprain your ankle in a pothole, or you could get hit by a truck.

Yet far more often than not, a regular run is a health-enhancing activity that makes your heart stronger, lowers your blood pressure, and keeps your weight in a good range.

Indeed, in an era of rampant obesity, it's increasingly clear that those who exercise a moderate amount are far healthier than those who don't exercise at all, and those who exercise a lot are somewhat healthier than the moderate exercisers. Pheidippides and Jim Fixx were among the unlucky. Most runners count themselves lucky to have found a sport that improves their health in so many different ways.

Index

Boldface page references indicate illustrations. <u>Underscored</u> references indicate boxed text.